WORKING IN
COMMUNITY
HEALTH
Foundations for a Successful Career

Karen Marie Perrin, PhD, MPH, CPH

**Associate Professor, University of South Florida,
College of Public Health, Tampa, Florida**

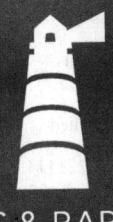

JONES & BARTLETT
LEARNING

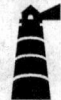

World Headquarters
Jones & Bartlett Learning
25 Mall Road
Burlington, MA 01803
978-443-5000
info@jblearning.com
www.jblearning.com

Jones & Bartlett Learning books and products are available through most bookstores and online booksellers. To contact Jones & Bartlett Learning directly, call 800-832-0034, fax 978-443-8000, or visit our website, www.jblearning.com.

Production Credits

Vice President, Product Management: Marisa R. Urbano
Vice President, Content Strategy and Implementation: Christine Emerton
Director, Product Management: Matthew Kane
Product Manager: Sophie Fleck Teague
Director, Content Management: Donna Gridley
Content Strategist: Tess Sackmann
Director, Project Management and Content Services: Karen Scott
Manager, Project Management: Jackie Reynen
Project Manager: John Coakley
Program Manager: Alex Schab
Senior Digital Project Specialist: Angela Dooley
Senior Marketing Manager: Susanne Walker

Content Services Manager: Colleen Lamy
Vice President, Manufacturing and Inventory Control: Therese Connell
Composition: Straive
Project Management: Straive
Cover Design: Briana Yates
Text Design: Briana Yates
Media Development Editor: Faith Brosnan
Rights & Permissions Manager: John Rusk
Rights Specialist: Maria Leon Maimone
Cover Image (Title Page, Part Opener, Chapter Opener):
   © pedrosala/Shutterstock
Printing and Binding: Gasch Printing

Library of Congress Cataloging-in-Publication Data
Names: Perrin, Karen M., author.
Title: Working in community health : foundations for a successful career /
   Karen (Kay) Marie Perrin, PhD, MPH, RN, CPH, Associate Professor,
   University of South Florida, College of Public Health, Tampa, FL.
Description: First edition. | Burlington, Massachusetts : Jones & Bartlett
   Learning, [2023] | Includes bibliographical references and index.
Identifiers: LCCN 2022037273 | ISBN 9781284234862 (paperback)
Subjects: LCSH: Community health services–Vocational guidance–United
   States. | BISAC: MEDICAL / Public Health
Classification: LCC RA440.9 .P47 2023 | DDC 362.2/2–dc23/eng/20221114
LC record available at https://lccn.loc.gov/2022037273

6048

Printed in the United States of America
28 27 26 25   10 9 8 7 6 5 4 3 2

Thanks to all Community Health Workers across the globe for your dedication to service for those individuals in need.

Brief Contents

Contents

SECTION 1 Community Health Workers in the Community   1

SECTION 3 **Aspects of Aging**   **139**

CHAPTER 8 **Safety for the Aging Population, Elderly, and Community Health Workers** **141**

CHAPTER 9 **Aspects of Aging** **169**

Foreword

Dr. Kay Perrin brings a wealth of experience and expertise to this important new textbook, *Working in Community Health*. Dr. Perrin's career has deep roots in nursing and in public health. Her interest in community health goes back at least 3 decades and includes an early focus on patient advocacy, health literacy, and the role of spirituality in health.

Her career in nursing has spanned the life cycle from birthing to geriatrics. She brings extensive personal and professional experience about the inner workings of health care systems and the need for assistance in navigating the complexities of those systems. She is the perfect professional to speak to the growing importance and roles of Community Health Workers (CHW).

Dr. Perrin's textbook reflects the competencies required for CHW. It starts with a section on the roles of CHW, grounding the book in public health, health literacy, health equity, and the social determinants of health. Section two recognizes that CHW need a basic understanding of the biological, infectious, and environmental causes of disease.

Section three draws on her deep understanding of geriatrics and aging, focusing on the roles that CHW can play in addressing the needs of this rapidly growing segment of our population.

Section four brings the text together by providing an overview of health insurance, health facilities, and patient rights and responsibilities—all key to the day-to-day efforts of CHW.

The text concludes with a chapter on the Community Health Worker profession, providing those new to the field with important guidance on the roles, opportunities, and responsibilities of this important and emerging profession.

Working in Community Health is an ideal textbook for the education of Community Health Workers whether they receive their education and training in Community Colleges, Health Department training programs, or on the job. As with all her writing, the book is clear, to the point, and filled with an abundance of realistic examples that bring the text to life.

I have seen firsthand Dr. Perrin's commitment and competence as an educator and author. I am confident that *Working in Community Health* will play an important role in the development of the Community Health Worker profession.

Richard Riegelman MD, MPH, PhD
Professor and Founding Dean
Milken Institute School of Public Health
The George Washington University

Preface

Community Health Workers (CHWs) are front-line public health workers that act as a link between health care providers, social service providers, and health care consumers. CHWs build individual and community capacity by increasing health knowledge and self-sufficiency through a range of activities such as outreach, community education, informal counseling, social support, and advocacy.

Working in Community Health: Foundations for a Successful Career is written to prepare and educate community health workers for employment with the potential of a career ladder. This book provides specific knowledge required for effective employment skills, understanding basic anatomy and physiology of the most common chronic diseases, teaching how to access and understand health knowledge, as well as resume development and interview proficiency.

The book contains four sections. The first section contains Chapters 1, 2, 3, and 4 and includes the synopsis of public health as related to community health workers (CHWs). Chapter 1 provides an overview of the CHW profession. Chapter 2 covers the topic of adult learning and all levels of health literacy, including verbal, written, and numerical. The awareness and understanding of literacy are essential for CHWs in all aspects of their employment and practice. Chapter 3 presents and defines the concept of health equity and social determinants of health. Health equity explores the cultural disparities of access to health care. Social determinants build on the aspect of cultural diversity by exploring race, ethnicity, poverty, education, housing, job opportunities, and neighborhoods. Chapter 4 defines and explores social justice and advocacy, including both self-advocacy and community advocacy.

The second section includes Chapters 5, 6, and 7 and introduces causes of disease. Chapter 5 explores environmental sources of various diseases, such as mold, mildew, insects, rodents, smoke, chemicals, water, and air pollutants. Chapter 6 examines the human body systems and the interactions between systems. In addition, the types of chronic diseases are defined and explained, including heart disease, type 2 diabetes, and osteoporosis. Chapter 7 investigates infectious diseases with a discussion about routes, vectors, common contagious diseases, and vaccines.

The third section consists of Chapters 8, 9, and 10 and focuses on the aspects of aging. Chapter 8 begins this section by discussing client safety, including body mechanics, fall risks, balance, and types of abuse. Chapter 9 explores the effects of aging on the body systems as well as diet, exercise, vision, hearing, and dental issues. Chapter 10 explores quality of life, advance directives, and end-of-life planning from the perspective of the elderly client as well as their family and friends.

The fourth section focuses on the CHW profession. Chapter 11 discusses types of health insurance, and Chapter 12 covers healthcare facilities as well as employment opportunities at various facilities. Chapter 13 discusses ethics, rights, and responsibilities related to CHWs. Finally, Chapter 14 provides information about various CHW curriculum and certification as well as resume writing and interviewing skills.

About the Author

Kay Perrin, PhD, MPH, RN, CPH

After working as a nurse for 17 years in hospitals and clinics, Dr. Perrin obtained her MPH and PhD. During her 25 years as faculty at the University of South Florida College of Public Health, she focused her research on maternal and child health and home visiting, initiated the successful Bachelor of Science in Public Health, and served as a Fulbright Scholar in Pune, India. Later, she served as the Associate Dean of Academic and Student Affairs for the college. Over the years, Dr. Perrin has taught numerous undergraduate and graduate courses.

She has published several textbooks with Jones & Bartlett Learning on the topics of evaluation, research, and health navigation. Currently, her research is in palliative support, hospice, elder care, and end-of-life decisions as a focus while volunteering at Sarasota Memorial Hospital and Tidewell Hospice in Sarasota, Florida.

Reviewers

Anna Torrens Armstrong, PhD, MPH, MCHES®, CPH
University of South Florida

Amy L. Bernard, PhD, MCHES®
University of Cincinnati

Ni Bueno, EdD
Health Education Department Chair
Cerritos College

Marcia Butler, RDH, MPH, DrPH
Assistant Dean Healthcare Professions; Chair, Department of Health Care Management
Clayton State University

Dolores E. Caffey-Fleming, MS, MPH
Charles R. Drew University of Medicine and Science

Amanda M. Carpenter, PhD
Arkansas State University

Dean Chiarelli, MA, RDN, CEP, CHES, REHS
Arizona State University

Elisa F. Correia-Dasalla, MA, CMA-AAMA

Sara K. Daniel, MS, CHES, RHIA
Arkansas Tech University

Dr. Laura Dowling, MBA, CHFP, CRCR, CSBI, NLPMP, ETFTFTMP
Gwynedd Mercy University

Susan Mayo Duett, MBA, PhD
Program Director for Health Administration, Associate Professor
Belhaven University

Shawn Ekwall, MBA, FACHE, PTL
Edward J. Bloustein School of Planning & Public Policy
Rutgers University

David Flint, MEd, MPH
Idaho State University College of Technology

Deborah Franklin, NHA, MHA

Anita Franzione, DrPH, MPA, CPH
Edward J. Bloustein School of Planning & Public Policy
Rutgers University

Tanisha Garcia, PhD, MHA
Department of Public Health
California State University, Fresno

Dr. Laurel A. Glover
Charleston Southern University

Dr. Shelly Gompf
Professor
Concordia College

Marzell Gray, DrPH, MBA
Assistant Professor
University of Minnesota Duluth

Mckelle Hamson, PhD candidate, MPH, CHES
Lecturer
Utah Valley University

Karen Harouse-Bell MS, RDN, LDN, CDCES
Seton Hall University

Pamela M. Hobbs, MS, MPH
Associate Lecturer of Health Sciences
Lee University

Ada Boone Hoerl, MEd, COTA/L
Program Director, Chair, Professor
Occupational Therapy Assistant Program
Sacramento City College

Lakesha Kinnerson, MPH, RHIA
Assistant Professor, Health Informatics and Analytics
Samford University

Jerome E. Kotecki, PhD
Professor of Health Science
Ball State University

Garry Ladd, DHSc
Professor, Chair
Health and Exercise Science Department
Southwestern Illinois College

Kim LeBard-Rankila, PhD
Assistant Professor
University of Wisconsin, Superior

Anna K. Leal, PhD
Assistant Professor of Biology
Centenary College of Louisiana

Charl Mattheus, DBA Healthcare Management
Assistant Professor, Program Internship
  Coordinator
Department of Public Health
California State University, Sacramento

Mary McMullen, MS, RD
Arizona State University

Marshae A. McNeal, PhD, MPH, CHES
Assistant Professor
Louisiana State University, Shreveport

Kathleen Montella, MPH, CHES
Public Health Program Director
School of Nursing and Health Professions
Langston University

Brandon A. Moton, DrPH, MPH

Lien Nguyen, MPH, PhD(c)
University of Wisconsin-Milwaukee

Brandye Nobiling, PhD, CHES, CSE
Salisbury University

Mark Popovitz, MBA, MPH
University of Cincinnati Blue Ash

Wendy Potratz, PhD, CHES
Program Director
Northwest Technical College

Brent Powell, PhD, CHES
Professor of Public Health Promotion
California State University, Stanislaus

Elbina Rafizadeh, PhD, MSN, RN
Associate Faculty
Mission College

Regina M. Riccioni, EdD, MBA, MPH, CHES

Clarence E. Riley, Jr., PhD
Associate Professor of Health and Physical
  Education, School Counselor Education
Fort Valley State University

April Rogers, MD, MPH, MBA
Assistant Professor, Program Director
St. John's University

Oreta M. Samples, BS, MPH, DHSc
Department of Veterinary Science and Public
  Health
Fort Valley State University

Hans Schmalzried, PhD
Professor Emeritus of Public Health
Bowling Green State University

Richard Silberman, MD
Adjunct Professor, Cardiologist
University of Wisconsin-Milwaukee

Jazmyne Simmons-Bryant, PhD, MPH
Florida A&M University

Lillian Upton Smith, DrPH, MPH
Professor and Divisional Dean
Public Health and Population Science, College of
  Health Sciences
Boise State University

Ellen Sobota, MS, RD, LDN, NBC-HWC
Seton Hall University

Joan Thoman, RN, PhD, CNS
Associate Dean of Research and Collaborative
  Partnerships, Director Community Health
  Worker Program
School of Nursing
Cleveland State University

Maka Tsulukidze, MD, PhD, MPH
Assistant Professor
Florida Gulf Coast University

Jessica K. Washington, PhD, CSCS
Berry College

Anita Walters, MS
Instructor and Coordinator of Personal Wellness
Fort Hays State University

Janice Dansby Washington, RHIA
Shelton State Community College

Jeffrey S. Wolf, MSM
Adjunct Professor
Franklin University

Sandra Dale Woodruff, MSPH
Instructor
Edson College of Nursing and Health Innovation
Arizona State University

Catherine Zeman, PhD, MS, RN
University of Northern Iowa

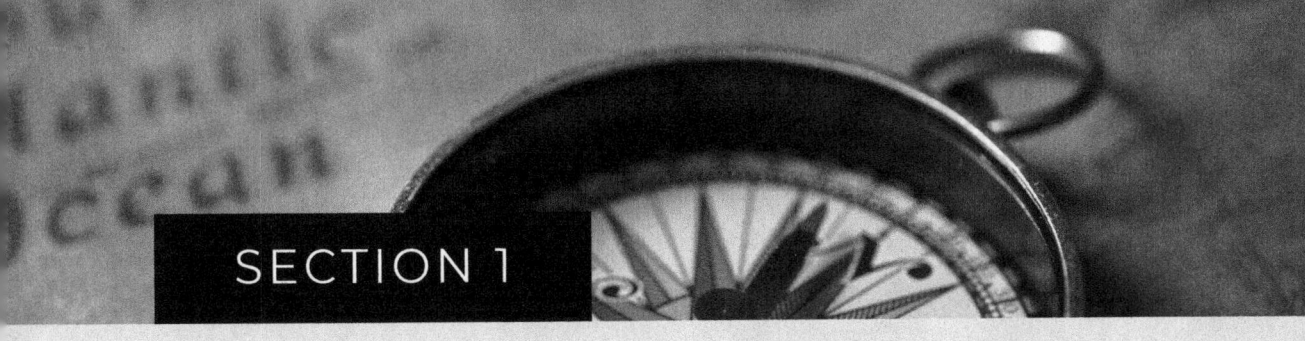

Community Health Workers in the Community

CHAPTER 1

What Is a Community Health Worker?

LEARNING OBJECTIVES

1. Define public health and individual health.
2. Describe the history of community health workers.
3. Explain the roles, skills, and responsibilities of community health workers.

KEY TERMS

community health workers (CHWs)
health
individual health

public health
health equity

Introduction

This chapter introduces the difference between population health and individual health. Next the discussion presents the history of **community health workers (CHWs)** and the roles, skills, and responsibilities of CHWs. Also, the chapter identifies various types of places for employment, including wages and geographical locations in the United States. Last, the chapter introduces how to search for job descriptions when seeking CHW positions.

Definition of Individual Health and Public Health

Before delving into the topic of community health work, it is important to examine the definition of **health**. According to the World Health Organization (WHO), health is defined as "a state of complete physical, mental, and social well-being and not merely the absence of disease or infirmity."[1–2] For example, even when individuals do not have an active disease diagnosis, it is not to be assumed that those individuals live in a complete state of health. They may be coping with social or financial issues that are causing sleepless nights. Their housing may be in a location where environmental or industrial pollution is causing poor outdoor air quality. Since everyone's life situation is different, it is important to consider the whole person when examining their health conditions, not merely their current medical diagnosis.[1–2] There are two broad categories of health: individual health and public health.

Individual Health. Individual health relates to health care and clinical disciplines (i.e., medicine, nursing, pharmacy, physical therapy, clinical psychology, dental, vision, hearing, and others) in which licensed professionals examine, diagnosis, and treat the health of one person at a time. When an individual is experiencing an illness,

the individual seeks health care to determine the cause of the symptoms and to create a tailored treatment plan. Public health professionals investigate the health needs of the entire community.[1,3]

Public Health. Public health considers all aspects of health in an entire community including social, education, economic, housing, environmental, etc. A community (population) may be as small as a faith-based community or as large as a country, continent, or the entire globe.[1,3] Population health is focused on the health of the public. See **Figure 1.1**. The outer circle shows the three core functions of public health: assurance, assessment, and policy development. The inner circle defines the three core functions into the 10 essential services of public health. Last, it is important to notice that equity is at the center of the circle.[5]

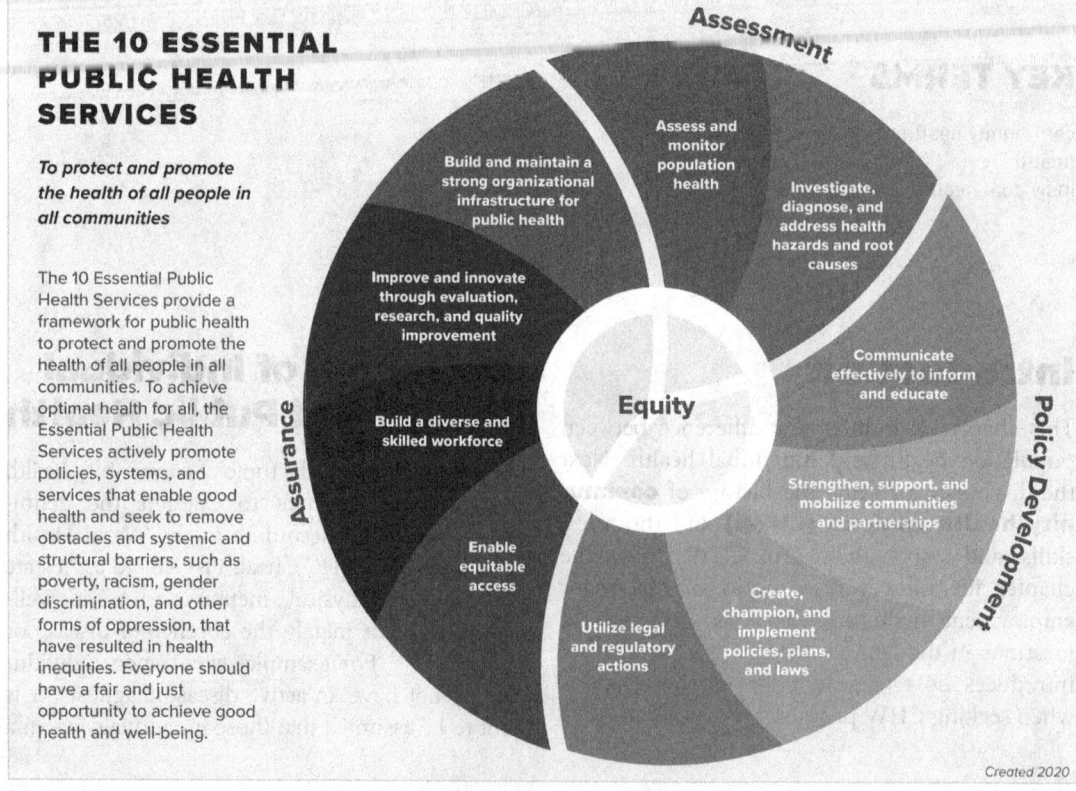

Figure 1.1 Core Functions of Public Health and 10 Essential Public Health Services

Figure from Centers for Disease Control and Prevention. 10 essential public health services. https://www.cdc.gov/publichealthgateway/publichealthservices/essentialhealthservices.html#:~:text=The%2010%20Essential%20 Public%20Health%20Services%20describe%20the,identify%20and%20solve%20health%20problems%20More%20items...%20. Accessed January 8, 2021. Reference to specific commercial products, manufacturers, companies, or trademarks does not constitute its endorsement or recommendation by the U.S. Government, Department of Health and Human Services, or Centers for Disease Control and Prevention.[4]

The simple definition of **health equity** is when everyone has the opportunity to be as healthy as possible.[3]

For some examples of how the role of CHWs fit into the big picture of public health service in their community, it is useful to begin with a definition of a CHW. Although there are various definitions for CHWs, the definition provided by the American Public Health Association states:

> *A community health worker is a frontline public health worker who is a trusted member of and/or has an unusually close understanding of the community served. This trusting relationship enables the worker to serve as a liaison/link/intermediary between health/social services and the community to facilitate access to services and improve the quality and cultural competence of service delivery. A community health worker also builds individual and community capacity by increasing health knowledge and self-sufficiency through a range of activities such as outreach, community education, informal counseling, social support, and advocacy.*[16]

Next, to understand how the definition and role of CHWs fits into the core functions and services of public health, see **Table 1.1**.

History of CHWs

1930: The first CHWs were "Farmer Scholars" who were trained in China in the 1930s and were the forerunners of the Barefoot Doctors, of whom there were more than one million from the 1950s to the 1970s.[5]

1960: In the 1960s, small CHW programs began to emerge in various countries, particularly in Latin America. The CHWs began to provide basic frontline health care in rural areas.[5] Since CHWs lived in the areas in which they worked, the community trusted them.[6]

1970: By the 1970s, the term CHW was used to describe a variety of individuals working to improve the health of their communities.[5–6] These individuals are knowledgeable of the local language, societal norms, cultures, and customs. There is no exact skill set for CHWs, and their demographics include all ages, levels of education, gender, and backgrounds. Their roles cover a broad spectrum of health topics, including prevention of disease, improvement of health outcomes through education, implementation of health interventions, and expansion of healthcare access.[5–6] Also, their community knowledge allows them to become essential workers in assisting with emergencies and disaster management due to their knowledge of the community.[6]

1980: By the 1980s, many impoverished healthcare systems around the world recognized the challenges in providing adequate healthcare services, and thus governments explored a flexible approach to adopt CHWs into the health systems to improve health. Although CHWs do not provide direct patient care, they offer limited services rather than no services.[6]

1990: In the 1990s, following the failure of many of the programs in the 1980s, new highly successful programs have emerged and as a result of research findings demonstrating the effectiveness of community-based programs in improving child health in particular, there is now a resurgence of interest and growth of CHW programs around the world.[5] CHW services were acknowledged as an important component within the health system and not as a separate unit. Along with this inclusion came questions about how to standardize the training, scope of services, and supervision of CHWs.[6–7] By 1998, the National Community Health Advisor Study provided guidance to improve the status of CHWs and identify the roles and competencies for CHWs.[7–8]

2000: In 2006, the CHW Special Primary Interest Group of the American Public Health Association strengthened the role

Table 1.1 Three Core Functions and 10 Essential Services of Public Health for CHWs

Three Core Functions	Ten Essential Services	Role of CHW
Assurance	1. Enable equitable access.	Assist individuals struggling to access healthcare services.
	2. Build a diverse and skilled workforce.	Incorporate cultural diversity.
	3. Improve and innovate through evaluation, research, and quality improvement.	Collect community data to improve health education efforts.
	4. Build and maintain a strong organizational infrastructure for public health.	Network with public health, clinical, and social service agencies.
Assessment	5. Assess and monitor population health.	Understand and monitor community health data to improve population well-being.
	6. Investigate, diagnose, and address health hazards and root causes.	Explore possible environmental or systemic causes of adverse health conditions.
Policy Development	7. Communicate effectively to inform and educate.	Create health education programs in common language and literacy level of the community.
	8. Strengthen, support, and mobilize communities and partnerships.	Network with community to maximize services and decrease duplicative resources.
	9. Create, champion, and implement policies, plans, and laws.	Identify need for changing in policies to improve health and safety of community.
	10. Utilize legal and regulatory actions.	Investigate legal and regulatory actions for greater understanding of services.

Data from Centers for Disease Control and Prevention. 10 essential public health services. https://www.cdc.gov/publichealthgateway/publichealthservices/essentialhealthservices.html#:~:text=The%2010%20Essential%20Public%20Health%20Services%20describe%20the,identify%20and%20solve%20health%20problems%20More%20items...%20. Accessed January 8, 2021. Reference to specific commercial products, manufacturers, companies, or trademarks does not constitute its endorsement or recommendation by the U.S. Government, Department of Health and Human Services, or Centers for Disease Control and Prevention.[4]

of a CHW by stating that a CHW is "a frontline public health worker who is a trusted member of and/or has an unusually close understanding of the community served."[9] Within a year, the Health Resources and Services Administration (HRSA) published a national report on CHWs. This study showed that CHWs provided a cost-effective way to address health concerns in underserved communities. This research provided needed information to private insurers, corporations, and the federal government as a possible way to change delivery and financing of health care[10] by employing CHWs as a complement service rather than a replacement of health and social service care.[11]

2010:   In 2010, the Bureau of Labor Statistics assigned an occupational code of 21-1091 to Community Health Workers.[12] Also, in 2010, CHWs were identified as an important component of the health workforce and were cited in the Patient Protection and Affordable Care Act (PPACA) as a health industry professional with a variety of new employment pathways.[13]

2013:   The Centers for Medicare and Medicaid Services (CMS) created a new rule that allows state Medicaid agencies to reimburse for preventive services provided by professionals that may fall outside of a state's clinical licensure system if the services have been initially recommended by a physician or other licensed practitioner. This new rule for the first time offers state Medicaid agencies the option to reimburse for more community-based preventive services, including those of CHWs.[14] As a result of the Medicaid reimbursement option, several states took initiatives to advance the CHW infrastructure, professional identity, workforce development, and financing. These initiatives opened new employment opportunities for CHWs.[14]

2014:   The Center for Disease Control and Prevention (CDC) identified 14 CHW policy components.[15]

See **Critical Thinking 1.1**.

Critical Thinking 1.1 What Is a CHW?

Review roles and skills of CHWs in Table 1.2 and answer the following questions.

1. How would you summarize the main role of the CHW? Why?
2. Which of your current skills will be most beneficial for your career as a CHW? Which of your skills might need improvement?

A CHWs Career

CHWs are recognized as an integrated model across different healthcare systems.[16] In some communities, the CHWs work to increase health screenings and use of health services, while in other communities, the CHWs focus on the enhancement of communication between community members and health providers. The community needs vary, but the services provided by CHWs are focused on creatively improving the overall health of the population.[16] CHWs are lay members of the community who work in close association with the local healthcare system in both urban and rural environments. CHWs usually share ethnicity, language, socioeconomic status, and life experiences with the community members they serve.[16] CHWs have numerous titles, roles, and skills in their various positions. See **Table 1.2**.

The CHWs achieve their goal of improving health for the population or an individual by working in community agencies, healthcare offices, county health departments, and nonprofit organizations.[16–17] Working under supervision of senior staff, CHWs add support to numerous healthcare providers including physicians, nurse practitioners, physician assistants, nurses, dietitians, certified health education specialists, lactation consultants, doulas, allied health professionals, school nurses, language interpreters, and last, they improve the overall patient experience.[17–18]

If CHWs are interested in direct patient contact, there are CHW roles within clinical settings:

- Conduct saliva-based HIV testing and counseling.
- Perform basic cholesterol or blood pressure screenings.
- Teach patients how to use asthma inhalers.
- Teach patients with diabetes how to test their blood glucose levels with a glucometer.
- Explain the patient's body mass index (BMI) in relationship to prescribed weight loss exercise, and healthy eating programs.
- Participate in COVID screening testing and contact tracing activities.

Table 1.2 Titles, Roles, and Skills of CHWs

Titles
Community health advisor
Lay health advocates
Promotors
Outreach educators
Health liaison
Community health representatives
Peer health promoters
Peer health educators
Health navigators
Health advocates

Data from U.S. Department of Health and Human Services, Health Resources and Services Administration, Bureau of Health Professions. Community health worker national workforce study. https://bhw.hrsa.gov/sites/default/files/bureau-health-workforce/data-research/community-health-workforce.pdf. Accessed January 8, 2021.[16]

Roles
Advocate for individual and community health needs.
Receive training to conduct clinical screenings and teach how to use medical equipment, such an asthma inhaler or diabetic glucose monitor.
Offer interpretation and translation services.
Provide culturally appropriate health education, promotion, and information.
Improve access to healthcare services for people in need.
Give informal health education, counseling, and guidance on health behaviors.
Assist in accessing medical and nonmedical service and health programs.
Provide some direct services such as basic first aid and blood pressure screening.
Increase health screening and healthcare services.
Provide a better understanding between community members, health providers, and social service systems.
Advocate for specific populations in the community.
Improve understanding and adherence to health recommendations.
Reduce the need for emergency and specialty services.

Data from U.S. Department of Health and Human Services, Health Resources and Services Administration, Bureau of Health Professions. Community health worker national workforce study. https://bhw.hrsa.gov/sites/default/files/bureau-health-workforce/data-research/community-health-workforce.pdf. Accessed January 8, 2021.[16]

Skills
Communication skill
Interpersonal and relationship-building skills
Service coordination and navigation skills

(continues)

Table 1.2 Titles, Roles, and Skills of CHWs   *(continued)*

Skills
Capacity building skills
Advocacy skills
Education and facilitation skills
Individual and community assessment skills
Outreach skills
Professional skills and conduct
Evaluation and research skills
Knowledge on diverse health topics

Reproduced from The Community Health Worker Core Consensus Project. C3 Project Findings: Roles & Competencies. https://www.c3project.org/roles-competencies. Accessed May 25, 2021.[17]

- Participate in community vaccine clinics with the eligibility, registration, and screening process.
- Assist community nurses during community blood drives by conducting the eligibility screenings.
- Assist school nurses by conducting the children's eyesight exams and tracking mandatory student vaccine records.

Because CHWs live in the community, they speak the same language, know the cultural beliefs, and recognize health barriers.[18] CHWs are likely to receive their own health care in the community; therefore, they know how to connect people to health services.[19] CHWs understand the needs of their community, so they are able educate about how to reduce the symptoms of chronic disease and improve medication compliance[20] and reduce health care costs.[21–22] Furthermore, when CHWs are integrated into the community's health care system, the clients receive a greater understanding of the services. CHWs provide a holistic and culturally sensitive approach that enhances the effectiveness of the care provided. For example, if a homeless individual is seeking care, the CHW can directly assist the homeless individual to provide a variety of needed services, such as food banks, shelters, employment services, and health care.[19–23] See **Critical Thinking 1.2**.

Critical Thinking 1.2 CHW **Promotes Heart Health in Community**

Jasmine has been working for 3 years as a CHW in an inner-city clinic. During February, the clinic decided to focus on promoting heart health in the community. Jasmine volunteered to chair this committee and design activities for February. She created a list of tasks, including recruit clinic staff to participate, plan the parking lot family kick-off event for the first Saturday in February, and develop patient activities in the clinic for each week of February.

Answer the following questions:

1. How would you recruit the staff to participate? What staff would you target for participation?
2. Make a list of tasks required for the kick-off event.
3. What types of patient activities would be suitable for each week of February?

CHW Professional Profile Examples

The CHW career spans a lifetime of interest. Here are a few examples:

Example One: Patricia was 18 years old and struggled to complete high school. After graduating a semester late, she was not ready for community college but knew that she enjoyed helping people. She saw a flyer at the local national chain drug store about a 6-week course to become a pharmacy technician. During the application process, Patricia learned that her $500 tuition would be waived if she worked full-time for the company for 6 months. She was excited to learn that she was on a path for full-time employment. Patricia enjoyed her job and worked for the national chain drug store for more than 5 years. Two years after she became a pharmacy technician, she learned that the company would pay her tuition at the local community college. She started taking one course at a time until she gained confidence in her study skills. After her third semester, her advisor suggested that she take a few health education courses and explore the CHW certificate. Patricia took the advice and graduated with an associate degree in health education with the CHW certificate. She was getting tired of the routine as a pharmacy technician, so she looked for a new position where she could use her education. She applied and received a CHW position at the local community hospital in the outpatient center. It was an excellent transition since Patricia had 5 years of customer service experience in the healthcare field.

Example Two: Soon after Maria graduated from high school, her grandmother, age 72, was diagnosed with cancer. Maria was the youngest of five children and had spent most of her childhood after school at her grandmother's house. She loved her grandmother. Her parents worked full-time at the local car dealership. Her dad worked in the service department, and her mom worked in the financial and loan office. Since she was not interested in college, Maria told her parents that she wanted to care for her grandmother. Her parents negotiated a salary for Maria for the caregiving role. Maria moved into her grandmother's home and assumed all care duties, including scheduling medical appointments, driving to the cancer treatments, purchasing groceries, cooking healthy meals, cleaning, and caring for her grandmother as the cancer progressed. Since Maria's

grandmother spoke only Spanish, Maria was able to become fluent again. She had let her Spanish lapse while she was in high school and was not spending much time with her grandmother until the cancer diagnosis. Two years into the diagnosis, the treatment was not working, and Maria's grandmother was admitted into home hospice. She died peacefully at home, as requested, with the family near her bed. Several months after Maria's grandmother died, Maria began looking online for some type of healthcare position. She found a position at a local retirement facility as a care coordinator for the assisted living wing of the facility. Maria was a perfect fit for the new position because of her extensive caregiver experience and ability to speak Spanish fluently.

Example Three: Arnie completed his bachelor of science in public health, but he was still not sure about the direction of his career. During his last year in college, the COVID pandemic hit, and he was stuck in his apartment taking classes online for most of the last semester. He was reading his email and noticed that the local health department was seeking students to become contact trackers for COVID. He could work from home with a flexible schedule, get paid, and gain experience for his resume. Arnie applied and was told that he could start immediately. He enjoyed calling and talking to the list of people on the email list that he received each day. After a few weeks, he was told that social distancing was adequate at the health department, so he could work from the call center. Arnie was tired of being home alone, so he worked half-time at the call center and half-time at home. After he completed his shift at the health department, Arnie asked his supervisor what other types of jobs were going to be available after COVID. His supervisor told him that there was a community health advocate position in the HIV/AIDS Clinic. Since Arnie is gay, he had always been interested in helping young gay males. He applied for the position after graduation. He was interviewed for the position and was hired to serve the LGBTQIA+ community and attend to various health needs.

Example Four: June, age 46, had spent most of her life raising her three children, working part-time at her church, and participating in school and sport activities with her children. She had been married to Gerald for 12 years. Soon after he was deployed to Afghanistan, Gerald was killed by a roadside bomb. Now that her last child had graduated from high school and was happily attending college out-of-state, June was ready to allow herself to explore career choices that may be of interest to her. Her other three children lived in the same city, but they were married and starting families of their own. June loved being a grandmother but had no desire in raising her grandchildren. Within a few weeks, June obtained a front receptionist position at the local health department clinic that served mainly elderly patients. She enjoyed talking to the elderly patients, but she soon she noticed that the patients needed more than her friendly greeting and big smile. She talked to the clinic supervisor and asked if she could get trained to be a CHW. June had lived in the community for the past 25 years. She knew many of the resources, services, and veteran benefits from her own experience after her husband passed. The supervisor told June that her ideas were good, but she needed to develop a job description for what she was proposing to do for the patients. Her supervisor admitted that she was not clear on the role of a CHW. June worked every evening for 2 weeks to develop the job description, duties, and average salary for this new position. She was asked to present her proposal at the monthly board meeting. Much to June's surprise, they approved her request. They hired a new front receptionist. June trained that person while she was preparing into her new role as the CHW.

Example Five: Robert, age 64, is a military veteran. While in the Army, he was trained to be a field medic. After discharge, he worked in the pharmaceutical industry for 25 years. After retirement, he and his wife of 34 years traveled and enjoyed spending time with their five grandchildren from their two daughters. When Robert's wife died suddenly of a stroke, he became lonely.

He recognized his depression when he no longer enjoyed playing golf. He scheduled an appointment with his long-term physician, Dr. Swanson. After a conversation, Dr. Swanson told Robert that he needed to find a new meaningful purpose in life before trying a prescription for anti-depression medication. Robert left the appointment a bit confused, but he remembered telling the same advice to wounded soldiers back when he was a medic. As he drove home, he thought about how much he enjoyed helping people. After a few days searching online for part-time employment, Robert concluded that he did not need income, but rather meaningful volunteer opportunities. He applied for a volunteer position at the large regional hospital near his home. The volunteer coordinator called Robert and scheduled him for an interview. He was excited to learn how he could contribute to the healthcare system. The volunteer coordinator provided a list of several open positions in various departments. Robert decided to volunteer two days per week: one shift in the rehabilitation unit and one shift in the patient discharge. The next day, he was excited to go to the uniform store to purchase his volunteer uniform. He attended the volunteer orientation later that week. Even before Robert's first shift, he felt that he had regained his sense of purpose by helping others. See **Critical Thinking 1.3**.

Critical Thinking 1.3 A Day in the Life of a CHW

Nancy was recently hired as the CHW in a rural clinic in Kentucky. She was born and raised in the community, so she knows many people in the area. During her first week of employment, she encountered two challenges: (1) assisting Mrs. Johnson, a 50-year-old woman, to understand her health insurance documents and (2) bridging the gap between the clinical staff and the patients. Answer the following questions:

1. How could Nancy begin to work with Mrs. Johnson?
2. How could Nancy begin to define her role in the clinic?

CHW Employment Outlook, Job Satisfaction, Salary, Place of Employment, and Training

Employment Outlook

According to O*Net in 2021, the occupation of CHW is an emerging profession, is expected to grow rapidly within the next several years, and will have large numbers of job openings.[24]

The list of the top five tasks for CHW employment included the following:

- Maintain updated client records with plans, notes, appropriate forms, or related information.[25]
- Advise clients or community groups on issues related to improving general health, such as diet or exercise.[25]
- Identify or contact members of high risk or otherwise targeted groups, such as members of minority populations, low-income populations, or pregnant women.[25]
- Contact clients in person, by phone, or in writing to ensure they have completed required or recommended actions.[25]
- Distribute flyers, brochures, or other informational or educational documents to inform members of a target community.[25]

Job Satisfaction

The job satisfaction is high among CHWs, and the U.S. Department of Labor Statistics expects the CHW profession to grow approximately 16 percent by 2026.[26] See **Box 1.1**.

Salary

As of 2019 in the United States, the average hourly wage for CHWs was $22.12 or approximately $46,000. However, keep in mind that the wages ranged from $13.47 per hour ($28,010 annually) to $34.03 per hour ($70,790 annually).[26] Another source reported the median wages in 2020 was $20.19 hourly or $42,000 annually.[25] See **Figure 1.2**.

Box 1.1 Pros and Cons of CHW Job Satisfaction

Pros of being a CHW
- Provides an opportunity to help individuals in the community
- Assists individuals seeking health care resources
- Offers a chance to work as a member of the healthcare team
- Provides ways to further education
- Offers an adequate salary along with benefits in most locations
- Presents ways to get acquainted with members of the community

Cons of being a CHW
- Does not appeal to individuals desiring a set work assignment and schedule
- Limited number of CHW positions in most communities
- Must positions require that bilingual applicant match the community
- Applicant needs be familiar with the community
- Applicant needs a flexible schedule and enjoy a variety of duties
- Salary may not be adequate, but advancement usually possible

Place of Employment

When exploring where CHWs are most likely to work, the U.S. Bureau of Labor Statistics show the following information. See **Table 1.3** and **Figure 1.3** to see the distribution of CHWs across the United States.

Training for CHW

While there are no universal training requirements for entry-level positions, CHWs are required to have at least a high school diploma or equivalent. For more advanced or specialized positions, employers may require an associate degree or higher in health or human services. After CHWs are hired, the employer may provide training and mentoring. Customer service

Annual mean wage of community health workers, by state, May 2020

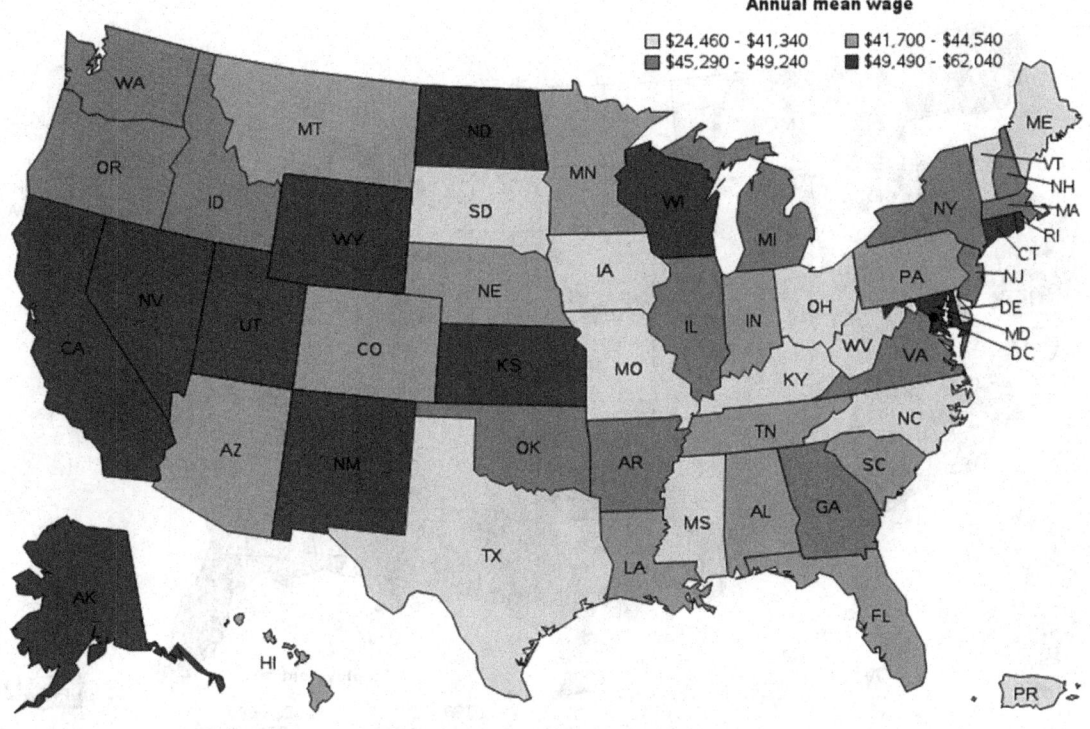

Blank areas indicate data not available.

Figure 1.2 Annual Mean Wage of CHWs by State

Figure from U.S. Bureau of Labor Statistics. Occupational employment and wages, May 2020, 21-1094 community health workers. https://www.bls.gov/oes/current/oes211094.htm#(1). Accessed on January 8, 2021.[26]

Table 1.3 Location and Wage Information for CHWs

Place of Employment	Percentage of Employment	Average Hourly Wage	Annual Mean Wage
Outpatient care centers	54%	$21.10	$43,880
Individual, family, community, and vocational rehabilitation services	43%	$20.19	$41,990
State and local government, excluding schools and hospitals	7%	$25.44	$52,920
Offices of physicians	14%	$20.24	$42,100
State, local, and private hospitals	9%	$24.62	$51,200

Data from U.S. Bureau of Labor Statistics. Occupational employment and wages, May 2020, 21-1094 community health workers. https://www.bls.gov/oes/current/oes211094.htm#(1). Accessed on January 8, 2021.[26]

Employment of community health workers, by state, May 2020

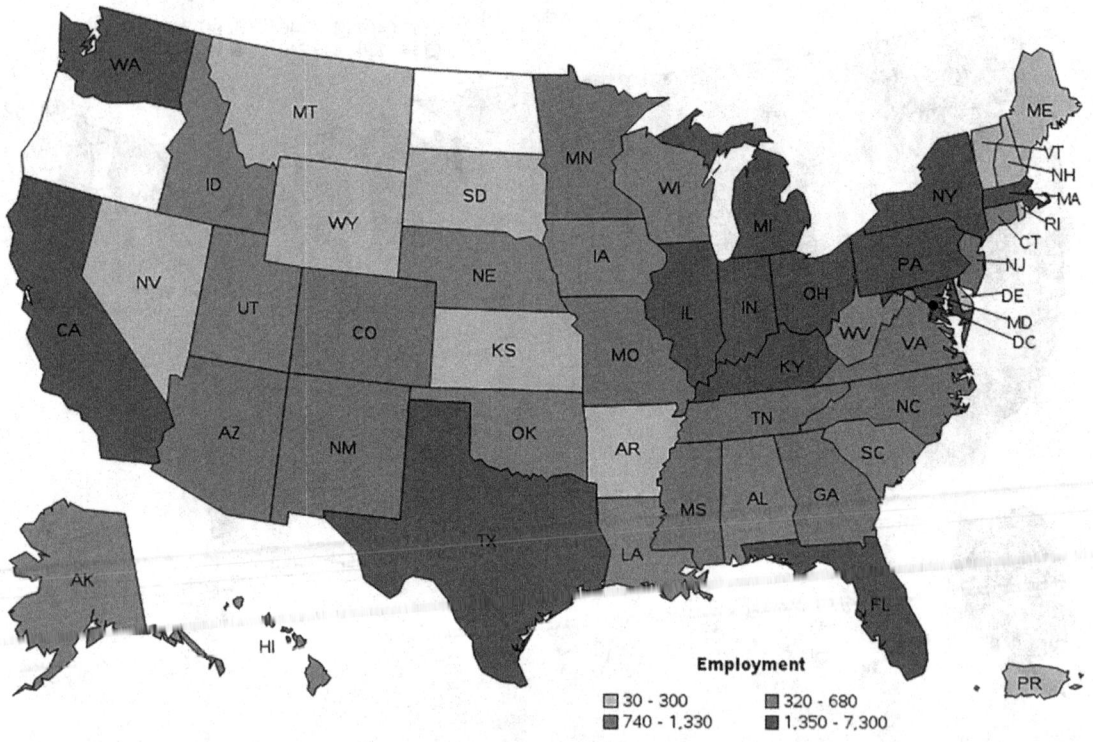

Employment

■ 30 - 300   ■ 320 - 680
■ 740 - 1,330   ■ 1,350 - 7,300

Blank areas indicate data not available.

Figure 1.3 Employment of CHWs by State

Table 1.4 States with Highest Employment, Hourly Mean Wage, and Annual Mean Wage for CHWs

State	Hourly Mean Wage	Annual Mean Wage
California	$25.45	$52,940
New York	$22.18	$46,130
Massachusetts	$22.26	$46,300
Texas	$19.75	$41,070
Washington	$22.33	$46,300

Data from U.S. Bureau of Labor Statistics. Occupational employment and wages, May 2020, 21-1094 community health workers. https://www.bls.gov/oes/current/oes211094.htm#(1). Accessed on January 8, 2021.[26]

experience is valuable because CHWs work in the community with a diverse population. In addition, CHWs with additional language and cultural skills will have a major advantage when applying for CHW employment opportunities.[27] See **Table 1.4**.

Since the CHW profession is an emerging profession and the career information changes rapidly, here are two helpful links:

- https://www.cdc.gov/dhdsp/pubs/docs/chw _state_laws.pdf shows the requirements for CHWs in most states.[28]

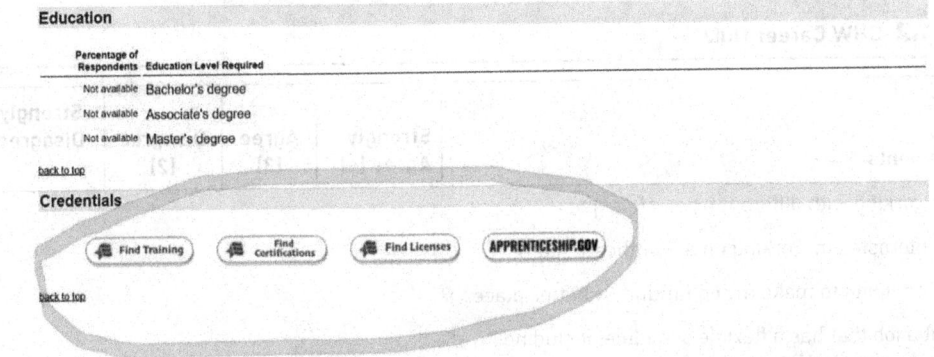

Figure 1.4 O*Net CHW Credentials

Figure from O*Net OnLine. Summary Report For: 21-1094.00- Community Health Workers. https://www.onetonline.org/link/summary/21-1094.00. Accessed October 23, 2021.[25]

- O*NET Online has searchable information about credentials and certifications (https://www.onetonline.org/link/summary/21-1094.00#Credentials).[25] For example, Arizona has a certification that is optional and not required; however, the benefits of certification versus noncertification are still being explored (https://human-resources-health.biomedcentral.com/track/pdf/10.1186/s12960-020-00487-7.pdf).[29] See **Figure 1.4**.

Examples of CHW Careers

Additionally, CHWs emphasize advocacy work among specific populations. For example, the LGBTQIA+ population advocates for equality and improved access to healthcare providers. CHWs join in such advocacy efforts, while focusing on numerous aspects of chronic disease, including access to health care and health insurance, understanding a diagnosis, taking medications correctly, communicating with healthcare providers, and other such topics. For example, if a CHW works with individuals in a rural area who have a chronic disease, the focus would be different than for a CHW serving elderly individuals who reside in a low-income housing community.

Now that you have learned what CHWs do in their community, it is time to think about if you would enjoy this career. By taking the 10-question career quiz in **Box 1.2**, you will discover if your responses match with the expectations of CHWs.

Now that you have an idea about whether you are suited for a CHW career, explore a sample job description for a CHW. See **Table 1.5**.

Would you apply for this position? You may wish to think about and consider the following questions:

- Would you get excited going to work each day if you were hired for this job?
- Do you know the healthcare resources in your community? If not, would you be willing to learn?
- Would you like to work with people and help them improve their health concerns?
- Would you like to help people to understand or resolve their health issues?
- Do you have the required qualifications? Do you have any of the preferred qualifications?

Now that you realize that becoming a CHW matches your desires and your experience, it is time to read through descriptions of available jobs. When you begin this process, it is not necessary to focus on geographical location of the position. Review Table 1.2 to remember the various titles given to CHWs. If you only search for CHWs positions, it is likely that you will skip over many other appropriate positions with

Box 1.2 CHW Career Quiz

Statements	Strongly Agree (4)	Agree (3)	Disagree (2)	Strongly Disagree (1)
I like working with different types of people.				
I am interested in working on a healthcare team.				
I enjoy helping to make my community a better place.				
I want a job that has a flexible schedule, including some evenings and weekends.				
I do not mind driving around the community if I am reimbursed for the mileage.				
I like researching topics to discover community resources for individuals in need.				
I enjoy getting involved with community committees to solve problems.				
I like to be creative at work to design or improve healthcare brochures.				
I am interested in a position that offers opportunities for advancement.				
I prefer a job I enjoy with adequate pay rather than a higher salary in a job that I do not enjoy.				
Total Score				

Results: The higher the score, the more likely you would enjoy a CHW position.

You would like a career in CHW: Score: Over 30
You would like portions of CHW: Score: 29–20
You would generally not like this work: Score: Under 20

difference titles. This type of search is for you to focus on the qualifications and skills required to apply for each position.[30] The question to keep in mind is:

Which qualifications and skills do I have, and which qualifications and skills do I need to acquire?

As you browse through the available positions, make a list of qualifications and skills requested that you may need to develop as preparation for becoming a CHW. This purpose of this chapter is to introduce the role of CHWs rather than present the details of resume writing and interviewing skills.

Chapter Summary

This chapter started with a description of public health by defining the three core functions and 10 essential services as well as the difference between public health and individual health. Next the discussion moved to the history of CHWs and the various roles, skills, and responsibilities of a CHW in the community including duties, wages, and places of employment.

Table 1.5 Example of Job Description for a CHW

Category	Duties
Summary	We are looking for a person who is a community-minded and interested in teaching classes about nutritious eating and exercise to promote healthy lifestyles. This job position is responsible for creating and integrating health-based programs, while partnering with various health organizations. It will be necessary to be familiar with community resources and understand effective program planning. Besides physical health, it is necessary to know about services for mental health and addiction services. Bilingual applicants will receive top priority for this position. If you enjoy helping others improve their lives and health, submit your application.
Responsibilities	Develop and maintain a client database including contact information, forms, notes, and supplementary information.
	Host neighborhood meetings to determine health program needs for individuals in the community.
	Participate in weekly community outreach events to raise awareness among special interest groups, such as the elderly, pregnant women, individuals with disabilities, and individuals with low incomes seeking health care in the community.
	Contact (in-person, phone, or virtual media) clients in existing programs to ensure their health and safety, answer questions, provide resources, and update their current concerns.
	Complete administrative tasks to keep records organized, update the client database and calendar for community events, upcoming client visit schedules, and other duties as assigned.
	Coordinate and schedule staff meetings and the agenda for the administrative management team.
Leadership and Advancement	Manage "train-the-trainer" opportunities as CHW increases in size and scope of responsibilities.
	Teach basic clinical skills (e.g., glucose monitoring, blood pressure screening, vaccine clinic participation) to new team members.
	Participate in opportunities to gain additional certifications and advanced skills.
Qualifications	Required
	■ High school diploma or its equivalent
	■ Basic computer skills for Microsoft Word, Zoom, and Facebook
	Preferred
	■ Experience in some aspect of the healthcare field
	■ Experience working with retired individuals and the Medicaid population
	■ Able to converse and write well in Spanish
	■ Customer service experience with the public
Application	Apply online at https//mycommunitycenter.com/application

Data from Livecareer. Community health worker job description writing and posting in 3 easy steps. https://www.livecareer.com/job-description/examples/social-services/community-health-worker. Accessed on January 18, 2021.[30]

CASE STUDY

Applying for a CHW Position

For the past 7 years, Brenda has been employed as a patient technician in a small, assisted living complex. She wants to explore how to become a CHW. She has an associate degree in health education and speaks fluent Spanish. Since she works full-time, she does not have much free time to investigate a career change to CHW.

1. Describe where Brenda should begin the process to become a CHW.
2. Identify places where Brenda might find employment as a CHW.
3. List ways to assist Brenda to update her resume prior to applying for CHW jobs.

References

1. World Health Organization (WHO) definition of health. Public Health Nigeria Web site. https://www.publichealth.com.ng/world-health-organizationwho-definition-of-health/. Accessed January 8, 2021.
2. The 1st International Conference on Health Promotion, Ottawa, 1986. World Health Organization Web site. https://www.who.int/teams/health-promotion/enhanced-wellbeing/first-global-conference. Accessed October 22, 2021.
3. What is health equity? Centers for Disease Control and Prevention Web site. https://www.cdc.gov/healthequity/index.html. Accessed October 22, 2021.
4. 10 essential public health services. Centers for Disease Control and Prevention Web site. https://www.cdc.gov/publichealthgateway/publichealthservices/essentialhealthservices.html#:~:text=The%2010%20Essential%20Public%20Health%20Services%20describe%20the,identify%20and%20solve%20health%20problems%20More%20items...%20. Accessed January 8, 2021.
5. Perry H. A brief history of community health worker programs. https://www.mchip.net/sites/default/files/mchipfiles/02_CHW_History.pdf. Accessed October 22, 2021.
6. Lehmann U, Sanders D. Community health workers: What do we know about them? https://www.who.int/hrh/documents/community_health_workers.pdf. Published January 2007. Accessed January 8, 2021.
7. Gilson L, Walt G, Heggenhougen K, Owuor-Omondi L, Perera M, Ross D, Salazar L. National community health worker programs: how can they be strengthened? *Journal of Public Health Policy.* 1989;10(4):518–532.
8. Summary of the national community health advisor study. University of Arizona Web site. https://crh.arizona.edu/sites/default/files/pdf/publications/CAHsummaryALL.pdf. Published 1998. Accessed on January 8, 2021.
9. Rosenthal LE, Heer HD, Rush CH, Holderby LR. Focus on the future: A community health worker research agenda by and for the field. *Progress in community health partnerships: research, education, and action.* 2008;2(3):183–184, 225–235.
10. Health Resources and Services Administration, Bureau of Health Professions. *Community Health Worker National Workforce Study.* Washington DC: US Dept of Health and Human Services; 2007.
11. Spencer MS, Gunter KE, Palmisano G. Community health workers and their value to social work. *Soc Work.* 2010;55(2):169–180.
12. Community health workers (CHWs). Rural Health Information Hub Web site. https://www.ruralhealthinfo.org/toolkits/care-coordination/2/care-coordinator-model/community-health-workers#:~:text=Community%20Health%20Workers%20(CHWs)&text=%E2%80%9CAssist%20individuals%20and%20communities%20to,improve%20individual%20and%20community%20health. Accessed on January 8, 2021.
13. Shah M, Heisler M, Davis M. Community health workers and the Patient Protection and Affordable Care Act: An opportunity for a research, advocacy, and policy agenda. *J Health Care Poor Undeserved.* 2014;25(1):17–24.
14. Legal Information Institute. 42 CFR § 440.130—Diagnostic, screening, preventive, and rehabilitative services. https://www.law.cornell.edu/cfr/text/42/440.130. Accessed May 26, 2021.
15. Policy evidence assessment report: community health worker policy components. Centers for Disease Control and Prevention Web site. https://www.cdc.gov/dhdsp/pubs/docs/chw_evidence_assessment_report.pdf. Accessed January 8, 2021.
16. U.S. Department of Health and Human Services, Health Resources and Services Administration, Bureau of Health Professions. Community health worker national workforce study. https://bhw.hrsa.gov/sites/default/files/bureau-health-workforce/data-research/community-health-workforce.pdf. Accessed January 8, 2021.
17. The Community Health Worker Core Consensus Project. C3 project findings: roles & competencies. https://www.c3project.org/roles-competencies. Accessed May 25, 2021.
18. Witmer A, Seifer DS, Finocchio L, Leslie J, O'Neil, HE. Community health workers: integral members

of the health care work force. *Am J Public Health.* 1995;85(8 Pt 1):1055–1058.

19. Balcazar H, Rosenthal L, Brownstein JN, Rush CH, Matos S, Hernandez L. Community health workers can be a public health force for change in the United States: three actions for a new paradigm. *Am J Public Health.* 2011;101(12):2199–220.

20. Allen JK, Dennison-Himmelfarb CR, Szanton SL, et al. Community Outreach and Cardiovascular Health (COACH) Trial: a randomized, controlled trial of nurse practitioner/community health worker cardiovascular disease risk reduction in urban community health centers. *Circ Cardiovasc Qual Outcomes.* 2011;4(6):595–602.

21. Whitley EM, Everhart RM, Wright RA. Measuring return on investment of outreach by community health workers. *J Health Care Poor Underserved.* 2006;17(1 Suppl):6–15.

22. Martinez J, Knickman JR. *Community Health Workers: A Critical Link for Improving Health Outcomes and Promoting Cost-Effective Care in the Era of Health Reform.* New York: New York State Health Foundation; 2010.

23. Integrating behavioral health with primary medical care. Health Resources and Services Administration Web site. https://www.hrsa.gov/behavioral-health. Accessed on January 8, 2021.

24. Bright outlook occupation: 21-1094.00-community health workers. O*Net OnLine. https://www.onetonline.org/help/bright/21-1094.00. Accessed October 23, 2021.

25. SummaryrReport for: 21-1094.00-community health workers. O*Net OnLine. https://www.onetonline.org/link/summary/21-1094.00. Accessed October 23, 2021.

26. Occupational employment and wages, May 2020 21-1094 community health workers. U.S. Bureau of Labor Statistics Web site. https://www.bls.gov/oes/current/oes211094.htm#(1). Accessed on January 8, 2021.

27. Role of community health workers. National Heart, Lung, and Blood Institute Web site. https://www.nhlbi.nih.gov/health/educational/healthdisp/role-of-community-health-workers.htm. Accessed January 8, 2021.

28. State law fact sheet: A summary of state community health worker laws. Centers for Disease Control and Prevention Web site. https://www.cdc.gov/dhdsp/pubs/docs/SLFS-Summary-State-CHW-Laws.pdf. Accessed June 15, 2021.

29. Ingram M, Sabo S, Redondo F, et al. Establishing voluntary certification of community health workers in Arizona: A policy case study of building a unified workforce. *Hum Resour. Health.* 2020;18(46).

30. Community health worker job description writing and posting in 3 easy steps. Livecareer Web site. https://www.livecareer.com/job-description/examples/social-services/community-health-worker. Accessed on January 18, 2021.

CHAPTER 2

Adult Learning and Health Literacy

LEARNING OBJECTIVES

1. Define literacy.
2. Provide a definition and example for each of the five types of literacy: verbal, written/reading, digital, numerical, and health.
3. Create health documents that support plain language and lower literacy levels.
4. Explain effective listening skills.
5. Demonstrate teaching techniques for the learning styles including visual, auditory, reading/writing, and kinesthetic.

KEY TERMS

literacy	plain language	personal health literacy
functional literacy	digital literacy	organizational health literacy
verbal literacy	digital learning gap	productive health communication
reading literacy	numerical literacy	VARK

Introduction

This chapter introduces an overview of literacy, including reading, writing, verbal communication, understanding basic numbers, application of digital and technology skills, and health literacy. All forms of literacy affect an individual's health outcomes.[1] The next section describes how to create documents in plain language with appropriate readability levels. This information is followed by effective listening skills. Lastly, the chapter introduces style of learning including visual, auditory, reading/writing, and kinesthetic (VARK).

Overview of Literacy

Literacy is defined as the capacity to communicate through verbal, written, numeric, reading, and digital/technological formats.[2] Let's consider how a child progresses from sound to language to reading literacy. First, the parents talk to the baby, and after a few months the baby begins to babble while trying to form words. The parents praise the child's attempts and soon the baby makes sounds. The first sounds might emerge as mama and dada. Next, the parents begin to read alphabet books to the baby, and as the child grows the sounds emerge into saying the alphabet in their language of origin. Upon saying the alphabet, the child recognizes the letters. By combining the letters, the child forms one-syllable words. For some children, the progression of language acquisition is delayed due to a disability, lack of exposure, or low literacy of the parents or guardians. When the child enters school, these delays may be noticed through testing and corrected with tailored education or speech therapy to meet the child's unique capabilities.

According to the National Center for Education Statistics, about four out of five U.S. adults (79 percent) have medium to high English literacy skills.[3] However, 21 percent of U.S. adults have difficulty completing these simple tasks, such as reading a short sentence to locate information or completing simple forms due a language barrier, lack of adequate education, enrollment in poor quality schools, cognitive disability, or physical disability.[4] In addition, the National Center of Education Statistics and the Program for the International Assessment of Adult Competencies (PIAAC) conducts a 23-country comparative study of adult literacy across three domains: literacy, numeracy, and problem solving in technology. In each of these domains, adults perform tasks with different levels of complexity. Their proficiency skills were ranked as "below level 1," which represents the lowest literacy level, and up to "level 5" as the highest literacy proficiency level. Only 12 percent of U.S. adults scored in the highest literacy proficiency levels, and only 9 percent scored in the highest numeracy levels.[5] See **Figure 2.1** and **Figure 2.2**.

U.S. literacy statistics indicate that approximately 50 percent of adults cannot read a book written at the eighth-grade level. Surveys show that the average reading level of the top 40 books read by teens within the United States in grades 9–12 is 5.3, barely above the fifth-grade level. An individual who has achieved a level of level 1 **functional literacy** is able to read the signs showcased in **Figure 2.3**.

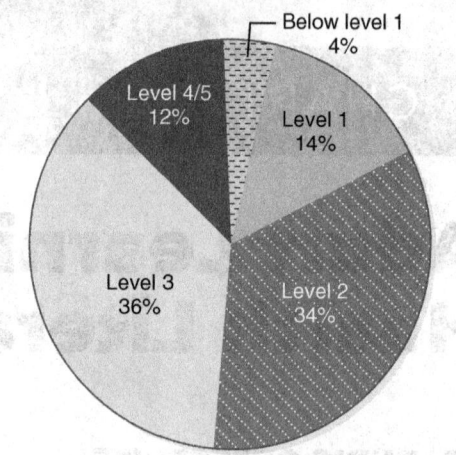

Figure 2.1 Percentage of U.S. Adults Aged 16 to 65 at Each Level of Proficiency on Literacy Scale

Centers for Disease Control and Prevention. Understanding literacy and numeracy. https://www.cdc.gov/healthliteracy/learn/understandingliteracy.html. Accessed April 6, 2021. Reference to specific commercial products, manufacturers, companies, or trademarks does not constitute its endorsement or recommendation by the U.S. Government, Department of Health and Human Services, or Centers for Disease Control and Prevention.

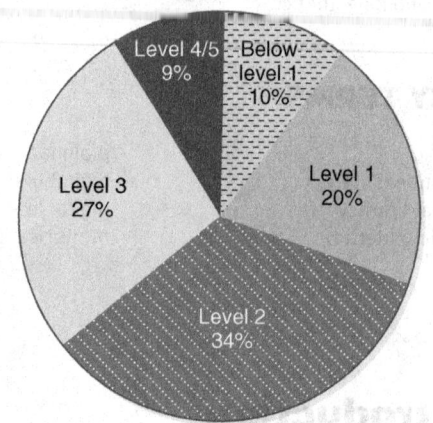

Figure 2.2 Percentage of U.S. Adults Aged 16 to 65 at Each Level of Proficiency on the Numerical Scale

Centers for Disease Control and Prevention. Understanding literacy and numeracy. https://www.cdc.gov/healthliteracy/learn/understandingliteracy.html. Accessed April 6, 2021. Reference to specific commercial products, manufacturers, companies, or trademarks does not constitute its endorsement or recommendation by the U.S. Government, Department of Health and Human Services, or Centers for Disease Control and Prevention.[6]

After reviewing the two pie charts in Figure 2.3 and reviewing the level 1 functional literacy sign examples, it is evident that many adults are lacking basic levels of proficiency in reading and understanding numeracy.[6] See **Figure 2.4**.

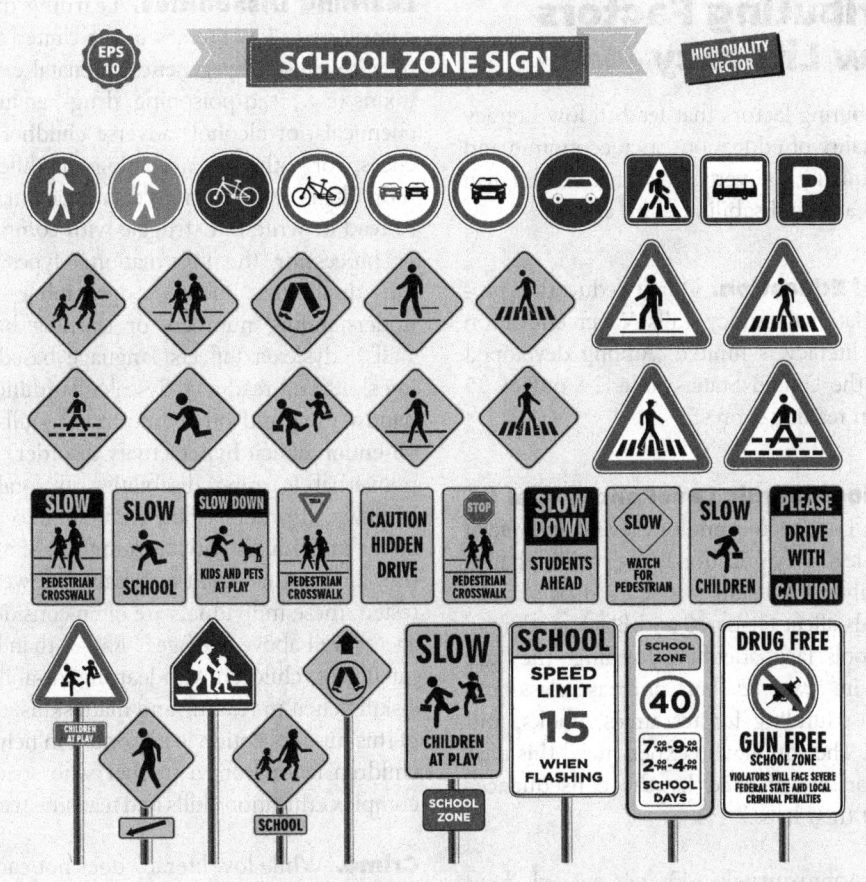

Figure 2.3 Level 1 Functional Literacy Example

© Albert Stephen Julius/Shutterstock.[7]

When adults learn how to read, write, do basic math, and use computers, they have the power to lift themselves out of poverty, lower health care costs, find and keep sustainable employment, and ultimately change their lives.

43 Million

More than 43 million adults in the United States cannot read, write, or do basic math above a third-grade level.

Figure 2.4 The Numbers Do Not Lie

Reproduced from ProLiteracy Worldwide, "U.S. Adult Literacy Facts" (2021), https://hubs.la/Q01lbvkJ0. Data source U.S. Dept. of Education, "Adult Literacy in the United States" (2019), https://nces.ed.gov/pubs2019/2019179.pdf.

Contributing Factors to Low Literacy

The contributing factors that lead to low literacy include quality of education, socioeconomic and racial inequality, poverty, non-native English speakers, learning disabilities, and crime.[9]

Quality of Education. Quality education provides foundational literacy skills. When education is limited, literacy is limited. Among developed countries, the United States ranks 24 out of 35 countries in reading scores.[9]

Low Socioeconomic Level and Racial Inequality. Low socioeconomic levels and racial inequality lead to educational inequality that is most heavily concentrated in U.S. urban areas. These trends affect Hispanic and Black students.[9] When schools lack adequate funding, they are forced to hire fewer teachers, increase class size, and decrease funding for resources, books, and computers. The adults who experienced this type of education are affected by the consequences throughout their lives.[9]

Poverty. Approximately 43 percent of low-literate adults live in poverty, compared to only 5 percent of people at the highest literacy level.[9–10] Also, low-income children are more likely to not attend preschool, attend low-funded schools, struggle with emotions, and develop learning challenges. These students are more likely to drop out of school to support their family, which leads to difficulty finding work due to a lack of qualification and low literacy.[9]

Non-Native English Speakers. Many non-native English speakers are literate in their native language but are illiterate in English. Approximately 64 percent of adult immigrants perform at low literacy levels compared to 14 percent of native-born Americans.[9] Many non-native English speaking adult immigrants and refugees seek out English education to become literate; however, developing reading proficiency takes time.[9]

Learning Disabilities. Learning disabilities contribute to low literacy in the United States and may be caused by genetics, prenatal exposure to toxins (e.g., lead poisoning, drugs, environmental chemicals, or alcohol) adverse childhood experiences, or other neurobiological differences.[9,11] Individuals with learning disabilities may be able to read or write but struggle with comprehension or processing the information.[9] Types of learning disabilities include dysgraphia (difficulty understanding numbers or learning basic math skills), dyslexia (affects language based processing skills and reading), dyscalculia (difficulty with handwriting and other fine motor skills), ADHD (attention deficit hyperactivity disorder) and other nonverbal learning disabilities, or oral/ written language disorders.[11] One common misconception about individuals with learning disabilities is that they are less intelligent or capable. However, when tested, these individuals are often considered average or well above average.[11] Rather than being less intelligent, children with learning disabilities have a skill deficit in reading and math skills. Awareness of this misconception is important in helping these children learn from a teacher who specializes in complex education skills and teaching techniques.[9]

Crime. While low literacy does not cause criminal behavior, low literacy may contribute to criminal behavior, which could lead to incarceration.[12] Racial inequality, poverty, poor education, and unsafe environments make individuals more vulnerable to crime and illiteracy.[9,12] Health literacy and educational opportunities prevent chronic disease and poor health outcomes. However, an absence of health literacy presents as a high risk for poor health outcomes among individuals released from incarceration.[12] Former convicts are more likely to work at a low-wage job and remain uneducated, unemployed, and in poverty.[9]

All the factors discussed intersect and contribute to low literacy across generations.[9] For example, poverty overlaps with discrimination toward racial minorities and non-native English speakers.[9,12] Poverty leads to attending low-funded schools that initiates low-income employment and thus creates an intergenerational cycle with little chance of escape.[9] See **Box 2.1**.

Box 2.1 How to Identify Adults with Low Health Literacy Skills

Low literacy seems invisible.[13] However, it is present among many of the patients seeking care. The healthcare system is complex and difficult to understand, especially for adults with low literacy levels.[13] In addition, these patients feel a sense of shame and attempt to hide their struggles with reading, writing, numbers, and technology.[13] The following list identifies ways to identify patients are at higher risk for low literacy:

- Misses appointments frequently[13]
- Unable to complete the registration forms
- Unable to name medications, explain purpose and dosage[13]
- Identifies pills at color and shape rather than reading the label
- Unable to provide a personal medical history[13]
- Shows a lack of follow-up on tests, scans, and referrals as prescribed[13]

States phrases such as:

"I forgot my reading glasses."[13]

"I will read it when I get home."

"I am too tired to read it now."[13]

Here is an appropriate statement to begin this conversation:

"A lot of people have trouble reading and remembering health information because it is difficult. Is this ever a problem for you?"[13]

When the CHW recognizes these phrases or actions from a patient several times, it is time to explore ways to assist them with their health information.

Data from Center for Health Care Strategies, Inc. How Is Health Literacy Identified. https://www.chcs.org/media/How_is_Low_Health_Literacy_Identified.pdf. Accessed October 31, 2021.[13]

Types of Literacy

This section describes the types of literacy including verbal, reading, digital, numerical, and health.[14–15]

Verbal Literacy

Verbal literacy includes speaking and listening that occurs in every aspect of daily life.[15] Communication includes sharing information, acquiring knowledge, seeking directions, providing emergency or weather warnings, or merely for enjoyment and socialization. Once individuals understand verbal communication, they begin to analyze and interpret the information presented.[14] For example, think about the list of new words that were acquired during the COVID-19 pandemic. Many new phrases became commonplace over a few weeks as the population learned the meaning of flattening the curve, proper handwashing techniques, social distancing, wearing a face mask properly, and sanitizing personal space.

Over time, individuals learn that each discipline has a unique language. If the individual wants to communicate with professionals within that discipline, it is necessary to learn the vocabulary necessary for productive verbal communication. For example, there are unique literacy demands whether it is health care, banking, credit reports, car maintenance, legal documents, or an apartment lease. In every phase of life, individuals learn to say and understand the meaning of new words to communicate in society.[14] See **Case Study 2.1**.

Case Study 2.1 Communication with a Healthcare Provider

Mrs. Williams, age 78, went to the neighborhood walk-in clinic because of her persistent pain in her left hip and leg. Since she was new to the community, she took the first available appointment with Dr. Bauman. Upon arrival, the receptionist asked Mrs. Williams to complete the intake medical history form. Mrs. Williams completed the form and returned it to the receptionist. Julie, the community health worker (CHW), called Mrs. Williams from the waiting room and led her to an exam room. After getting her blood pressure and weight, Julie said that Dr. Bauman would be in soon. Dr. Bauman came in within about 5 minutes. She seemed in a hurry and started asking questions after a brief introduction. She glanced at Mrs. Williams medical history and started the following conversation:

DR. BAUMAN: How long have you had this left hip and leg pain?

MRS. WILLIAMS: About 3 months.

DR. BAUMAN: Why did you wait so long?

MRS. WILLIAMS: I was moving from another state.

DR. BAUMAN: Let's examine your leg. Please remove your shorts.

Mrs. Williams struggles to remove her sandals and stretchy shorts.

DR. BAUMAN: Have you been taking any OTC pills?

MRS. WILLIAMS: No.

DR. BAUMAN: Are you experiencing any neuropathy type pain?

MRS. WILLIAMS: No.

DR. BAUMAN: When was the last time you had a DEXA scan?

MRS. WILLIAMS: I do not know.

DR. BAUMAN: When do you experience the most discomfort? Is it intermittent?

MRS. WILLIAMS: Nighttime.

DR. BAUMAN: I will order a series of radiology tests to rule out any abnormalities. There is no need for a diagnosis or treatment yet. I will see you again after you obtain the tests. Do you have any other questions?

When Julie came back into the exam room, Mrs. Williams looked upset. Julie helped Mrs. Williams with her shorts and sandals prior to getting off the exam table. They went to Julie's office, and she offered Mrs. Williams a bottle of chilled water. Before starting to schedule that Dr. Bauman ordered, she asked Mrs. Williams if she had any questions.

Questions

1. How would you rewrite Dr. Bauman's conversation using lower literacy words?
2. Why did Mrs. Williams answer "no" to most of Dr. Bauman's questions?
3. What actions did Julie perform to help Mrs. Williams?

As illustrated by Case Study 2.1, for individuals to understand what is being communicated, it is essential that the speaker uses the appropriate level of literacy. Otherwise, there is no interaction and understanding happening between the two

individuals. For example, a new hospital volunteer works in the Dispatch Department and delivers various items to different departments. On day he asks for directions to the Pathology Department to deliver a small clear bag containing the paper orders along with the surgical specimen. The hospital employee providing the directions is trying to be helpful but uses words unfamiliar to the volunteer by stating: "Go to the end of the corridor and turn left at the ED sign. Take the first elevator that you see to the third floor. When you get off, turn right, and look for the ICU signs. Walk past the ICU entrance, and Pathology will be on your left. Open the Pathology door, sign-in, and deliver the bag." Even though the hospital volunteer has adequate literacy skills, he does not recognize the directions due to lack of adequate hospital vocabulary. This example shows that everyone can experience verbal literacy challenges in unfamiliar situations.

Reading and Written Literacy

Reading literacy is defined as the ability to understand and use the written language required by society.[15–16] Reading includes many traditional written forms of paper (books, newspapers, documents, billboards, menus, etc.) to the internet and digital formats on a variety of screens including cell phones, tablets, kiosks, laptops, desktops, and virtual shared screens. Regardless of the format, reading is the essential format by which individuals acquire and exchange information for communication.[17]

Writing in Plain Language with Lower Literacy

As a CHW, it is important that documents, forms, brochures, pamphlets, and signs are created using plain language. **Plain language** is grammatically correct language that includes complete sentence structure and accurate word usage.[15] Writing that is clear and to the point helps improve communication and takes less time to read and understand. Clear writing states exactly what the reader needs to know without using unnecessary words or expressions.[17] Communicating saves time and money. It also improves how the reader responses to messages. Using plain language avoids creating barriers with the people with whom the communication is intended.[17]

CHWs have many opportunities convert or create health documents that focus on simple language for greater understanding and comprehension regardless of health literacy proficiency. When writing low literacy documents, it is useful to know a few basic concepts.[17]

1. Use a simple writing style. Each sentence contains only a few words.
   Example: Normal blood pressure is 120/80.[18]
2. Use one-syllable words when possible.
   Example: Three ways to lower your blood pressure:
   a. Take a brisk walk each day.[18]
   b. Stop smoking.[18]
3. Write in active voice.
   Examples:
   Active voice: Walking keeps weight in control.
   Passive voice: A healthy weight may be achieved with regular exercise.
4. Write information in a logical format. Put the most important information near the beginning of the document.
   Example: (Prescription label)
   Take one pill every morning.
   Eat breakfast after taking this pill.
5. Select a simple font. Use a font size of at least 12 points. Do not use several fonts in order to avoid confusion.
   Example:

Too small:	This font is too small to read.
Difficult to read:	*This font is too fancy to read.*
ALL CAPITALS:	**AN ALL CAPITAL FONT IS DIFFICULT TO READ.**
Simple:	**This font is easy to see and read.**

6. Select illustrations appropriate for the age of the audience, place the illustrations near the text, and always show the whole body rather than only the organ.
   Example: Which illustration of the kidneys is easier to understand?

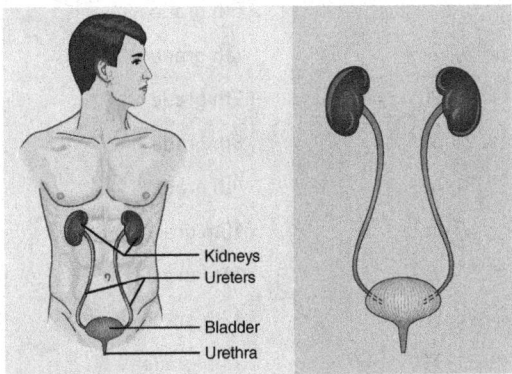

Left figure from KidsHealth. Urinary Reflux. https://www.kidshealth.org.nz/urinary-reflux. Accessed October 31, 2021.[19]

Right figure from BlogSpot. Writing and Diagram Explained. https://antasyaalinda.blogspot.com/2018/07/diagram-of-urinary-system-with-labels.html. Accessed October 31, 2021.[20]

7. Estimate the reading level of the document by following the steps in **Box 2.2**.

Box 2.2 Instructions for Measuring Readability

Using an abbreviated version of the SMOG reading formula,[21-22] follow these steps to estimate the reading level of a document.

1. Choose a single block of 30 sentences in a row from a document or combine three blocks of 10 sentences each.
2. Count the number of words with three or more syllables. Circle each word.
   a. Count one syllable for each letter or number in an acronym or symbol.
   b. For example, the year 2022 = four syllables; 10 minutes = four syllables (one for each number and two for the word minutes); CHW = six syllables (certified = three syllables, health = one syllable; worker = two syllables).

3. Use this SMOG table[2] to estimate the reading grade level.

Words with 3+ Syllables	Approximate Grade Level
0–2	4th grade
3–6	5th grade
7–12	6th grade
13–20	7th grade
21–30	8th grade
31–42	9th grade
43–56	10th grade
57–72	11th grade
73–90	12th grade
91–110	13th grade
111–132	14th grade
133–156	15th grade
157–182	16th grade
183 or more	17th grade

Data from U.S. Department of Health and Human Services, Centers for Medicare & Medicaid Services. TOOLKIT for Making Written Material Clear and Effective Part 7 Using Readability formulas: A Cautionary Note. https://www.cms.gov/Outreach-and-Education/Outreach/WrittenMaterialsToolkit/Downloads/ToolkitPart07.pdf. Accessed October 31, 2021.[21] Readability Formulas. The SMOG Readability Formula. https://www.readabilityformulas.com/smog-readability-formula.php#:~:text=SMOG%20Readability%20Formula%201%20Step%201.%20%3A%20Take,4%20Step%204.%20...%205%20Step%204.%20. Accessed November 1, 2021.[22]

Now practice the information in Box 2.1. When a CHW is learning to decrease the reading level of a printed document, it helps to start the process by reading the document aloud. After becoming familiar with the content, start by circling every word that is three or more syllables. Calculate the reading level. Use the computer to find a synonym to replace the multi-syllable word. For example, to replace the four-syllable word "medication," the suggested synonyms are drug or pill. After replacing the multi-syllable words with simple words, go back

to the document and examine the long sentences. Rewrite the long sentences into short and simple sentences. Practice these skills on the following original statement. Revise the paragraph in simple, plain language.[17,21]

Original Statement:
Chronic obstructive pulmonary disease (COPD) is a chronic inflammatory lung disease that causes obstructed airflow from the lungs.[23] Symptoms include breathing difficulty, cough, mucus (sputum) production, and wheezing. It is typically caused by long-term exposure to irritating gases or particulate matter, most often from cigarette smoke.[23] People with COPD are at increased risk of developing heart disease, lung cancer, and a variety of other conditions. Although COPD is a progressive disease that gets worse over time, COPD is treatable.[23] With proper management, most people with COPD can achieve good symptom control and quality of life, as well as reduced risk of other associated conditions.[23] (105 words in the sample)

Revised Statement:
COPD is a lung disease. People with COPD have a hard time breathing, and they may cough often.[23] COPD begins when a person is exposed to cigarette smoke or factory fumes. This disease increases the risk of getting lung cancer, heart disease, and other illnesses.[23] COPD gets worse over the years. Most people control COPD by going to the doctor often. The doctor provides ways to treat COPD. If the person follows the treatment plan, they will reduce the risk of getting other diseases.[23] (85 words in the revised sample)

Digital (Technology) Literacy

Digital literacy is defined as the knowledge and ability to use computers and related technology devices efficiently.[24–25] The utilization of digital literacy often depends on one's knowledge, skill, and comfort level with technological devices. Computer skill levels range from basic to advanced computer programming.[24–25] Prior

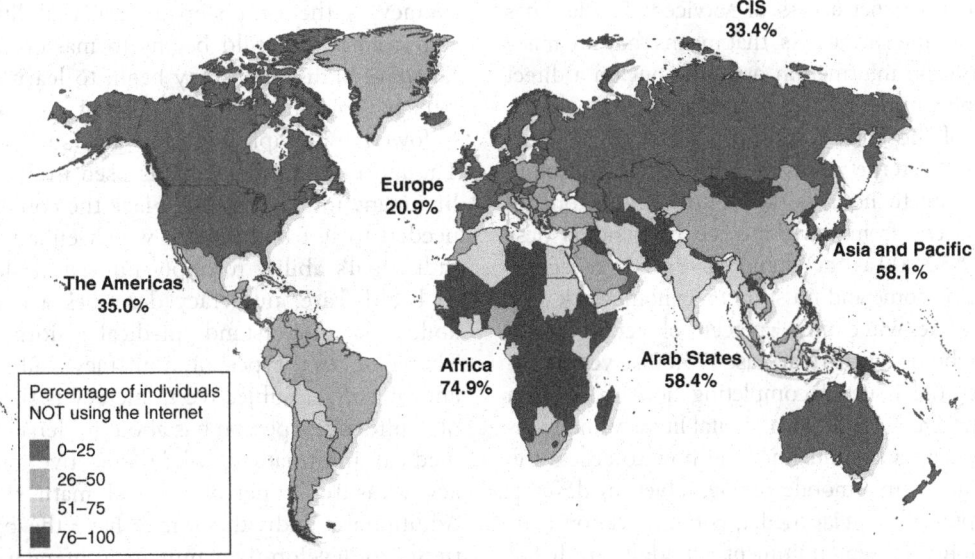

Figure 2.5 World's Offline Population in 2016

Reproduced from Ortiz DN. Digital health literacy. https://www.statista.com/statistics/1155552/countries-highest-number-lacking-internet/ Accessed September 5, 2022.[24]

to the COVID-19 pandemic, there were arguments about the pros and cons of using digital technology in classroom settings. Due to COVID-19, virtual learning has become recognized as a valuable tool for communication among all ages. Individuals develop virtual communication skills to stay connected in education, employment, telehealth, and especially with family. However, access to digital literacy varies widely across the globe.[24–25] See **Figure 2.5**. Though the continents with limited computer access are evident, it is useful to note that up to 25 percent of the United States and Canadian population does not have internet access. See **Box 2.3** to explore why this may be the case.

Last, the **digital learning gap** is causing distinct differences in how individuals in the United States access and use technology to improve learning opportunities and outcomes. The digital learning gap presents three parts of the problem: lack of access and participation which are described next.[27]

Lack of Access

In 2018, 2.3 million families living in rural and remote communities did not have access to

Box 2.3 Reasons Why Individuals in United States May Not Use the Internet

Economic: Poverty; cannot afford to buy a computer or internet service or Wi-Fi contracts; intermittent ability to pay monthly electric bill.

Education: Limited knowledge on how to learn computer skills; not taught in school.

Housing: Homeless; living conditions are not wired for internet access.

Geographical Location: Rural or remote locations lack reliable internet access; limited access to adult education; not all inner-city housing is wired with internet access; mobile home parks may not have reliable internet services.

Literacy: Embarrassed to admit low literacy; cannot read information on computer screen.

Age and Disabilities: Feeling too old to learn computer skills; disabilities such as limited vision to see the screen; low hearing to attend a class; limited hand/finger movement; inability to sit for long periods of time at a desk; limited cognitive ability to learn and retain new skills and knowledge.

Data from Zickuhr K. Who's not online and why? https://www.pewresearch.org/internet/2013/09/25/whos-not-online-and-why/. Accessed November 1, 2021.[26]

reliable internet access or service.[27] For families without internet access, that means they are missing out on information or losing out on a direct line of communication with schools and teachers. One of the biggest problems faced by students without internet access at home is their inability to complete homework.[28] Furthermore, one in four teens from lower-income households (less than $30,000 a year) do not have access to a computer at home and must do their homework on a cellphone, while only 4 percent of teens living in households that earn at least $75,000 a year experience the issue of completing homework on a cell phone.[27] In addition, digital literacy and technology goes beyond knowing how to access the internet from a mobile phone, tablet, or desktop computer for social media, communication connections, and entertainment. In addition, digital literacy allows individuals to learn, understand, access resources, and solve problems.[27]

Participation

Despite how almost every American has access to the internet, approximately 7 percent do not use it.[29] According to the Pew Internet and American Life Project, age, income level, and educational attainment were all strongly tied in with usage patterns. Among those 65 and older, 44 percent do not use the internet. They account for just about half (49 percent) of the offline adult population in America.[30] In addition, individuals living in rural parts of the United States are more than twice as likely not to use the internet compared to individuals living in suburbs and cities.[27] For example, if a CHW assists 15 people in a health clinic each day, there is a good chance that each day one of those individuals does not use the internet.

Numerical (Numeracy) Literacy

Numerical literacy is defined as the ability to use and understand mathematics to solve basic problems in real-world situations.[31] Numerical literacy is the next step after verbal literacy. For example, a child begins to master simple language skills, then they begin to learn numbers by counting. The concept of counting is followed by simple addition and subtraction. Though numerical literacy is used in everyday life, many individuals often lack the confidence needed to use basic math, which enhances an individual's ability to apply numerical skills.[32] In health care, numeracy describes a person's ability to understand medical information. There are two types of numeracy: subjective and objective. Subjective numeracy is the level of confidence a person has about understanding medical information, while objective numeracy measures a person's actual math skills.[33] Additionally, individuals may have the opportunity to develop their numerical literacy skills through employment or daily experiences.[34] **Box 2.4** showcases some of the general numerical skills used in daily life.

Box 2.4 Examples of General Numerical Skills

- Budgeting: relationship between salary and cost of basic needs (food, shelter, health care, transportation); saving money for unexpected expenses
- Money: simple and compound interest rates on credit card bills, discount rates, counting correct amount of change, balancing a checkbook
- Driving: speed limit, time, and distance to destination, gallons of fuel per mile
- Health: healthy numbers for weight, blood pressure, glucose level, pulse, body mass index (BMI)
- Medications: understanding dosage, time to take medication, before or after meals, measuring insulin in the syringe
- Cooking: time, temperature, and measuring ingredients
- Graphics: understanding bar graphs and pie charts

As noted by the previous list, it is easy to see that individuals need numerical skills. It is important to be familiar with the numerical skills that are required for a CHW whether the individual is employed in a clinical setting, home health agency, or a community service agency. See **Case Study 2.2**.

Health Literacy

The U.S. Department of Health and Human Services (HHS) has published the new *Healthy People 2030*, which includes a focus on improving personal health literacy and organizational health literacy.[37] The goal of *Healthy People 2030* is to establish specific goals and objectives related to the improvement of current areas regarding the nation's health. Improving health literacy can lead to disease prevention and health promotion and allow individuals to better understand their health and communicate with healthcare providers. **Personal health literacy** is defined as the degree to which individuals can find, understand, and use information and services to inform health-related decisions and actions for themselves and others.[37] In addition, **organizational health literacy** is defined as the degree to which organizations equitably enable individuals to find, understand, and use information and services to inform health-related decisions and actions for themselves and others.[37] This section focuses on the patient's health literacy as well as the healthcare provider's health communication skills.

Case Study 2.2 Utilizing Basic Numerical Skills

Debra, the CHW, is planning a basic 60-minute class on the topic of carbohydrate consumption when eating vegetables. She divides the information into four topics.

1. Definition of carbohydrates: Carbohydrates are essential nutrients that include sugars, fibers, and starches.[35] They are found in grains, vegetables, fruits, and in milk and other dairy products. They are one of the basic food groups that play an important role in a healthy life. The food containing carbohydrates are converted into glucose or blood sugar during the process of digestion by the digestive system. Consuming excess carbohydrates increases the body's glucose level.[35] The body utilizes glucose as a source of energy for the cells, organs, and tissues. The extra amount of glucose (sugar) is stored in the muscles and liver. If the individual does not use the stored energy from glucose, it is stored as excess weight.[35]
2. Types of carbohydrates: There are three types of carbohydrates: sugars, starches, and fiber.[35]
   a. Sugars: healthy sugars are found in natural fruit and milk. Less healthy sugars as found in sodas, baked goods, and many packaged foods, such a cookies, candy, spaghetti sauce, ketchup, and salad dressings. When reading food labels, if the ingredients include any word that ends in "-ose" (i.e., fructose), corn syrup, or juice, the product contains added sugar.[35]
   b. Starches: Examples of starches are wheat, oats, grains, corn, potatoes, dried beans, lentils, and peas.[35]
   c. Fiber: Fiber is found in plant foods, such as fruits and vegetables. Fiber is healthy for digestions and provides a feeling of being full after eating.[35]
3. Carbohydrates can be found in vegetables. Review low carbohydrate vegetable chart in **Figure 2.6**.
4. As a CHW, you may have patients inquiring about eating healthier or reducing their intake of carbohydrates, such as individuals with type 2 diabetes who require glucose level monitoring. Therefore, it is important to be familiar with creative ways to assist and encourage your patients.

Question

Create a salad recipe for two servings by practicing your skills using the following sample recipe. Remember, each serving should be less than 8 carbohydrates (1 carbohydrate = 1 gram (g). How can you incorporate low carb vegetables into a meal, without exceeding 8 carbohydrates per meal in total? Use Figure 2.6 and the following sample recipe to help you.

A sample recipe:

1 cup spinach
1 cup romaine lettuce
½ stalk celery
½ cup cucumber
1 cup diced tomato
¼ cup diced onion
¼ cup diced bell pepper

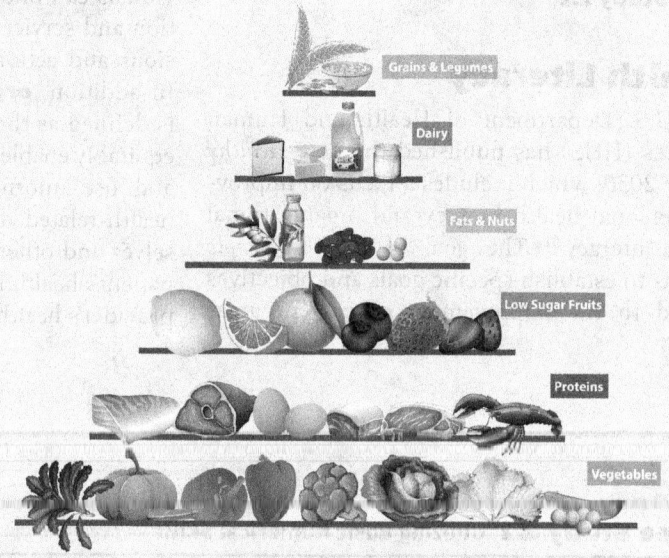

Figure 2.6 Low-Carb Vegetables

Figure from Ball J. How Many Carbs Are in Vegetables? https://www.eatingwell.com/article/290784/how-many-carbs-are-in-vegetables/. Accessed November 2, 2021.36
Data Ball J. How Many Carbs Are in Vegetables? https://www.eatingwell.com/article/290784/how-many-carbs-are-in-vegetables/. Accessed November 2, 2021.

Patient's Side of Health Literacy

For the patient, health literacy includes their ability to read, comprehend, and analyze health information. They must also understand instructions, symbols, charts, and diagrams. Finally, the patient and family need to explore risks and benefits, make decisions regarding their health care, and proceed to take necessary action toward that decision.[38] The two most important health literacy skills required to improve health outcomes are understanding directions and information recall.[39–40] Unfortunately, patients report understanding and retaining only about 50 percent of the information shared by their healthcare providers.[41–42] When patients have low health literacy, they are less likely to ask questions,[43] understand health information in printed or digital formats,[44] or remember verbally communicated medication instructions.[45]

Typically, adults 60+ years of age have the most difficulty with health literacy and are considered a large group with the lowest level of proficiency.[46] Among younger adults, the digital health literacy has significant potential for improving broad health literacy efforts and achieving relatability and further understanding of health information. However, the aging population remains at risk of being left behind because digital literacy often requires the use of technology, which can be particularly lacking among the aging population.[46]

As older adults learn new skills related to digital health technology, such as communicating with healthcare providers through a patient portal, their health outcomes improve along with their confidence. CHWs can assist older adults with improving their health literacy as time permits with each clinic visit. For example, after the patient has completed a visit with the healthcare provider, the CHW meets with the patient to review their prescriptions and schedule scans or lab tests. In this environment, the patient is more likely to ask questions without embarrassment to confirm that they understood the directions. At the same visit, the CHW may provide guidance to patients in understanding their insurance plans, co-payments, and benefits, especially for those that have not previously been insured.[38] Last, language barriers and the inability to read or understand health information poses serious health risks to individuals with limited English proficiency. Language is therefore a critical component of any effort to improve communication and access to quality health care for patients, their family members, caregivers, and friends.[38] See **Box 2.5**.

The individual must be able to understand what the healthcare provider is saying and ask appropriate questions to gain clarification. In addition, if the healthcare provider gives the patient a new prescription, the individual must understand if the new prescription replaces the current daily medication or is in addition to the daily medication, the possible side effects, when and how to ingest the new medication (i.e., with or without food, morning, or bedtime). If lab tests or radiology images (CT scan, MRI, or X-ray) are prescribed, the patient may become more confused. Scheduling the requested tests and follow-up appointments add to overall confusion. Last, on the way out, the patient may pull a few brochures from the wall display in hopes of gaining more information. However, the medical brochures are likely to add to the patient's confusion. For this common situation, ideally the clinic employs several CHWs. Before leaving the

---

Box 2.5 A Summary of Health Literacy Skills

When individuals receive a medical diagnosis, they face complex health information and treatment decisions.[38] If the individual lacks the needed health literacy skills, it is important that a CHW is available to assist with the following health literacy skills:

- Access healthcare services as appropriate for their health insurance coverage
- Analyze relative risks and benefits of proposed treatment options
- Understand when and how to take medications
- Learn to communicate with healthcare providers in person and through the digital patient portal system[38]
- Locate and evaluate health information in verbal, printed, and digital formats for quality and reliability
- Interpret lab and radiology test results[38]

Data from U.S. Department of Health and Human Services. Health literacy. National Institutes of Health Web site. https:// www.nih.gov/institutes -nih/nih-office-director/office-communications-public-liaison/clear -communication/health-literacy. Accessed November 2, 2021.

---

clinic, the patient and caregivers are given the opportunity to meet with a CHW to review and explain the new prescription, coordinate any radiology imaging, and schedule lab tests and follow-up appointments for convenient dates and times. Unfortunately, too often, clinics with limited budgets fail to acknowledge that hiring CHWs will ultimately save on healthcare costs and improve the overall health of the community through prevention and health promotion.

Health Professional's Communication

While the patient perspective of health literacy has been the focus, it is time to concentrate on the provider, including CHW, side of the conversation. Despite the importance of the verbal and written communication for patient understanding, more professional training is required to impact health outcomes.[47] **Productive health communication** occurs when both the healthcare provider and the patient discusses the plan for treating the patient's diagnosis.

The healthcare provider assumes the role as the listener, while the patient describes their symptoms. At this point, the roles then become reversed, as the patient listens, and the healthcare provider describes the diagnosis and treatment plan.[48] For the health communication to be effective, both providers and patients must listen and exchange information.[1, 47] To improve communication between healthcare providers and their patients, the conversation must include the ability to speak and listen, simplify understanding, answer questions, and interpret basic health information to facilitate health decision-making, teaching the patient to manage their disease, and assists with navigation through the healthcare system.[1] Even though patients prefer receiving health information through a conversation, studies show that most patients only retain about 50 percent of the information given by their provider.[1,49] As discussed earlier, many patients find it difficult to ask questions or admit not understanding the directions (i.e., English as a second language, hearing loss, low health literacy, disabilities, and age).[9] In this situation, the patient nods to respond to questions. When the healthcare provider asks if the patient has any questions, a common response is "no."[1] To avoid such situations, healthcare providers focus on patient-centered communication skills.[1] See **Box 2.6**.

Adult Learning Styles

Along with the various types of literacy, learning styles fall into four categories: visual, auditory, reading/writing, and kinesthetic.[51] The acronym for remembering the learning styles is **VARK**.[51–52] Everyone has a preferred learning style that allows for better understanding unique to their learning needs.[51–52] Because everyone is different, when CHWs are presenting health information, all four learning styles are incorporates. Often learners have a primary learning style, but they also use the concepts of information presented from one or two secondary learning styles.[51–52] Perhaps you aren't sure which learning style describes yourself best, visit this website and

---

Box 2.6 Effective Listening Skills

- Use common language instead of medical terms (e.g., high blood pressure instead of hypertension, high blood sugar instead of hyperglycemic, fast heart rate instead of tachycardia).[1]
- Speak slowly, clearly, and ask questions to verify understanding.[1]
- Ask questions to determine patient's level of health literacy.[1]
- Access the patient's level of emotional distress and their ability to understand health information given the present situation (e.g., emergency department, pain level, severity of diagnosis, absence of support person due to circumstances).[1]
- Ask for a return demonstration to verify the patient understood the directions.[1]
- Engage a person to translate or use computer-generated software to translate if the patient's first language is not English.[1]
- Install volume-controlled devices for hard-of-hearing patients.[1]
- Sit at the same level of the patients rather than standing while the patient is sitting.[1, 50]
- Address the patient, but also include the caregiver in the conversation.
- Face the patient while speaking. If the provider is looking away or at the computer, it sends a message that they are not paying attention to what is being said.[50]
- Be attentive, but relaxed. Make appropriate eye contact. Try to stay focused.[50]
- Keep an open mind. Avoid judging the patient or jumping to conclusions.[50]
- Do not interrupt the patient. Refrain from offering a solution until the patient has a chance to tell their whole story.[50]
- Provide feedback to the patient, including a nod, a smile, and briefly restating what was said. Be aware of making appropriate facial expressions to show that you understand what the patient is saying.[50]

Data from Harrington KF, Valerio, MA. A conceptual model of verbal exchange health literacy. *Patient Educ Couns.* 2014;94(3):403–410.[1]

Data from Schilling D. 10 Steps to Effective Listening. https://www.forbes.com/sites/womensmedia/2012/11/09/10-steps-to-effective-listening/?sh=2980f4a23891. Accessed April 26, 2021.[50]

complete the VARK questionnaire: https://vark-learn.com/the-vark-questionnaire/.[52] **Box 2.7** shows the characteristics of each specific learning style in greater detail. See **Case Study 2.3**.

Box 2.7 Describing VARK Learning Style Categories

Visual Learners
- Prefer to learn by seeing maps, diagrams, infographics, and colors[52]
- Use different color highlighters to take notes
- Create a chart to track progress
- Watch the teacher carefully to stay focused
- The ideal assignment is to make a poster illustrating the key concepts and present it to the other students
- Avoid: Clutter and too many posters in the classroom; distracting for the visual learner

Auditory Learners
- Prefer to learn by listening to what is being said (i.e., lectures, discussions and reading aloud; recorded lectures allow for later review)[52]
- Often ask questions in class and like to give speeches
- May talk aloud to themselves while studying; audiobooks are ideal
- Learn in study groups or leading a discussion group
- May appear as if they are not paying attention and looking around the room, but they are listening intently
- When writing, they can find errors by reading their essay aloud
- Avoid: Posting PowerPoint slides with narration

Reading/Writing Learners
- Prefer to learn by reading books and taking notes as they read the material[52]
- Read the PowerPoint slides on the screen while taking notes
- Rewrite class notes onto flashcards for studying
- Add diagrams to their notes for greater clarification
- Choose physical books over e-books and audiobooks

- Write vocabulary words with definitions and take-home hand-outs for review
- Avoid: Finishing a PowerPoint slide before these learners have finished writing the information from the slide in their notes

Kinesthetic Learners
- Prefer to learn by doing, touching, and solving real problems[52]
- Write and physically manipulate information to retain knowledge (i.e., labs, art studios, computer labs)
- Learn through demonstrations, experiments, live videos, physical props, field trips, and "learn by doing" or through emphasis on application
- Teach principles, show a demonstration, and have learners demonstrate technique to show thorough understanding

Data from Loveless B. Discover Your Learning Style—Comprehensive Guide on Different Learning Styles. https://www.educationcorner.com/learning-styles.html. Accessed April 29, 2021.[52]

Case Study 2.3 Application of Adult Learning Styles

When Belinda, a CHW, teaches adult learners in the clinic, it is not possible for her to know the learning style of each student prior to the beginning of the class. Therefore, she plans the class around all four learning styles to accommodate various student needs. In this example, Belinda is teaching in the meeting room at the neighborhood clinic. There is no charge for this class. Students are encouraged to register, but walk-in students may attend. The 60-minute class is offered at 4:00 p.m., so patients may schedule a late afternoon healthcare visit and then stay for this class. Belinda encourages caregivers and family members to attend the class along with the patients, so everyone hears the same information.

As the students enter the meeting room, Belinda greets each participant and completes a name tag to create a sense of community. Also, Belinda has prepared plastic envelope packets that contain a pen, a small notebook to taking notes, take-home worksheets that participants can fill-in the blanks during the class for reviewing after class, and copies of the PowerPoint slides written in plain language and large font. The topic of today's class is "Exercise."

Since the class is 60 minutes, Belinda presents the material in 10-minute segments using the PowerPoint slides on the screen. This method allows everyone the time to take notes and ask questions. She asks a few general questions in the presentation to determine if the participants are understanding the material. She never calls on a student to answer the question, but rather lets the students volunteer to respond to avoid any embarrassment. If Belinda calls on a specific participant to answer a question, it is likely that participants will not attend any of the other classes that Belinda offers out of fear of embarrassment after being asked to answer a question and not knowing the correct response.

Near the middle of the class, Belinda allows the students to form groups of three or four individuals per group. In their packets is a list of possible topics for the short 20-minute group discussion, such as finding time to exercise, lack of motivation, exercises for sore joints, exercise buddies, etc. Each group selects a topic, and Belinda tells the class that it is fine if all groups select the same topic to discuss. After the discussion, each group shares with the class what they discussed. During this sharing time, if Belinda recognizes any myths or incorrect information, she politely corrects the information. If some participants do not wish to talk that is fine. In the last 10 minutes of the class, Belinda distributes the correct answers for the take-home worksheets, so the students leave with the correct answers to review. She stays after class to answer any specific questions that participants did not feel comfortable asking during class.

Questions

1. Name the type or types of learning styles used in two activities.
2. How would you improve this class?

Chapter Summary

This chapter introduces an overview of literacy, including reading, writing, verbal communication, understanding basic numbers, application of digital and technology skills, health literacy. All forms of literacy impact an individual's health outcomes.[1] The next section describes how to create documents in plain language with appropriate readability levels. This information is followed by effective listening skills between patients and their health care providers to enhance understanding and communication. Lastly, the chapter introduces style of learning including visual, auditory, reading/writing, and kinesthetic (VARK). Examples of each learning style were provided to enhance the knowledge and understanding.

References

1. Harrington KF, Valerio MA. A conceptual model of verbal exchange health literacy. *Patient Educ Couns.* 2014;94(3):403–410.
2. Foley, MJ. Literacy. *Encyclopedia Britannica.* https://www.britannica.com/topic/literacy. Accessed April 6, 2021.
3. U.S. literacy rates by state. World Population Review Web site .https://worldpopulationreview.com/state-rankings/us-literacy-rates-by-state. Accessed October 31, 2021.
4. Organization for Economic Cooperation and Development. *OECD Skills Outlook 2013: First Results from the Survey of Adult Skills.* Paris: OECD Publishing. http://dx.doi.org/10.1787/9789264204256-en. Accessed April 6, 2021.
5. Program for the International Assessment of Adult Competencies (PIAAC): What is PIAAC? National Center for Education Statistics Web site. https://nces.ed.gov/surveys/piaac/. Accessed April 6, 2021.
6. Understanding literacy and numeracy. https://www.cdc.gov/healthliteracy/learn/understandingliteracy.html. Centers for Disease Control and Prevention Web site. Accessed April 6, 2021.

7. American English Doctor. Four Levels of Literacy. https://americanenglishdoctor.com/four-levels-of-literacy/. Accessed October 31, 2021.

8. The numbers don't lie. ProLiteracy Web site. https://www.proliteracy.org/home/adult%20literacy%20facts. Accessed October 31, 2021.

9. Haderlie C, Clark C. Illiteracy among adults in the US. https://www.ballardbrief.org/our-briefs/illiteracy-among-adults-in-the-us. Accessed October 31, 2021.

10. Why does literacy matter? Literacy Alliance of Northeast Florida Web site. https://literacyallnefl.org/why-does-literacy-matter. Accessed October 31, 2021.

11. Types of learning disabilities. Learning Disabilities Association of America Web site. https://ldaamerica.org/types-of-learning-disabilities/. Accessed October 31, 2021.

12. Hadden KB, Puglisi L, Prince L, Aminawung JA, Shavit S, Pflaum D, Calderon J, Wang EA, Zaller N. Health literacy among a formerly incarcerated population using data from the Transitions Clinic Network. *Journal of Urban Health.* 2018;95(4):547–555.

13. How is health literacy identified? Center for Health Care Strategies, Inc. Web site. https://www.chcs.org/media/How_is_Low_Health_Literacy_Identified.pdf. Accessed October 31, 2021.

14. What is literacy? Alberta Education Web site. https://education.alberta.ca/literacy-and-numeracy/literacy/everyone/what-is-literacy/. Accessed April 6, 2021.

15. An introduction to health literacy. National Library of Medicine Web site. https://new.nnlm.gov/guides/intro-health-literacy. Accessed October 31, 2021.

16. TIMSS & PIRLS International Study Center, Boston College Lynch School of Education. A definition of reading literacy. http://pirls2021.org/frameworks/home/reading-assessment-framework/a-definition-of-reading-literacy/. Accessed April 6, 2021.

17. Plain language at NIH. National Institutes of Health Web site. https://www.nih.gov/institutes-nih/nih-office-director/office-communications-public-liaison/clear-communication/plain-language. Accessed October 31, 2021.

18. Blood pressure readings explained. Healthline Web site. https://www.healthline.com/health/high-blood-pressure-hypertension/blood-pressure-reading-explained. Accessed April 29, 2021.

19. Urinary reflux. KidsHealth Web site. https://www.kidshealth.org.nz/urinary-reflux. Accessed October 31, 2021.

20. Writing and diagram explained. BlogSpot Web site. https://antasyaalinda.blogspot.com/2018/07/diagram-of-urinary-system-with-labels.html. Accessed October 31, 2021.

21. U.S. Department of Health and Human Services. TOOLKIT for making written material clear and effective part 7 using readability formulas: a cautionary note. Centers for Medicare & Medicaid Services Web site. https://www.cms.gov/Outreach-and-Education/Outreach/WrittenMaterialsToolkit/Downloads/ToolkitPart07.pdf. Accessed October 31, 2021.

22. Readability Formulas. The SMOG Readability Formula. https://www.readabilityformulas.com/smog-readability-formula.php#:~:text=SMOG%20Readability%20Formula%201%20Step%201.%20%3A%20Take,4%20Step%204.%20...%205%20Step%204.%20. Accessed November 1, 2021.

23. COPD lung symptoms, diagnosis, and treatment. MedicineNet Web site. https://www.medicinenet.com/copd_pictures_slideshow/article.htm. Accessed November 1, 2021.

24. Ortiz DN. Digital health literacy. https://www.who.int/global-coordination-mechanism/working-groups/digital_hl.pdf#:~:text=%EF%80%ADDigital%20health%20literacy%20%28or%20eHealth%20literacy%29%20is%20the,gained%20to%20addressing%20or%20solving%20a%20health%20problem. Accessed April 6, 2021.

25. Tobin CD. Developing computer literacy. *The Arithmetic Teacher AT.* 1983;30(6):22–60.

26. Zickuhr K. Who's not online and why? https://www.pewresearch.org/internet/2013/09/25/whos-not-online-and-why/. Accessed November 1, 2021.

27. Cator K. Closing the digital learning gap. https://digitalpromise.org/2019/01/09/closing-the-digital-learning-gap/. Accessed April 10, 2021.

28. Lynch M. The absence of internet at home is a problem for some students. https://www.theedadvocate.org/the-absence-of-internet-at-home-is-a-problem-for-some-students/. Accessed November 1, 2021.

29. Perrin A, Atske S. 7% of Americans don't use the internet. Who are they? https://www.pewresearch.org/fact-tank/2021/04/02/7-of-americans-dont-use-the-internet-who-are-they/. Accessed April 10, 2021.

30. Nagel D. Who Doesn't Use the Internet: The Elderly, the Poor, and the Uneducated. https://campustechnology.com/articles/2013/09/25/who-doesnt-use-the-internet-the-elderly-the-poor-and-the-uneducated.aspx. Accessed November 1, 2021.

31. Parker S. What is numerical literacy? https://saraparker.weebly.com/definition.html. Accessed April 13, 2021.

32. What does math literacy mean? Oxford Learning Centres, Inc. Web site. https://www.oxfordlearning.com/what-does-math-literacy-mean/. Accessed April 13, 2021.

33. Numeracy. Center for Disease Control and Prevention Web site. https://www.cdc.gov/healthliteracy/researchevaluate/numeracy.html. Accessed November 1, 2021.

34. Valchev M. Job interview skills & techniques to help get you a job. https://www.businessphrases.net/job-interview-skills/. Accessed April 13, 2021.

35. Carbohydrates. https://byjus.com/biology/carbohydrates/. BYJUs Web site. Accessed November 2, 2021.

36. Ball J. How many carbs are in vegetables? https://www.eatingwell.com/article/290784/how-many-carbs-are-in-vegetables/. Accessed November 2, 2021.

37. U.S. Department of Health and Human Services. Health literacy in Healthy People 2030. https://health.gov/our-work/national-health-initiatives/healthy-people/healthy-people-2030/health-literacy-healthy-people-2030. Accessed November 2, 2021.

38. U.S. Department of Health and Human Services. Health literacy. National Institutes of Health Web site. https://www.nih.gov/institutes-nih/nih-office-director/office-communications-public-liaison/clear-communication/health-literacy. Accessed November 2, 2021.

39. Martin LT, Schonlau M, Haas A, Derose KP, Rudd R, Loucks EB, Rosenfeld L, Buka SL. Literacy skills and calculated 10-year risk of coronary heart disease. *J Gen Intern Med.* 2011;26(2):45–50.

40. Rosenfeld L, Rudd R, Emmons KM, Acevedo-Garcia D, Martin L, Buka S. Beyond reading alone: The relationship between aural literacy and asthma management. *Patient Educ Couns.* 2011;82(1):110–116.

41. Kessels RP. Patients' memory for medical information. *J Royal Soc Med.* 2003;96(5):219–222.

42. Schillinger D, Piette J, Grumbach K, Wang F, Wilson C, Daher C, Leong-Grotz K, Castro C, Bindman AB. Closing the loop—Physician communication with diabetic patients who have low health literacy. *Arch Intern Med.* 2003;163(1):83–90.

43. Katz MG, Jacobson TA, Veledar E, Kripalani S. Patient literacy and question-asking behavior during the medical encounter: a mixed-methods analysis. *J Gen Intern Med.* 2007;22(6):782–786.

44. Koo M, Krass I, Aslani P. Enhancing patient education about medicines: factors influencing reading and seeking of written medicine information. *Health Expectations.* 2006;9(2):174–187

45. Rigotti N, Munafo M, Stead L. Smoking cessation interventions for hospitalized smokers: a systematic review. *Arch Intern Med.* 2008;168(18):1950–1960.

46. Xie B. Improving older adults' e-health literacy through computer training using NIH online resources. *Library Information Sciences Research.* 2012;34(1):63–71.

47. Kennedy A, Gask L, Rogers A. Training professionals to engage with and promote self-management. *Health Ed Res.* 2005;20(5):567–578.

48. Centers for Disease Control and Prevention. Vital signs: Asthma prevalence, disease characteristics, and self-management education—United States, 2001–2009. *MMWR Weekly.* 2011;60(17):547–552.

49. Brown CJ, Peel C, Bamman MM, Allman RM. Exercise program implementation proves not feasible during acute care hospitalization. *Journal of Rehabilitation and Research Development.* 2006;43(7):939–946.

50. Schilling D. 10 steps to effective listening. https://www.forbes.com/sites/womensmedia/2012/11/09/10-steps-to-effective-listening/?sh=2980f4a23891. Accessed April 26, 2021.

51. Loveless B. Discover your learning style—comprehensive guide on different learning styles. https://www.educationcorner.com/learning-styles.html. Accessed April 29, 2021.

52. The VARK questionnaire. VARK Learn Limited Web site. https://vark-learn.com/the-vark-questionnaire/. Accessed April 29, 2021.

Appendix

1. Literacy Is the Answer: https://www.youtube.com/watch?v=z-h-BhcV7DM

2. The Power of Literacy: https://www.youtube.com/watch?v=83DO0POacCE

3. Digital Literacy—Closing the Divide: https://www.youtube.com/watch?v=apcYBGInXps

4. How Is Literacy Measured: https://www.youtube.com/watch?v=HwUcl1H8Y9Q

5. Basic Mathematical Literacy and Numeracy:
   Video 1: https://www.youtube.com/watch?v=_ro2gtO4qqM
   Video 2: https://www.youtube.com/watch?v=MI7PiD3XLFg.
   Video 3: https://www.youtube.com/watch?v=YIEmJXqEnD4

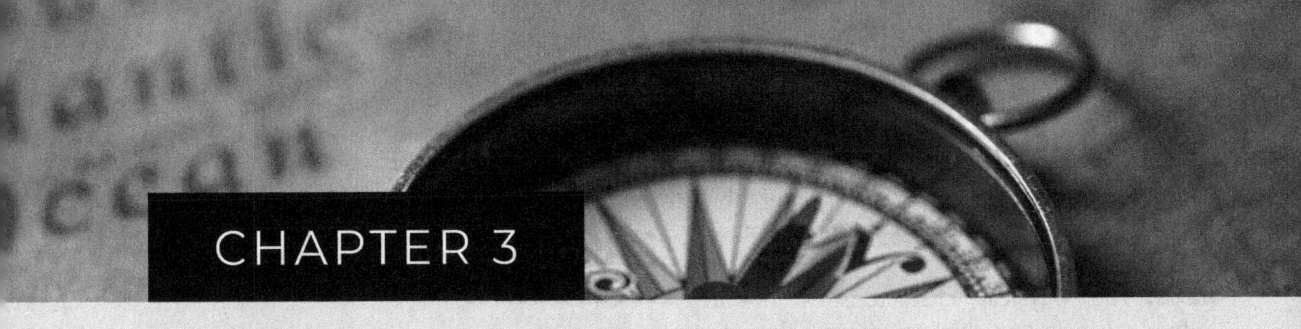

CHAPTER 3

Health Equity and Social Determinants of Health

LEARNING OBJECTIVES

1. Define the terms: health equity, health inequities, race, and ethnicity.
2. Describe the terms: equality, diversity, and inclusion.
3. Explain the five categories in the social determinants of health.
4. Illustrate examples of cultural competencies.
5. Demonstrate the link between cultural competencies and health literacy.

KEY TERMS

health equity
health inequities
race
ethnicity
equality

diversity
inclusion
social determinants of health
discrimination
social cohesion

adverse childhood experiences (ACEs)
cultural competency

Introduction

This chapter begins by defining the differences between health equity and health inequity, race, ethnicity, and examines the importance of equality, diversity, and inclusion. The conversation continues by providing a detailed overview of social determinants of health, including topics on economic stability, access to educational opportunities, healthcare access and quality, the built environment, and health related to social and community contexts.[1] The chapter ends with a discussion about cultural competency.

Health Equity and Health Inequities

According to the Center for Disease Control and Prevention (CDC), **health equity** is defined as the opportunity for every individual to attain their full health potential.[2] Individuals are not disadvantaged due to their race, ethnicity, education, income, geographical location, or social status. **Health inequities** are reflected in many ways, such as an individual's quality and length of life, rate and severity of disease, disability, and death, and access to health care and treatment.[2]

Race and Ethnicity

Race and ethnicity are often used interchangeably.[3] However, these words have separate definitions.

Race. The physical characteristics of an individual including skin color, eye color and shape, facial structure, and hair color, texture, and curl. **Race** refers to the diverse qualities or attributes among populations, including evident genetic differences.[3]

Ethnicity. The cultural identity of an individual, which includes language, religion, nationality, ancestry, dress, and customs. The members of a particular **ethnicity** tend to identify with each other based on these shared cultural traits.[3]

While there is an apparent overlap across race and ethnicity, it is important to recognize the distinct differences. For example, two individuals may identify their ethnicity as American, yet their races may be Asian and Black. In addition, individuals may share the same race but have separate ethnicities. For example, individuals identify as White, but have unique ethnicities, such as Israeli, Russian, Italian, or Canadian. Over time people move around the globe due to war, displacement, political unrest, religious persecution, famine, earthquakes, and other natural disasters. As groups of people move, the definitions of race and ethnicity change, which affects how some cultural groups are treated differently.[3]

For example, the mistreatment and derogatory labels placed upon the communities of color in the United States has led to decades of racism that continues into the present. According to the American Public Health Association (APHA), racism promoted unequal opportunities and assigns value based on how a person looks.[4] Racism results in conditions that unfairly advantage some and unfairly disadvantage others. Racism hurts the overall health of the United States by preventing some people the opportunity to attain their highest level of health. Racism is active at all levels of society including, but not limited to, access to health care, education, housing, finance, and employment. Racism is intentional or unintentional depending on the situation. To address racism, it is important to address injustices caused by racism.[3–4]

Equality, Diversity, and Inclusion

Now it is time to understand the differences between the terms of equality, diversity, and inclusion.

Equality provides equal opportunities and protects individuals from discrimination due to various reasons including age, sexual orientation, disability, race, ethnicity, religion, marital status, and pregnancy.[5] Here are several examples of gender discrimination: (1) An individual was not seriously considered for the position because she wore a hijab (headscarf) to the interview; (2) a qualified individual was not hired because his religion does not allow working on Saturdays; (3) some individuals continue to believe that people from specific ethnic backgrounds are inferior; and (4) sexual orientation may be used as an excuse not to promote a highly qualified individual.[5]

Diversity is about empowering people by respecting, recognizing, and appreciating what makes them different, in terms of age, sexual orientation, ethnicity, religion, disability, education, and national origin.[6]

Inclusion is an individual's experience in the workplace, community, and society. Inclusion is viewed as the extent to which the individual feels as an active participant rather than merely invited, but not given an equal voice.[5] Inclusion makes people feel respected and valued for who they are as an individual. The process of inclusion engages individuals as being essential to the success of the organization.[6]

In summary, equality provides equal opportunities, while diversity refers to traits that make individuals unique, and inclusion refers to behaviors and social norms that make certain for individuals to feel welcome.[6]

Social Determinants of Health

With an understanding of race, ethnicity, equality, diversity, and inclusion, it is important to apply this knowledge to the concept of social determinants of health. **Social determinants of health** are defined as the conditions in which individuals are born, grow, live, work, and age.[1] These circumstances are shaped by the distribution of wealth, power, and resources across global, national, and local levels. The social determinants of health include economic stability, education access and quality, healthcare access and quality, neighborhood and built environment, and social and community context.[1] In other words, health starts at home and then branches out to communities including schools, workplaces, healthcare facilities, neighborhoods, and communities.[7] Many changes must occur to provide health equity for the population. The changes required to improve social determinants of health for everyone involves working together at the local, county, state, and federal level.[7]

These changes are not limited to health care but may also include education, childcare, housing, business, law, media, community planning, transportation, clean air and water, and agriculture. Resources are needed to implement the appropriate changes to enhance quality of life.[7] These essential changes can have a significant influence on population health outcomes.[7] Five domains represent the social determinants of health.[1,7] These domains are healthcare access and quality, education access and quality, social and community context, economic stability, and the neighborhood and other parts of the built environment.[7] See **Figure 3.1**.

According to *Healthy People 2030,* the main social determinants of health include economic stability, education access and quality, healthcare access and quality, neighborhood and built environment, and social and community context.

Health Care Access and Quality

In the United States, health and health care are influenced by geographical location, race and ethnicity, age, income, education, and health literacy attainment.[1,8] These health differences are called health disparities. These differences are not a result of the individual or group behaviors but rather reflect the decades of systematic inequality across economics, housing, and within healthcare systems. The

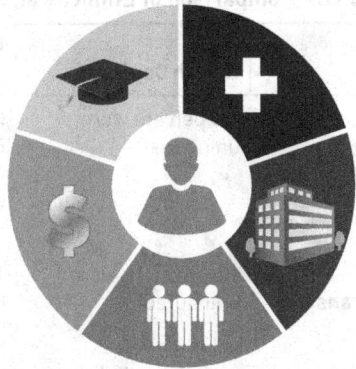

Social determinants of health

Figure 3.1 Social Determinants of Health (SDOH)

Social determinants of health. Healthy People 2030. U.S. Department of Health and Human Services, Office of Disease Prevention and Health Promotion Web site. https://health.gov/healthypeople/objectives-and-data/social-determinants-health. Accessed November 5, 2021

elimination of health disparities requires sustained effort to address multiple social determinants of health, such as poverty, segregation, environmental degradation, and racial discrimination.[8] **Table 3.1** showcases the unequal access to health care across multiple races and ethnicities, including Asian Americans, Black Americans, Hispanic Americans, Native Hawaiian and other Pacific Islander Americans, and White Americans to compare health coverage, chronic health conditions, mental health care, and data on infant mortality.[8]

As shown in Table 3.1, approximately 1 in 10 individuals in the United States do not have health insurance.[9] The absence of health insurance leads to a cascade of issues. For example, individuals without insurance are less likely to have a primary care provider and may be unable to afford the healthcare services and medications they need. Strategies to increase insurance coverage are critical for ensuring that persons receive healthcare services, like preventive care, cancer screenings, and treatment for chronic illnesses.[19]

Social and Community Context

Social and community connections are shown to improve and sustain the health and well-being of a community.[20] Without support, when individuals face challenging circumstances (i.e., unsafe

Table 3.1 Comparison of Ethnicity and Health

Topic	Health Coverage	Chronic Health Conditions	Mental Health	Infant Mortality
Asian Americans	7.3 percent were uninsured[9]	Reported having nearly twice the incidence of liver and inflammatory bowel disease cancer[10]	6.3 percent of adults received mental health services compared[11]	3.8 infant deaths per 1,000 live births[12]
Black Americans	14.3 percent were uninsured[13]	13.8 percent reported having fair or poor health[14]	8.7 percent of adults received mental health services[15]	11 infant deaths per 1,000 live births[13]
Hispanic Americans	16.1 percent of were uninsured[9]	10 percent reported having fair or poor health[14]	8.8 percent of adults received mental health services[16]	5.1 infant deaths per 1,000 live births[8]
Native Hawaiian or Pacific Islander Americans	8.3 percent were uninsured[17]	Reported having higher rates of smoking, alcohol consumption, and obesity[8]	10.9 percent of adults received mental health services[8]	7.6 infant deaths per 1,000 living births [18]
White Non-Hispanic Americans	5.9 percent were uninsured[17]	8.3 percent reported having fair or poor health[14]	18.6 percent of adults received mental health services[16]	5.8 infant deaths per 1,000 living births[13]

housing, discrimination, unemployment, natural disasters, or disease), the impact leads to adverse outcomes. However, individuals with social and community support have better health outcomes and coping mechanisms.[20] In the following section, social and community context will be thoroughly discussed to include the following domains: civic participation, discrimination, and social cohesion.[20]

Civic Participation

There are numerous examples of civic participation that improve quality of life for the community.[20] First, when a natural disaster hits a community, the news sends journalists to the field to report on community action. Reports often include or show-case scenes of neighbors gathering to help each other clear the debris and establish places for food and clothing distribution.[20] Second, civic participation is noted during the holidays, summer, and before school starts including toy drives and food donations during the winter holidays, summer camps that provide meals to the participating children, and groups that fill new backpacks with

the required school supplies.[20] Third, civic participation spans across all age groups, and some specialize in elderly populations by including home visiting programs, meals on wheels and elderly day care centers for engagement and activities.[20]

Discrimination

Discrimination is defined as understanding the distinction between one topic in two different ways (i.e. positive and negative).

Positive example: The chef has discriminating taste when identifying differences between two nearly identical red wines.

Negative example: Prior to the 1970s, U.S. universities were able to deny admission to student applicants based on their gender, race, or ethnicity.

Furthermore, over the years, discrimination has been a socially structured word or action that is unfair, unjustified, or harms individuals and groups.[21–22] Many acts of discrimination negatively affect the health of an individual, community, or a population.[21-22] Unfortunately, discrimination is a common experience. Approximately, 31 percent of U.S. adults report at least one major discriminatory occurrence in their lifetime, and 63 percent report experiencing discrimination everyday.[23]

There are two types of discrimination: individual and structural.

Individual discrimination: Negative interactions between individuals, (e.g., health care provider and patient, student and teacher, or salesperson and customer) based on the individual's characteristics (e.g., race, ethnicity, gender, disability, age, language, or clothing).[24] Over time, discrimination causes physical and mental health symptoms, such as irregular heartbeat, anxiety, depression, obesity.[25]

Structural discrimination: Less privileged groups with conditions that limit their opportunities, resources, economic status, education, and access to health care (e.g., neighborhoods with poor air and water quality due to location near factories, residential segregation, low-funded schools, poor housing options) which limit "opportunities, resources, and well-being" of less privileged groups.[26]

Some examples of discrimination include unfair dismissal from a job, poor customer service, denied access to housing because the owner or bank refuses request from specific types of individuals contingent on their color of skin, sexual orientation, gender identity, disability, age, or religious beliefs.[25-26] See **Box 3.1** for a break down on how discrimination influences specific populations.

Box 3.1 Impact of Discrimination on Different Populations

Communities of color, racial and ethnic minorities: Linked to health disparities including low birth weight, high blood pressure, and poor health status.[27-29] Social determinants of health including poorer housing, lower-level education, exposure to poor air and water quality, and lack of access to health care.[1]

Gender: Linked to negative health impacts for women.[30-32] These negative impacts include levels of unhappiness, loneliness, and depression. For example, women reported discrimination due to physical appearance and gender were strongly related to reduced self-reported receipt of Pap smears, mammography, and clinical breast exams.[32]

LGBTQIA+ (lesbian, gay, bisexual, transgender, queer (or questioning), intersex, and asexual (or allies): Linked to a lifetime of discrimination across multiple domains along with and day-to-day experiences.[33] Adolescents who identify as LGBTQIA+ exhibit symptoms of emotional distress, depressive symptoms, suicidal ideation, and self-harm due to social rejection and isolation,[34] decreased social support, and verbal or physical abuse.[34-36]

Disabilities: In 2016, approximately 61.4 million individuals or 25.7 percent of the population within the United States reported having a disability or limitation.[37] Adults with disabilities are more likely to report their health to be fair or poor due to complex activity limitations (e.g., work, self-care, movement, cognitive function, vision and hearing).[38] Adults with disabilities are 2.5 times more likely to report skipping or delaying health care because of the cost.[39] People with disabilities consistently report higher rates of obesity, lack of physical activity, and smoking.[38] These disparities in health contribute to the result of insufficient health insurance coverage, patient choice of care, or inaccessible transportation.[40]

Elderly individuals and ageism: Ageism is discrimination against anyone due to their age from young to old. There are four types of ageism: *Personal Ageism* is a bias against individuals based on their older age. *Institutional Ageism* is related to missions, rules, and practices that discriminate against individuals or groups because of their older age. *Intentional Ageism* are practices that take advantage of the vulnerabilities of older individuals. *Unintentional Ageism* are practices in which perpetrators unaware of bias against persons based on their older age.[41] Everyday discrimination affects emotional health.[23] Perceived discrimination among the aging population impedes overall health status and increases emotional distress. The health vulnerabilities of older adults amplify the health effects of discrimination.[23]

Another form of structural discrimination involves incarceration and the criminal justice system, including rates at which racial/ethnic minorities are arrested, convicted, and incarcerated for criminal offenses.[42-44] Due to the state and federal policies that impact incarceration rates for racial/ethnic minorities, there are negative impacts on families, housing, employment, political participation, and health.[44, 45-48] Routine discrimination can be a chronic stressor and increase vulnerability to physical illness.[49] As with other forms of sustained stress, discrimination "may lead to wear and tear on the body."[49-50] Also, sustained stress is called "weathering."[49-50]

Social Cohesion

Social cohesion is defined as the strength of relationships and the sense of community among the members.[51] The strength of relationships includes social capital (resources), social networks (interwoven safety net), and social support (friend-to-friend). There are multiple links in social cohesion, such as social networks influence the spread of social capital.[51] This influence is called "social contagion" and may be positive or negative.[51]

> Negative example: If an individual's friend, sibling, or spouse is obese, the individual's likelihood of also becoming obese increases. Similar patterns are seen for smoking and drinking behaviors.[51]

> Positive example: For a positive example, social support may help people stick to healthier diets and reduce emotional stress.[51]

Additionally, support groups such as Alcoholics Anonymous (AA), help individuals abstain from alcohol consumption. Social support can therefore directly benefit people and indirectly buffer them from risk factors that might otherwise damage health.[51] Social support is important for minority populations. One study involving African American adults found that social support acted as a barrier against the harmful health effects of discrimination.[52] See **Case Study 3.1**.

Case Study 3.1 Community Senior Day Care Facility

Recently, Shannon started her new position as a community health worker (CHW) at the local community senior day care facility. She has 5 years of CHW experience at an assisted living residence for elderly in a nearby town. She spent the first week reviewing files, getting to know the staff and the seniors that attend the adult day care daily. As a CHW, one of Shannon's many roles and responsibilities is to promote inclusivity and social cohesion. Social cohesion is an important component to consider for aging adults. By the end of the second week, Shannon had a few questions.

Questions

1. How would you advise Shannon on how to creatively improve social cohesion among the elderly individuals that routinely come to the senior facility?
2. A CHW at the neighborhood clinic walked over to the senior day care facility to introduce herself to Shannon. What ideas might you suggest on ways that the two of CHWs might improve elderly health outcomes between the two facilities?
3. Shannon reviewed the intake forms of the elderly who participate regularly at the senior day care facility. From reviewing the intake forms, Shannon realized that many participants live in a large apartment complex near the facility. What would you suggest to Shannon do with this information to enhance social networks?

Education Access and Quality

There are numerous connections between education and health including early childhood education through high school graduation.[53] For example, children from low-income families, children with disabilities, and children who routinely experience bullying are more likely to struggle with math and reading and are less likely to graduate from high school or go to college. The results suggest that their incomes are lower and thus they will have less access to health care.[53] In addition, the stress of living in poverty affects the brain development of children, thus leading to poor academic performance. As noted previously, the connection between education and health is important.[53]

Without high literacy performance, the individual is less likely to obtain a living wage, have adequate access to health care, and basic understanding of health concepts for well-being. For example, people with higher levels of education are more likely to live healthier and longer lives.[53] See **Box 3.2**.

Box 3.2 **Adverse Childhood Experiences (ACEs)**

Adverse childhood experiences (ACEs) are defined as traumatic experiences in childhood and throughout the teenage years that increase the child's risk of exposure to violence, chronic health problems, mental illness, and substance abuse in adulthood.[54-56] These experiences can affect children for years and impact their emotional, physical, and mental well-being across the lifespan.[54-56]

ACEs include many forms, such as experiencing violence, abuse, or neglect, witnessing violence in the home or community, divorce, poverty, and having a family member attempt or die by suicide.[55-56] Also included are aspects of the child's environment that can undermine their sense of safety, stability, and bonding such as growing up in a household with substance use problems, mental health problems, instability due to parental separation, or instability due to incarceration of a parent, sibling, or other members of the household being in jail or prison.[55-56]

Children growing up with toxic stress may have difficulty forming healthy and balanced relationships. They may also have unstable work histories as adults and struggle to maintain economic stability, pursue an education, secure a job, and experience depression or anxiety throughout life.[54-56] These effects can also be passed on to their own children. Some children may face further exposure to toxic stress from historical and ongoing traumas due to systemic racism or the impacts of poverty resulting from limited educational and economic opportunities.[54-56]

Though challenging, ACEs can be prevented. Several factors may increase or decrease the risk of perpetrating and/or experiencing violence.[56] To prevent ACEs, the contributing factors must be understood and addressed to adequately prevent the risk:

- Creating and sustaining safe, stable, nurturing relationships and environments for all children and families[57]
- Raising awareness of ACEs[57]
- Early interventions[57]
- Shifting the focus from individual responsibility to community solutions[55-57]
- Reducing stigma around seeking help with parenting challenges or seeking care related to substance misuse, depression, or suicidal thoughts[57]
- Promoting safe, stable, nurturing relationships and environments where children live, learn, and play[55-57]

Data from Preventing adverse childhood experiences. Centers for Disease Control and Prevention Web site. https://www.cdc.gov/violenceprevention/aces/fastfact.html. Accessed November 17, 2021. Reference to specific commercial products, manufacturers, companies, or trademarks does not constitute its endorsement or recommendation by the U.S. Government, Department of Health and Human Services, or Centers for Disease Control and Prevention.

Economic Stability

According to *Healthy People 2030,* in the United States, 1 in 10 individuals live in poverty.[57] Within the United States, some people are unable to afford the necessities of life, including sufficient healthy food, employment, health care, transportation, childcare and housing.[57-58] It is important to recognize how the definition of poverty can slightly differ depending on the geographical location. For example, poverty in the United States relates to individuals who earn an income of less than $36 a day or an income of less than $72 a day for a family of four. In comparison, underdeveloped countries with an income of less than $1.90 a day is considered extreme poverty as defined by the World Bank standards.[59] Individuals with steady employment are less likely to live in poverty thus adversely affecting their health. However, individuals with chronic illness and long-term disabilities are limited by the work that they can perform, such as lifting, standing, sitting for long periods of time, and constraints due to mental health issues. Even individuals with a steady income of minimum wages do not earn enough to afford their basic needs. Some communities offer short-term programs and policies that assist individuals with temporary needs such as paying past due rent, electrical, and water bills. Most communities have food bank services in local faith-based communities or neighborhood service centers. Since CHWs will encounter many types of individuals with immediate needs, it is essential that the CHW maintain an up-to-date list of nearby services available. Lastly, once the immediate needs are met, the CHW begins to focus on long-term needs, such as employment training programs, career counseling, budget advising, childcare services, and free healthcare and mental health services.[57–58]

Neighborhood and Built Environment

In the United States, there is a need to focus on improving health and safety where individuals and their families live, work, learn, and play.[60] It is recognized that communities and neighborhoods have a major impact on health and wellness.[60] For example, in the United States, many individuals live in neighborhoods with high rates of violence, unsafe air or water, and other health and safety risks. Individuals from racial/ethnic minorities, or with low incomes are more likely to live in unsafe environments. Lastly, individuals may live in a safe environment, but they may be employed in an industry where they are exposed to a harmful environment, such as fumes, particles, secondhand smoke, or loud noises. This exposure over time may be harmful to their health.[60] Interventions and policy changes at the local, state, and federal level can help reduce these health and safety risks and promote health. For example, when a community adds sidewalks and bike lanes, the change improves the overall health, safety, and quality of life of the population.[60] CHWs should be aware of environmental exposures and unsafe living conditions in the communities where they live and work. CHWs maintain lists of services, agencies, and nonprofit organizations that strive to reduce hazardous environmental conditions and promote healthy environments for living and working.

Cultural Competency

The discussion of social determinants is closely linked to cultural competency.[61] An exploration of cultural competency begins by defining each word separately. First, culture is defined as a collection of behaviors including language, thoughts, communications, actions, customs, beliefs, values, and considers institutions such as racial, ethnic, religious, or social groups.[61] Second, competence is defined as the capacity to function effectively as an individual within the context of the cultural beliefs, behaviors, and needs presented by individuals and their communities.[61] Now put the words back together. **Cultural competency** is the capacity to value, understand, and consider diversity across various domains, learn about cultural knowledge, adapt to diverse cultures, and incorporate all cultural aspects into community practice and policies.[61] Here are four examples of cultural competency.

Example 1: Recently, six families were allowed political asylum from their country of origin to the United States. The local Lutheran Church is serving as their sponsor and translators while helping the families get settled with food, clothing, housing, and access to health care. The families are required to get physical exams and vaccination within the first 14 days after arrival. The Lutheran sponsors schedule the clinic appointments and accompany the families to the clinic. During each appointment, the translator teaches the clinic staff and providers about the culture of the families. The CHW is involved with providing additional community services and resources. The clinic administration involves the community to address the health, social, educational, economic needs of the six families.

Example 2: A faith-based community may have a unique culture in terms of how the members dress, their dietary habits, and their healthcare practices and beliefs. The clinic staff notices that members of this community schedule appointments but often cancel the appointments without providing a reason. The CHW reaches out to this faith-based community to learn about their cultural, faith-based beliefs, and healthcare needs. This effort is the first step in understanding the cultural practices and forming a partnership regarding their health care needs.

Example 3: A social LGBTQIA+ community may have a unique culture regarding how they support common activism topics related to policies, such employer benefits and legally recognized marriage and spousal rights. Recently, the clinic had a position open for a finance manager. The top candidate asked at his interview if the clinic healthcare benefits allowed his partner to be recognized for equal healthcare benefits. The Clinic Administrator was pleased to say to the candidate that the clinic's health benefits would meet his needs and the needs of his partner. The candidate accepted the position knowing that he and his partner would be professionally accepted by the clinic staff.

Example 4: Most individuals may not be familiar with the Indian Health Service (IHS) that serves the Indigenous population of American Indians and Alaska Natives. The IHS aims are to improve the health of the Indigenous population by enhancing preventive efforts at local, regional, and national levels.[62] The IHS Health Promotion and Disease Prevention develops and implements effective health promotion and chronic disease prevention programs to increase the health of individuals, families, and communities. Their initiatives concentrate on the following focus areas: diabetes, nutrition, obesity, physical activity and exercise, and tobacco cessation.[62] For CHWs interested in learning more about Indian Health Services, please go to these two websites:

1. https://www.ihs.gov/forproviders/health andwellness/.[63]
2. https://www.ihs.gov/chr/.[64]

Indian health programs employ health professionals who are passionate about practicing within a unique, interdisciplinary team-based environment and one that embraces the mission: "To raise the physical, mental, and spiritual health of American Indians and Alaska Natives throughout the continental United States and Alaska."[66] A career in Indian health offers clinicians an extraordinary opportunity to provide the highest level of comprehensive, patient-centered care. Serving these important, diverse, and culturally rich patient populations enable our clinicians to distinguish themselves in fulfilling ways both personally and professionally.[66]

There is another way to examine cultural competence, using a national service called Culturally and Linguistically Appropriate Services (CLAS).[66] It is a way to improve the quality of services provided to all individuals to help reduce health disparities and achieve health equity. CLAS is about respect for the entire individual (e.g., physical, mental, emotional, economic, educational, and spiritual) while responding to the individual's health needs and preferences. Using CLAS is one way to reduce health inequities.[66–67] By personalizing services to each patient, healthcare providers achieve improve positive outcomes for diverse populations regardless of culture, language, literacy level, age, or disability. Excellence in health care is a right for all.[66–68] For more information on the National CLAS Standards, check out this website: https://www.minorityhealth. hhs.gov/Default.aspx.[68] See **Case Study 3.2**.

Case Study 3.2 Institutionalize
Cultural Competence for a Clinic Setting

The Southwest Community Clinic determined that too many of their patients failed to show up for appointments. The office manager and her team analyzed the missed appointment data to see if there was a pattern. They looked at the following variables: time of appointment, day of appointment, age, gender, ethnicity, healthcare provider, and purpose of appointment. After analyzing the data, the manager was able to categorize the potential cause for the missed appointments. Here were the results:

1. There were no significant differences between healthcare providers and purpose of appointment related missed appointments.
2. Time of appointment show the most results:
   a. Younger patients missed appointments scheduled before 3:00 p.m. especially if the appointment was for wellness check-up or sports physical rather than a brief follow-up.
   b. Older patients missed early morning appointments.
   c. Working patients missed midday appointments.
3. The clinic has one Spanish-speaking healthcare provider. The Spanish-speaking patients always scheduled their appointments with Dr. Maria Lopez. It was noted that those patients missed a low number of appointments because they wished to see Dr. Lopez.

The team concluded that the most missed appointments occurred during the early to mid-morning time. As a result, the team recommend that the clinic change their hours of operation from 9:00 a.m. to 4:30 p.m. to 10:30 a.m. to 7:00 p.m. This change would accommodate the elderly patients, the working patients and parents, and the school-age patients. In addition, the Spanish-speaking patients demonstrated that they appreciated having a Spanish-speaking front office clerk and a healthcare provider. The appointment was easily scheduled for a convenient time with the clerk, and therefore the patients made the effort not to miss their appointments.

The Southwest Community Clinic showed cultural competence toward the community in additional ways through analyzing the missed appointment data, showcasing respect for their busy patient's schedules by changing the clinic hours of operation, and adapting to the diversity and cultural context of the community they serve by hiring a Spanish-speaking front office clerk and healthcare provider. In addition, the clinic practiced cultural competence by hiring the front office clerk from the community, invited community members to join the clinic board for local input on policies and practices, and converted all patient documents and office posters into low literacy text in larger fonts in both English and Spanish versions.

Culture and Health Literacy

It is important to explore the link between culture and health literacy. Culture is one important aspect of promoting health literacy.[66,69] For individuals from different cultural backgrounds, health literacy is affected by belief systems, communication styles, clarity, and a community's response to health information. For example, if the health information is not communicated in the preferred language and at the appropriate literacy level, the individuals receiving the information may not know how to ask questions, communicate their symptoms, and understand the treatment plan, which contributes to a lack knowledge and inability to apply the health information.[69]

CHWs take an active role by working together to ensure effective communication between individuals and their healthcare providers. Even though individuals must take an active role in health decisions, the CHW can facilitate the development of health information skills for the individual. In addition, the CHW may assist healthcare providers to utilize effective health communication skills including, printed, digital and verbal information using plain language.[69] See **Case Study 3.3**.

Case Study 3.3 Culture and Health Literacy

Several years ago, Don and Pete moved to New York City to Florida. Don, age 72, is a retired gentleman who worked in finance for most of his long career. His partner, Pete, age 77, is retired after working in the university budget office for over 20 years. Pete is experiencing some early signs of dementia, and his hip joint has severe arthritis, but he refuses a hip replacement. They have been in a committed relationship for more than 40 years. They have adequate retirement savings, but they live on a strict monthly budget to extend their savings. They have Medicare health insurance with a supplemental policy. They have a few new friends in Florida, but no long-term friendships. Don has one sister in California, but they are not close. Pete's only sibling died 5 years ago.

Out of fear, denial, finances, and inconvenience, Don put off having an annual physical examination. Recently, he decided that it was time to schedule a physical exam due to persistent pain in his lower abdomen and problems emptying his bladder. During the physical exam, Dr. McCormick, internal medicine physician, found that Don's prostate gland was enlarged. The physician told Don that he needed a surgical prostate biopsy. Dr. McCormick told Don that his enlarged prostate was a positive sign of cancer, and the biopsy would determine the stage of the cancer.

Given the size of the enlarged prostate, the physician wanted Don to be admitted to the hospital for the surgical biopsy and possible removal of the prostate. However, before they left the exam room, Dr. McCormick looked at Pete's electronic health record (EHR) and noted that Pete's last physical exam was 2 years ago, so he suggested that they schedule a physical exam appointment today for Pete to be evaluated.

While they returned to the office clerk, Dr. McCormick dictated Don's exam and prognosis into the EHR. Don appreciated that Pete had come to the appointment today because he investigated his symptoms on the internet prior to the appointment. As Don was checking out, the office clerk said that the CHW, Marjorie, was available to provide additional information about his upcoming surgery if they were available to extend their visit. Even though Don and Pete have extensive knowledge about finance and economics, they consider themselves to be in good health, exercise daily, eat a healthy diet, and have never had been hospitalized for any major health issues. Additionally, Don had no family history of cancer. They were grateful to meet with Marjorie, the CHW, to get some immediate answers about Don's upcoming surgery.

While Don and Pete waited for a few minutes, the office clerk scheduled Pete's appointment for a physical exam for the following week. In the meantime, Marjorie reviewed Don's EHR, read Dr. McCormick's dictation from today, learned about Don's symptoms and need for a surgical biopsy, and noted his high literacy level and that he had no prior surgeries except his fractured tibia (lower leg bone) while playing soccer in college. She prepared a plastic file envelop filled with useful information for Don and Pete. The packet included the contact information for three urology (bladder/prostate) surgeons with a specialty in cancer surgery that accept Don's health insurance coverage, several informational booklets about prostate cancer and treatment options, coping with a cancer diagnosis, and one booklet focused on the role of the caregiver. Since they had excellent internet skills, she included a laminated page of websites pertaining to prostate cancer information. Last, since the large plastic envelope would contain a few small, useful items, Marjorie added several pocket size notepads, a small calendar, two pens, and a few bite-size snacks. Since Don and Pete were able to meet with Marjorie, she was able to go through the packet of information and answer a few basic questions. Before Don and Pete left the office, they scheduled another appointment with Marjorie. She happened to be available on the same day as Pete's physical next week. It was not necessary for Don to see Dr. McCormick until after the surgery, but they took advantage of back-to-back appointments with Dr. McCormick and Marjorie.

Don and Pete left the office with the envelope of valuable information and feeling a bit more in control about taking the next steps related to Don's prostate cancer diagnosis. As Don drove, his thoughts spiraled between fearing his surgery and dreading what Dr. McCormick may uncover regarding Pete's health especially his severe limp from hip pain and his inability to follow a long conversation. At home, they took a nap, had a late lunch, and reviewed the information in the envelope. Don called two of the three urology offices and scheduled the first available appointment with both offices. The third surgeon was not in a convenient location. They wanted to compare the treatment plans between the two surgeons before consenting to have the surgery.

Questions

1. What questions may Don and Pete ask at their next appointment?
2. What community resources should Marjorie have available for their next appointment?
3. Since Pete no longer drives and Don will not be able to drive for several weeks, what services are Don and Pete going to need when Don is discharged from the hospital?
4. What questions should Marjorie ask Don and Pete at their next appointment?

Chapter Summary

This chapter begins by defining the differences between health equity and health inequity, race, and ethnicity and, last, equality, diversity, and inclusion. Then the discussion moves into a detailed explanation of the social determinants of health economic stability, education access and quality, healthcare access and quality, neighborhood and built environment, and social and community context.[1] Next the chapter explored the importance of cultural competency to value diversity, learn about cultural knowledge, adapt to the diversity in different cultures, and incorporate all aspects into community practice and policies. Last, the link between health literacy and cultural competency illustrates that various belief systems and communication styles influence an individual's response to health information.

References

1. Social determinants of health. *Healthy People 2030*. U.S. Department of Health and Human Services, Office of Disease Prevention and Health Promotion Web site. https://health.gov/healthypeople/objectives-and-data /social-determinants-health. Accessed November 5, 2021.
2. Health equity. Centers for Disease Control and Prevention Web site. https://www.cdc.gov/chronicdisease /healthequity/index.htm. Accessed June 3, 2021.
3. Pariona A. What is the difference between race and ethnicity? World Atlas Web site. https://www.worldatlas .com/articles/what-is-the-difference-between-race-and -ethnicity.html. Accessed June 3, 2021.
4. Racism and health. American Public Health Association Web site. https://www.apha.org/topics-and-issues/health -equity/racism-and-health. Accessed June 3, 2021.
5. Hasa. Difference between equality diversity and inclusion. https://www.differencebetween.com/difference-between -equality-diversity-and-inclusion/. Accessed June 5, 2021.
6. What is diversity & inclusion? Global Diversity Practice Web site. https://globaldiversitypractice.com/what-is -diversity-inclusion/. Accessed June 5, 2021.
7. About social determinants of health (SDOH). Centers for Disease Control and Prevention Web site. https://www.cdc .gov/socialdeterminants/about.html. Accessed June 5, 2021.
8. Carratala S. Health disparities by race and ethnicity. https://www.americanprogress.org/issues/race /reports/2020/05/07/484742/health-disparities-race -ethnicity/. Accessed June 5, 2021.
9. Berchick ER, Hood E, Barnett JC. Health insurance coverage in the United States: 2017. https://www.census .gov/library/publications/2018/demo/p60-264.html. Accessed June 20, 2021.
10. Cancer and Asian Americans. U.S. Department of Health and Human Services Office of Minority Health Web site. https:// minorityhealth.hhs.gov/omh/browse.aspx?lvl=4&lvlid =46. Accessed June 20, 2021.
11. Mental and behavioral health—Asian Americans. U.S. Department of Health and Human Services Office of Minority Health. https://minorityhealth.hhs.gov/omh /browse.aspx?lvl=4&lvlid=54. Accessed June 20, 2021.
12. Infant mortality and Asian Americans. U.S. Department of Health and Human Services Office of Minority Health. https://minorityhealth.hhs.gov/omh/browse.aspx ?lvl=4&lvlid=53. Accessed June 20, 2021.
13. Health of Black or African American non Hispanic population. Centers for Disease Control and Prevention Web site. https://www.cdc.gov/nchs/fastats/black-health .htm. Accessed June 21, 2021.
14. Health of Hispanic or Latino population. Centers for Disease Control and Prevention Web site. https://www.cdc.gov/nchs/ fastats/hispanic-health.htm. Accessed June 21, 2021.
15. Mental and Behavioral Health—African Americans. U.S. Department of Health and Human Services Office of Minority Health Web site. https://minorityhealth.hhs.gov/ omh/browse.aspx?lvl=4&lvlid=24. Accessed June 21, 2021.
16. Mental and Behavioral Health – Hispanics. U.S. Department of Health and Human Services Office of Minority Health Web site. https://minorityhealth.hhs.gov/omh/browse.aspx ?lvl=4&lvlid=69. Accessed June 21, 2021.
17. Profile: Native Hawaiians/Pacific Islanders. U.S. Department of Health and Human Services Office of Minority Health. https://minorityhealth.hhs.gov/omh /browse.aspx?lvl=3&lvlid=65. Accessed June 21, 2021.
18. Ely DM, Driscoll AK. Infant mortality in the United States, 2017: Data from the period linked birth/infant death file. *National Report of Vital Statistics.* 2019;68(10):1–20.
19. Health Care Access and Quality. *Healthy People 2030*. Washington, DC: U.S. Department of Health and Human Services, Office of Disease Prevention and Health Promotion. https://health.gov/healthypeople/objectives -and-data/browse-objectives/health-care-access-and -quality. Accessed June 26, 2021.

20. Social and community context. *Healthy People 2030.* Washington, DC: U.S. Department of Health and Human Services, Office of Disease Prevention and Health Promotion. https://health.gov/healthypeople/objectives -and-data/browse-objectives/social-and-community -context. Accessed June 26, 2021.

21. Abramson, CM, Hashemi M, Sánchez-Jankowski, M. Perceived discrimination in US healthcare: charting the effects of key social characteristics within and across racial groups. *Prev Med Rep.* 2015;2:615–621.

22. Dovidio JF, Penner LA, Albrecht TL, Norton WE, Gaertner SL, Shelton JN. Disparities and distrust: the implications of psychological processes for understanding racial disparities in health and health care. *Soc Sci Med.* 2008:67(3):478–486.

23. Luo Y, Xu J, Granberg E, Wentworth WM. A longitudinal study of social status, perceived discrimination, and physical and emotional health among older adults. *Res Aging.* 2012;34:275–301.

24. Krieger N. Discrimination and health. *Social Epidemiology.* 2000;1:36–75.

25. Pascoe EA, Smart RL. Perceived discrimination and health: a meta-analytic review. *Psychol Bull.* 2009;135(4):531–554.

26. Lukachko A, Hatzenbuehler ML, Keyes KM. Structural racism and myocardial infarction in the United States. *Soc Sci Med.* 2014;103:42–50.

27. Shavers VL, Fagan P, Jones D, et al. The state of research on racial/ethnic discrimination in the receipt of health care. *Am J of Public Health.* 2012;102(5):953–966.

28. Cuffee YL, Hargraves JL, Rosal, M, et al. Reported racial discrimination, trust in physicians, and medication adherence among inner-city African Americans with hypertension. *Am J Public Health.* 2013;103(11): e55–e62.

29. Mustillo S, Krieger N, Gunderson EP, Sidney S, McCreath H, Kiefe CI. Self-reported experiences of racial discrimination and Black-White differences in preterm and low-birthweight deliveries: The CARDIA Study. *Am J Public Health.* 2004;94(12):2125–2131.

30. Pavalko EK, Mossakowski K.N, Hamilton VJ. Does perceived discrimination affect health? Longitudinal relationships between work discrimination and women's physical and emotional health. *J Health Soc Behav.* 2003;44(1):18–33.

31. Fazeli DS, Hall KS, Dalton VK, Carlos RC. The link between everyday discrimination, healthcare utilization, and health status among a national sample of Women. *J Women's Health (Larchmt).* 2016;25(10):1044–1051.

32. Jacobs EA, Rathouz PJ, Karavolos K, et al. Perceived discrimination is associated with reduced breast and cervical cancer screening: The Study of Women's Health Across the Nation (SWAN). *J Women's Health (Larchmt).* 2014;23(2):138–145.

33. Mays VM, Cochran SD. Mental health correlates of perceived discrimination among lesbian, gay, and bisexual adults in the United States. *Am J Public Health.* 2001;91(11):1869–1876.

34. Almeida J, Johnson RM, Corliss HL, Molnar BE, Azrael D. Emotional distress among LGBT youth: the influence of perceived discrimination based on sexual orientation. *J Youth Adolesc.* 2009;38(7):1001–1014.

35. Rosario M, Schrimshaw EW, Hunter J, Gwadz M. 2002 gay-related stress and emotional distress among gay, lesbian and bisexual youths: a longitudinal examination. *Journal of Consulting and Clinical Psychology.* 70(4), 967.

36. Wyss SE. 'This was my hell': the violence experienced by gender nonconforming youth in US high schools. *International Journal of Qualitative Studies in Education.* 2004;17(5):709–730.

37. Okoro CA, Hollis ND, Cyrus AC. Prevalence of disabilities and health care access by disability status and type among adults—United States, 2016. *MMWR Morbidity Mortality Weekly Report.* 2018;67(32):882–887.

38. Altman BM, Bernstein A. Disability and health in the United States, 2001–2005. Hyattsville (MD): National Center for Health Statistics; 2008.

39. Centers for Disease Control and Prevention. Quick-Stats: Delayed or forgone medical care because of cost concerns among adults aged 18–64 years, by disability and health insurance coverage status—National Health Interview Survey, United States, 2009. *MMWR.* 2010;59(44):1456.

40. Kirschner KL, Breslin ML, Iezzoni LI. Structural impairments that limit access to health care for patients with disabilities. *JAMA.* 2007;297(10):1121–1125.

41. Sporre K. Ageism: the four types. https://refinedbyage. com/2019/02/17/ageism-the-four-types/#:~:text= %20Ageism%3A%20The%20Four%20Types%20 %201%20Personal,are%20carried%20out%20 with%20the%20knowledge...%20More%20. Accessed November 13, 2021.

42. Freudenberg N. Adverse effects of U.S. jail and prison policies on the health and well-being of women of color. *Am J Public Health.* 2002;92(12):1895–1899.

43. The Pew Charitable Trusts. Collateral costs: incarceration's effect on economic mobility. Washington (DC): The Pew Charitable Trusts; 2010.

44. Travis J, Western B, Redburn FS. The growth of incarceration in the United States: exploring causes and consequences. Washington, DC: The National Academies Press; 2014.

45. Pager D, Shepherd H. The sociology of discrimination: racial discrimination in employment, housing, credit, and consumer markets. *Annu Review of Sociol.* 2008;34:181–209.

46. Pattillo M, Western B, Weiman D., eds. Imprisoning America: the social effects of mass incarceration. Russell Sage Foundation; 2004.

47. Manza J, Uggen C. Locked out: felon disenfranchisement and American democracy. Oxford University Press; 2008.

48. Pager D. Marked: race, crime, and finding work in an era of mass incarceration. University of Chicago Press; 2008.

49. Gee GC, Spencer M, Chen J, Takeuchi D. A nationwide study of discrimination and chronic health conditions among Asian Americans. *Am J Public Health.* 2007;97(7):1275–1282.

50. Geronimus AT, Hicken M, Keene D, Bound J. "Weathering" and age patterns of allostatic load scores among blacks and whites in the United States. *Am J Public Health.* 2006;96(5):826–833.

51. Social cohesion. *Healthy People 2030,* U.S. Department of Health and Human Services, Office of Disease Prevention and Health Promotion. https://health.gov/healthypeople/objectives-and-data/social-determinants-health/literature-summaries/social-cohesion. Accessed November 17, 2021.

52. Corral I, Landrine H. Racial discrimination and health-promoting vs damaging behaviors among African American adults. *J Health Psychol.* 2012;17(8):1176–1182.

53. Early childhood development and education. *Healthy People 2030.* U.S. Department of Health and Human Services, Office of Disease Prevention and Health Promotion. https://health.gov/healthypeople/objectives-and-data/social-determinants-health/literature-summaries/early-childhood-development-and-education. Accessed November 17, 2021.

54. Adverse childhood experiences (ACEs). Centers for Disease Control and Prevention Web site. https://www.cdc.gov/violenceprevention/aces/index.html. Accessed November 17, 2021.

55. Help youth at risk for ACEs. Centers for Disease Control and Prevention Web site. https://www.cdc.gov/violenceprevention/aces/help-youth-at-risk.html. Accessed November 17, 2021.

56. Preventing adverse childhood experiences. Centers for Disease Control and Prevention Web site. https://www.cdc.gov/violenceprevention/aces/fastfact.html. Accessed November 17, 2021.

57. Semega J, Kollar M, Creamer J, Mohanty A. Income and poverty in the United States: 2018. https://www.census.gov/content/dam/Census/library/publications/2019/demo/p60-266.pdf. Accessed June 28, 2021.

58. *Healthy People 2030.* Washington, DC: U.S. Department of Health and Human Services, Office of Disease Prevention and Health Promotion. https://health.gov/healthypeople/objectives-and-data/browse-objectives/economic-stability. Accessed June 28, 2021.

59. Poverty definition. Federal Safety Net Web site. https://www.federalsafetynet.com/poverty-definition.html. Accessed July 6, 2021.

60. Neighborhood and built environment. *Healthy People 2030.* Washington, DC: U.S. Department of Health and Human Services, Office of Disease Prevention and Health Promotion. https://health.gov/healthypeople/objectives-and-data/browse-objectives/neighborhood-and-built-environment. Accessed June 28, 2021.

61. Cultural competence in health and human services. Centers for Disease Control and Prevention Web site. https://npin.cdc.gov/pages/cultural-competence#1. Accessed June 29, 2021.

62. Best and promising practices. Indian Health Service Web site. https://www.ihs.gov/forproviders/bestpractices/. Accessed June 29, 2021.

63. Health and wellness programs. Indian Health Service Web site. https://www.ihs.gov/forproviders/healthandwellness/. Accessed June 29, 2021.

64. Community health representative. U.S. Department of Health and Human Services, Indian Health Services Web site. https://www.ihs.gov/chr/. Accessed November 18, 2021.

65. Careers@IHS. U.S. Department of Health and Human Services, Indian Health Services Web site. https://www.ihs.gov/careeropps/. Accessed November 18, 2021.

66. Think cultural health—what is CLAS? U.S. Department of Health and Human Services Web site. https://thinkculturalhealth.hhs.gov/clas/what-is-clas. Accessed June 28, 2021.

67. Our mission. U.S. Department of Health and Human Services Office of Minority Health Web site. https://www.minorityhealth.hhs.gov/. Accessed June 29, 2021.

68. The National CLAS Standards. U.S. Department of Health and Human Services Office of Minority Health Web site. https://www.minorityhealth.hhs.gov/Default.aspx. Accessed June 29, 2021.

69. Health literacy online: a guide to simplifying the user experience. U.S. Department of Health and Human Services, Office of Disease Prevention and Health Promotion Website. https://health.gov/healthliteracyonline/. Accessed June 29, 2021.

70. Poverty simulation. Spent Web site. http://playspent.org/html/. Accessed June 19, 2021.

Appendix: Educational Learning Exercise to Understand Social Determinants of Health

To further illustrate the impact of social determinants of health, visit the following link: http://playspent.org/.[70] The link leads to an interactive poverty simulation game where the player's goal is to utilize their last $1,000. Though difficult, this simulation takes the individual on a journey to showcase how challenging it is to live in poverty while considering insurance, income, medical expenses, housing, and other basic necessities. Can you survive?

Supplemental Learning Videos

1. What Is Health Equity? https://www.youtube.com/watch?v=ZPVwgnp3dAc
2. Social Determinants of Health: https://www.youtube.com/watch?v=CALj8t8EnD8
3. Surgeon General's Prescription for Happiness: https://www.youtube.com/watch?v=Fm388TS1WOM
4. Education & Health: https://www.youtube.com/watch?v=7AN13Tqd_M4
5. CLAS: https://www.youtube.com/watch?v=O6xOLto2t6w&t=317s
6. Health Literacy & Cultural Competency: https://www.youtube.com/watch?v=qXRJmu7eVks

Social Justice, Advocacy, and Community Resources

LEARNING OBJECTIVES

1. Define social justice.
2. Describe self-advocacy and community advocacy.
3. Categorize effective community resources.
4. Determine access and barriers to community resources.

KEY TERMS

advocacy
self-advocacy

community advocacy
social justice

personal barriers
societal barriers

Introduction

This chapter focuses on social justice, advocacy, and resources. To begin, social justice is defined with a historical perspective and includes examples. Second, the definition of **advocacy** is derived from the Latin language where "ad" = to, and "vocare" = means to call or speak for someone.[1] It is essential for community health workers (CHW) to understand how to appropriately advocate for diverse people groups. There are several types of advocacy categories, which include self-advocacy and community advocacy. **Self-advocacy** is speaking for yourself and

effectively communicating with others about your emotional, physical, and mental needs regardless of a known health condition.[2]

Community advocacy involves speaking for individuals or identifying an issue or cause to initiate the change of a policy or program to improve conditions for a specific people group or for the entire community needs related to age, race, ethnicity, disabilities, and sexuality. Additionally, community advocacy focuses on topics, such as equity in access to health care and health resources. Regardless of the advocacy category, the goal of advocacy is to speak on behalf of marginalized individuals and be a voice for the overlooked and underrepresented.[2] Third, CHWs are trained to teach individuals how to advocate for themselves as well as be an advocate for the community. This chapter introduces community resources, including how to develop a community resource map and create a community resource guide.[2] Once the guides are completed, CHWs learn to investigate, verify, and make a successful referral to a community service or resource for individuals in need of services and information. Lastly, the discussion explores the process of improving access by decreasing barriers to community resources.

Social Justice

The concept of social justice began in the early nineteenth century during the Industrial Revolution. This was a time of historical transition as Europe and the United States moved from making essential products one at a time by hand to expanding the mass production of manufactured goods by using steam power. This change caused a social stratification between the wealthy owners and the poor laborers. Early social justice advocates focused on capital, property, and the distribution of wealth.[3] By the twentieth century, social justice was expanded from focusing on economics to include other topics of social life, including age, race, ethnicity, disabilities, sexuality, and other issues of inequality.[3]

Currently, **social justice** is defined as equal rights, equal opportunities, and equal treatment for all.[4] By exploring a few examples, this broad definition becomes clear.

Age. Although ageism can apply to any age group, ageism in health care can be especially dangerous for seniors.[5] Some physician's prejudice against the elderly adults can lead to a poorer level of treatment, such as having lower expectations for the individual's ability to recover and might mean not receiving the necessary treatment.[5]

Race and Ethnicity. Racism directed toward diverse racial and ethnic minority groups,

throughout the United States, experience higher rates of illness and death across a wide range of health conditions, including diabetes, hypertension, obesity, asthma, and heart disease, when compared to their White counterparts.[6] Additionally, the life expectancy of non-Hispanic/Black Americans is 4 years lower than that of White Americans.[6] The COVID-19 pandemic and its impact regarding access and delivery of care among racial and ethnic minority populations is another example of these enduring health disparities.[6]

Disabilities. Though disability has a broad impact on population groups despite age, in the United States, two out of five adults over 65 live with a disability, and one in four women have a disability.[7] Many individuals with disabilities lack access to adequate health care to support their needs. Health disparities can be the result of inaccessible healthcare facilities and equipment, lack of knowledge among health professionals about specific differences among people with disabilities, transportation difficulties, and higher poverty rates among people with disabilities.[8] See **Figure 4.1**.

Sexuality. Individuals in the lesbian, gay, bisexual, transgender, questioning/queer, intersex, asexual, and allies (LGBTQIA+) within the community face significant disparities in access to health services and how informed care is delivered.[9] Thus, individuals experience poor physical and mental health outcomes. Sexual minority women report fewer lifetime Pap smear tests, transgender youth have less access to health care, and LGBTQ individuals are more likely to delay or avoid necessary medical care.[9] Perceived discrimination from healthcare providers and denial of health care altogether are common experiences among LGBTQQIA+ patients and have been identified as contributing factors to health disparities. Disparities in healthcare access and outcomes experienced by LGBTQ patients are compounded by vulnerabilities linked to racial identity, economic status, and geographic location.[9]

Disability and Healthcare
ACCESS

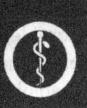

Healthcare access barriers for working-age adults include

1 in 3
adults with disabilities
(18–44 years)

do not have a **usual healthcare provider**

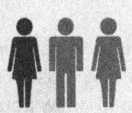

1 in 3
adults with disabilities
(18–44 years)

have an **unmet healthcare need because of cost** in the past year

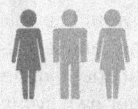

1 in 4
adults with disabilities
(45–64 years)

did not have a **routine check-up** in the past year

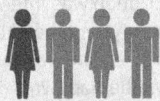

Figure 4.1 Disability and Healthcare Access

Figure from Centers for Disease Control and Prevention. Disability Impacts All of Us Infographic. https://www.cdc.gov/ncbddd/disabilityandhealth/infographic-disability-impacts-all.html#:~:text=26%20percent%20(one%20in%20 4)%20of%20adults%20in,South.%20Percentage%20of%20adults%20with%20functional%20disability%20types:. Accessed July 8, 2021. Reference to specific commercial products, manufacturers, companies, or trademarks does not constitute its endorsement or recommendation by the U.S. Government, Department of Health and Human Services, or Centers for Disease Control and Prevention.[7]

As CHWs learn about advocacy in the next section, it remains essential for social justice initiatives to be the foundation when advocating for equal rights, equal opportunities, access to community resources, and equal treatment for all individuals seeking health care.

Advocacy

Two types of advocacies are presented in this section: self-advocacy and community advocacy.

Self-Advocacy

Before CHWs advocate for community members, it is important that they learn to be an advocate

for their own health. After reading this case study, the discussion breaks down the segments for greater understanding about how to be an advocate for one-self and why this skill is important for CHWs. See **Case Study 4.1**.

Case Study 4.1 Brenda's Challenge of Self-Advocacy

Recently Brenda, age 51, was hired as a CHW for a downtown clinic located near two low-income senior housing apartments. She was raised in this city, so she is familiar with many resources for families and seniors. For the past 6 years, she was employed as the front desk receptionist

(continues)

in a private physician's office. Brenda is divorced and has two children ages 21 and 25 years old. They have completed 2-year technical degrees from the community college. Renee, age 25, works as a radiology technician at the city hospital. Her brother, Josh, age 21, works as an air conditioning technician. The siblings live together in a small home and share the rent to save money. Brenda is proud that her children are on their own.

While working at the medical office for many years and sitting most of the day, Brenda knew that she gained a few pounds. She realized that she was gaining weight, but she was stressed after her divorce due to limited finances. She assumed that when her life settled down, she would be able to lose some weight. She sold her house after the divorce and a rented a tiny apartment in the garden district. She loves having her own living space, and the rent allows her to get control of her financial situation. Life is improving.

Upon the advice of a friend who is a CHW, Brenda decided to apply for the CHW position because the description was interesting, she knows the community, and the salary would provide a $3,000 raise. She was hired shortly after the first interview. She had two weeks of vacation time left at the medical office, so she took those two weeks to schedule medical appointments that she had neglected for the last few years. Also, she wanted to take advantage of using her medical office health insurance since she purchased an extension on her insurance until the new health insurance is activated at her new position. She scheduled her annual physical exam, a dental appointment, and an ophthalmology appointment to obtain a new prescription for her reading glasses. Brenda was anticipating a fresh start when she started her position as a CHW.

Unfortunately, the 2 weeks of ongoing appointments increased Brenda's stress. The dentist found two cavities. One cavity required a root canal to save the tooth. She agreed to the recommended treatment even though the cost was beyond her budget. The dentist had her meet with the office manager, and they worked out a monthly payment plan with low interest. Her ophthalmology appointment determined that she had early stages of glaucoma (increased pressure of the eye), but medication was not required at this time. The

doctor recommended a follow-up appointment every 6 months to track Brenda's pre-glaucoma diagnosis. Also, she needed a new prescription for her reading glasses to reduce her eye strain, and the ophthalmologist gave her a discount coupon for her new glasses. She liked her fresh look when she wore her new glasses.

Last, Brenda had her physical exam. She dreaded the appointment because of her excessive weight gain. Since she had not had a physical for several years, Dr. Sylvia Richardson ordered lab tests prior to the appointment. Brenda complied with the fasting lab tests. When the medical assistant weighed her, Brenda was shocked that she weighed 227 pounds. She does not have a scale at home. The medical office where Brenda worked for years had a scale a few steps from her desk, but she never stepped on it. The medical assistant took her blood pressure and pulse. Both numbers were out of the normal range. She dreaded seeing the lab results. Dr. Richardson completed the physical exam including a Pap smear test. After Brenda got dressed, Dr. Richardson started the discussion by going over Brenda's lab tests. It was worse than Brenda had expected: fasting blood glucose was in the range of a type 2 diabetes diagnosis, hemoglobin and hematocrit showed mild anemia, and urine indicated a small amount of protein. Dr. Richardson explained that Brenda needed to improve her diet as the first step. After conducting a Pap smear, Dr. Richardson asked about Brenda's menstrual cycle. Brenda mentioned that her anemia might be due to excessive bleeding with her monthly periods. Dr. Richardson ordered a sonogram to determine if Brenda had uterine fibroids or endometriosis (abnormal growths in uterus) and a mammogram to detect breast cancer. She knew Brenda was overwhelmed and wanted to provide immediate health education, so she referred Brenda to the hospital diabetic center and made an appointment for Brenda to meet with the nurse practitioner in a few days to answer immediate questions. Dr. Richardson's next appointment was scheduled in 2 weeks. Brenda left with referrals for the uterine sonogram, breast mammogram, and diabetic education plus a prescription for hypertension.

When Brenda got into her car, she began to sob. She was trying to determine what to do

(continues)

first. Since it was early afternoon, she decided to drop the prescriptions off at the pharmacy located in her grocery store and purchase some healthy food. She went home and sat on her apartment balcony while she ate lunch. Later, Brenda explored reliable websites ending with .gov (governmental), .edu (educational), or .org (organizational). She knew the websites ending in .com or .net are commercial and less reliable. She started a list of questions for the nurse practitioner's appointment about type 2 diabetes, hypertension, and anemia.

Since Brenda's friend Kathy is a CHW, she called her for general guidance. Brenda was starting to panic about her new position as a CHW, since she does not know enough about her own health. Kathy walks Brenda through the steps to enhance her self-advocacy skills. Here are the steps:

1. Read your health insurance policy. You need to know what medical treatments, education classes (i.e., type 2 diabetes management classes), and prescriptions are and are not covered. Review the cost of your deductibles and maximum out of pocket expenses.

2. Communicate with your health providers and their office staff. Make a list of questions prior to each appointment. Ask a family member or friend to come with you to make sure that all questions are answered and understood. Also, your friend can take notes and ask for spelling of medical words. Add your friend's name and contact information to your electronic medical records, so the healthcare providers can communicate with that person if you desire. Take time to get acquainted with the office staff, so you know their names when you call to ask questions. Visit with your pharmacist. The pharmacist can answer questions about new prescriptions, whether a cheaper generic prescription is available, what side effects you might experience, and any medication interactions that may occur when adding a new medication.

3. Take the time to gain access to the electronic patient portal for each of your healthcare providers and pharmacy. Keep records of your login and password information. It is useful to print copies of prescription, lab, and test results even if the reports are stored in the patient portal. Providers at one office may not have access to electronic records in another office. If you have printed copies, it is easier to take copies to other providers and they will upload the copies to their electronic records. Providers need to know all health services that you are receiving including chiropractic adjustments, acupuncture, massage, and herbal supplements.

4. Learn about your diagnosis by searching reliable websites on the internet. Understanding the medical terminology and common treatment plans helps you to understand your diagnosis and ask more informed questions. Gaining knowledge is not meant for you to challenge your providers decisions, but rather to give you the tools to have a conversation with your providers.

5. Become a compliant patient by keeping your appointments, arriving on time, and writing questions for each appointment. You do not wish to waste time during your appointment, but you do want to understand the answers to your questions. Only change your appointment when necessary. If you miss, change appointments, or arrive late, the provider and staff begin to think that you are not taking your diagnosis seriously. Follow the prescribed treatment plan. If you are not taking the prescribed medications for any reason, inform your provider. Your healthcare provider may change your prescription to a less expensive generic medication. If you start taking herbal supplements, share the information. Do not alter your treatment plan without a discussion with your healthcare provider. To establish a trusting relationship with providers, you must maintain honesty on your side and except the same from the provider. No relationship is flawless, but trust must be established and maintained from both individuals.

After Kathy explained ways to establish self-advocacy skills, Brenda's confidence improved, and she felt empowered to improve her health. After meeting with the nurse practitioner and registering for a 6-week series of diabetic information classes, she knew that she was on a successful path. Brenda was thrilled to learn

(continues)

that she would receive a free glucose monitor and test strips at the first diabetic class.

She knew that she needed to learn how to monitor her blood glucose daily. Also, Brenda knows that sustaining a healthy behavior change is difficult, and she will encounter setbacks along the way. As a first step reward, Brenda purchased new walking shoes and began a daily routine of walking every morning for 20 minutes before going to work since her new position starts at 9:00 a.m. She intends to increase the time and distance over the next few weeks. Brenda likes the accountability aspect of the diabetic classes, plans to register for the second 6-week session, and expects to see her blood glucose levels decreasing gradually. Since her physical exam appointment, Brenda has lost 4 pounds. She keeps thinking that slow and steady is the success to better health.

Questions

1. What questions would you suggest that Brenda add to her list when she meets with the nurse practitioner?

2. Name a minimum of three types of medications used to treat hypertension. Explain how each medication reduces the blood pressure.

Community Advocacy

Before exploring community advocacy, it is essential to re-examine social justice with a focus on community advocacy. Social justice is fairness as it manifests in healthcare, employment, housing, and more. Social justice is not achieved without an emphasis on the following four principles: human rights, access, participation, and equity.[11]

Human Rights. Human rights reflect the privileges inherent to all human beings, regardless of race, sex, nationality, ethnicity, disability, language, religion, or other status.[12] Human rights include the right to life and liberty, freedom from slavery and torture, freedom of opinion and expression, the right to work and education, and many more. Everyone is entitled to these rights, without discrimination.[12]

Access. Access is the capacity to have essential food, clothing, shelter, education, and healthcare. In communities, access is equal opportunity to participate, such as having an equal vote and seat at the table of civic meetings. When access is denied due to gender, disability or race/ethnicity, it leads to discrimination and injustices across the community. For example, if some buildings fail to build ramps, any individual with a disability requiring a wheelchair is denied access. For another example, think of buildings that have revolving doors at the entrance. For individuals using a walker/crutches or pushing a baby stroller would find it nearly impossible to navigate the entrance. Even if there are swinging doors on each side of the revolving door, the side doors are not likely to have push plates to open the door automatically. Lastly, signage in buildings is important, especially for individuals without disabilities. They should not need to retrace their steps due to lack of signage showing the way to the elevator.

Participation. Social justice is not achieved if only some voices are heard and acknowledged. Participation is often linked to power structures.[14] When participation is marginalized, the vulnerable are silenced. Even when society tries to address problems, solutions will not work if those who are most affected are unable to participate in the process.[14] Participation must be encouraged and rewarded so that everyone has an equal chance at the table and an equal chance to speak.[14]

Equity. Equity is often believed to mean "equality." While equality is an important principle to social justice, the term to best describe the idea of fairness is "equality." What's the difference? Equity considers the effects of discrimination and aims for an equal outcome. See **Figure 4.2**.

The tallest individual is able to see over the fence to watch the baseball game, thus they represent the most privileged in society.[11] The individual in the middle can barely see over the fence, while the shortest individual cannot see over the fence at all. This individual represents the most vulnerable in society. "Equality" gives everyone a

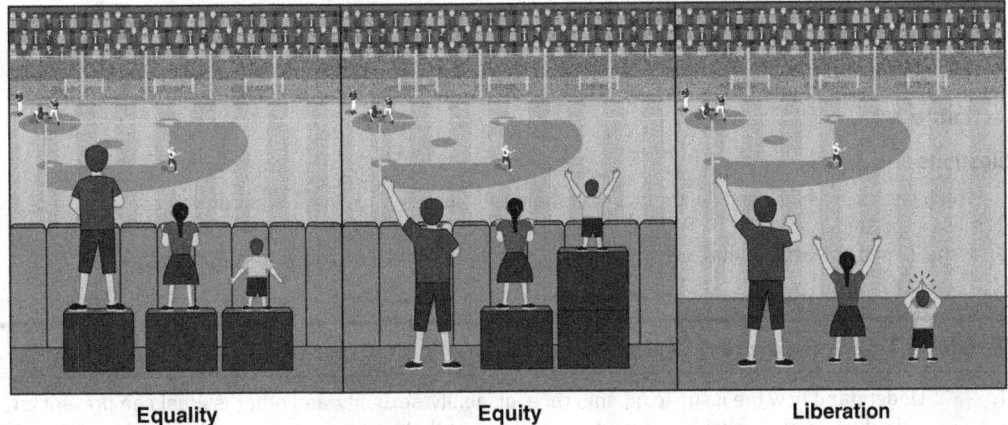

| Equality | Equity | Liberation |

Figure 4.2 Equality, Equity, and Liberation

Reproduced from WriteHear. What is Accessibility? Available at: https://www.seewritehear.com/learn/what-is-accessibility/. Accessed November 24, 2021. A collaboration between Center for Story-based Strategy & Interaction Institute for Social Change.

box to stand on, even though the tallest figure does not need it.[11] However, the shortest individual cannot see. "Equity" is defined as fairness to all, thereby a box is not provided to the privileged person, the middle person gets one box and the shortest person gets two. Now, everyone is at an equal level and can see over the fence to watch the game together.[11] Lastly, "Liberation" removes the fence, so everyone can participate without any barriers.

Community advocacy involves speaking for a group of individuals or identifying an issue or cause to propose a change to a policy or program to improve conditions for a specific people group or among the entire community.[2,11,13] While community advocacy may focus on topics, such as equity in access to health care and health resources, advocating for individuals from any marginalized group acknowledges the complexities associated with actively participating throughout a community as demonstrated through the difficulties navigating the healthcare system and outlining the structural and the social barriers that those individuals encounter daily.[2,11,13] See **Case Study 4.2**.

Case Study 4.2 Self-Advocacy for Individuals

Mark is a Black, 34-year-old CHW and has been employed in a 600-bed hospital outside of Lexington, Kentucky. During Mark's sophomore year in high school, he was a passenger in a multi-vehicle crash. He recovered but sustained serious spinal damage and uses a wheelchair. He drives a retrofitted van with hand controls that accommodates his wheelchair via a motorized ramp. Mark obtained his associate degree at a local community college and has worked as a CHW for the past 10 years. Mark has been married to his partner, Jamal, for 5 years. They met while Jamal, a Navy veteran, was hospitalized for complications from his military injury.

Mark has years of experience dealing with his own disability as well as providing valuable resources and services to individuals with disabilities and their families. Because Jamal's disability is not visible and connected to his military service, Mark has learned ways to advocate for veterans to obtain their entitled benefits. Whether the individual and their family has dealt with a disability for many years, recently acquired a disability, or is new to the community, they benefit from learning self-advocacy skills and becoming acquainted with available community services and resources.

In his hospital office, Mark has several large, framed motivational posters. He wants his patients and their families to feel comfortable asking questions about difficult times in their lives and understand how to self-advocate. In addition, Mark developed a booklet to teach individuals self-advocacy skills. People from all walks of life may benefit from learning how to advocate for themselves and others including situations related to age, race, ethnicity, disability, sexuality, or many other issues. See **Table 4.1**.

Questions

1. Which issues are Mark and Jamal facing in their self-advocacy journey? What do you consider to be the most important?
2. Of the 12 self-advocacy skills, which one is most important as a first step in your opinion?

Table 4.1 12 Self-Advocacy Skills

1.	Understand how the issue (e.g., age, race, disability, sexuality, and other issues) can prevent an individual from specific activities; however, accept that systemic discrimination and negative societal attitudes are far more limiting.
2.	Know that the rights of all individuals are the same. Rights are not diminished due to a specific issue (e.g., age, race, disability, sexuality, and other issues) such as the right to education, health care, food, safe housing, employment, happiness, and respect. The issue does not dictate a lesser quality of life.
3.	Assume that fighting for your rights is essential. Be aware of abusive individuals (e.g., caregivers, drivers, intimate partners, and employers) who may prey on vulnerable persons. Strive to maintain a high self-esteem, though difficult at times, to sustain a good quality of life. Learn the federal laws linked to your issue (e.g., American Disability Act, The Civil Rights Act of 1964,[15] Age Discrimination Act of 1975,[16] and for the LGBTQ+ community the Equal Protection Clause and the Due Process Clause in 2015).[17]
4.	Discover your advocacy style. You do not have to be the person on stage in front of the microphone. If you have writing skills, invite others to join a letter-writing campaign to advocate for an issue, policy, or organize data into create simple graphics. Do not be afraid to advocate among friends, family, and in various social settings when you feel comfortable.
5.	Conduct research to gain in-depth knowledge about the topic, issue, or policy prior to advocating.
6.	Remain polite, clear, professional, and direct when advocating for yourself or for your client. Try to learn something from every conversation. Reserve all assumptions. Stick to the facts and stay focused.
7.	Keep accurate notes for accountability of the date, time, individuals involved, and outcome. When you are working on complex issues, it is difficult to remember exactly what happened on each date.
8.	Be persistent. If the individual fails to return your calls, try again the next day. Always write down the name of the person that spoke to you. In some cases, it is effective to have a friend call for you. Do not give up. If one method did not work, change the approach, and try again.
9.	Always appeal any denial. Step back, regroup, and try again. In some cases, you may find help with your state rights organization. The government system is hoping that you will give up the fight.
10.	Always be polite and remain calm for the first few steps of your request. If the business or organization is not accommodating with your request, you may gather the information, write down the details of phone conversations with all individuals, dates, and time. If your request is not resolve, you may file a discrimination case. You can file a lawsuit or a complaint with your state civil rights commission or the Department of Justice.

(continues)

Table 4.1 12 Self-Advocacy Skills		*(continued)*
11.	Use social media. If you reach out to an establishment and they are not willing to accommodate your request, you may wish to leave a negative review on social media. However, if a business goes out of their way to adapt to your request and accommodate, you want to post an excellent review.	
12.	Practice self-care along the way including stress management, exercise, and meditation. Self-advocacy is a lifelong journey. Systems change slowly, so you must be persistent.	

Data from Willison K. The Ability Toolbox Blog. 12 Self-Advocacy Skills for Adults with a Disability or Chronic Illness. https://theabilitytoolbox.com /self-advocacy-skills-disability-chronic-illness/. Accessed July 8, 2021.[18]

The CHW in Community Advocacy

As discussed, advocacy is defined as the act of arguing in favor of a cause, issue, idea, or policy.[19] CHWs have the unique ability to draw attention to or advocate for an issue that is unnoticed or ignored among leaders or members of the community. CHWs investigate information to understand all aspects of the issue and provide the information to the attention of community leaders for action or change. In health care, CHWs advocate for individuals by assisting with access to care, navigating the healthcare system, and locating various resources.[2] After gaining experience, the CHWs address issues related to social determinants of health, such as inequities in health care, housing, education, and employment as well as injustices regarding language, literacy, gender, sexual orientation, disabilities, and faith-based communities.[2] See **Box 4.1**.

Whether it is for yourself, an individual, or the community, advocacy requires persistence, passion, determination, and focus to initiate change and educate others on the topic of interest. Self-advocacy is about trying to improve health, education, employment, or some other issue of concern.[2] Community advocacy is advocating for one individual or a group of people to initiate action toward that positive change, such as improving community

---

Box 4.1 What Are 2-1-1 Hotlines?

Each day thousands of individuals across the United States call 2-1-1 for information and support 24 hours a day, 7 days a week. The individuals who answer the calls provide a free, confidential referrals and information related to finances, health, veteran services, prevention/rehabilitation programs, food banks, animal rescues, housing, or disaster-related updates, such as evacuation routes. Some communities offer a community website in addition to the 2-1-1 phone hotline service. Do some general research about your local community's 2-1-1 hotline and answer the following questions to the best of your ability. You can view United Way's 2-1-1 website here: https://www.unitedway.org/our-impact/ featured-programs/2-1-1#.[20]

Questions

1. Does your community offer a 2-1-1 hotline service and a comprehension website of services?
2. Create a list of three questions. Call the 2-1-1 hotline and ask your questions.
3. Look on the 2-1-1 website and compare the responses provided on the hotline with the information on the website. What responses were the same and different? Why might there be differences?

Data from United Way. 2-1-1. https://www.unitedway.org/our-impact /featured-programs/2-1-1#. Accessed July 8, 2021.[20]

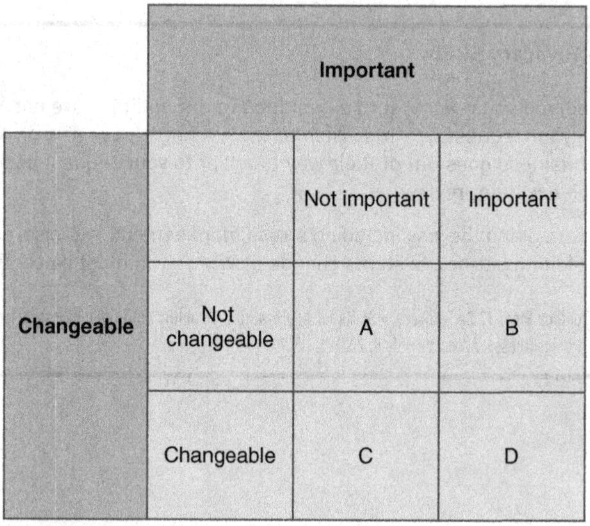

	Important		
Changeable		Not important	Important
	Not changeable	A	B
	Changeable	C	D

A = Not important and not changeable
B = Important and not changeable
C = Changeable and not important
D = Important and changeable

Figure 4.3 Decision Box

education opportunities, employment, civil and voting rights, inclusive transportation for individuals with disabilities, or other pertinent community issues.[2] When considering a topic or issue, it is useful to utilize the decision box. See **Figure 4.3**.

It is necessary to devote time, energy and funding to advocacy projects that are important and changeable (Box D). A simple way to determine if the proposed project is worthwhile to pursue is to use the decision box tool. If the project is not important and not changeable, it is likely going to be frustrating to accomplish. For example, adding sidewalks is important and changeable. It is good to start with a few big wins to show the community that it is possible to complete smaller projects prior to tackling major long-term projects, such as creating low-income housing. It is useful to review the characteristics of effective community advocacy prior to initiating any type of advocacy. See **Table 4.2**.

Table 4.2 Characteristics of Effective Community Advocacy

1.	Listen and learn. Approach the issue by looking at multiple sides and understand that there is never a clear *yes* or *no* related to community issues. It is important to hear all sides before proceeding to make decisions and plan accordingly.
2.	Focus on the long-term goals. Though it takes multiple small steps to achieve long-term goals, without organized planning, it is easy to become overwhelmed with the overall idea of the long-term goal rather than focusing on the importance of each small step.
3.	Support others. It is exhausting to make or propose change to any community. People are often excited and passionate in the beginning, but quickly lose momentum as the process slows down. This can breed frustration and disappointment. Thus, mutual support is vital to achieve success.

(continues)

Table 4.2 **Characteristics of Effective Community Advocacy** *(continued)*

4.	Find a variety of ways to share the message. The message must be delivered in many ways to capture the entire audience, including social media, radio, flyers, billboards, bus bench ads, bus posters, mailing, faith-based bulletin inserts, community forums, and county or city commissioner meetings.
5.	Collaborate with a wide selection of individuals to obtain a broad spectrum of opinions, beliefs, attitudes, and views. A diverse interdisciplinary team brings new ideas and insight across multiple professions which fuels creativity. A blended professional response is advantageous to advocacy efforts and community success.
6.	Review the available data available on the topic, including meeting minutes from past county commissioner meetings, newspaper articles and editorials, county data of demographics, cost benefit analysis, maps, and any other information available.
7.	Rebound from setbacks, negative pressure, and comments. Do not expect that everyone will understand or agree with the idea, concept, or proposed change.
8.	Connect all segments of the population to gain additional support. Identify the appropriate stakeholders from the beginning that will impact the neighborhood and the public.

Data from Blackburn BR, Blackburn R, Williamson R. 8 Characteristics of Effective Advocates. https://www.edcircuit.com/8-characteristics-of-effective-advocates-education/. Accessed July 12, 2021.[21]

Types of Resources

CHWs are involved in finding information and services, making referrals, and following-up to determine if an individual's needs were appropriately met. CHW are focused on the three basic types of resources: community, health, and social services.[22]

Community Resources. Community resources involve the organizations the serve a specific need for individuals or resources for a specific geographical area. Sources of funding include government, businesses, nonprofit groups, faith-based communities, cultural organizations, or private funds such as donations.[22]

Social Services. Social services are mostly funded by federal, state, or local programs.[22] Examples of social services include public schools, health department services and clinics, subsidized housing, disability services, public transportation, and public libraries.[22]

Healthcare Services. Healthcare services are essential and funded by federal, state, or local government agencies, corporations, institutions, or private nonprofit associations.[22] Communities strive to provide adequate health care for their vulnerable populations, such as individuals with disabilities, chronic illnesses, and those who lack adequate financial resources.[22]

When a CHW starts a new position, it is important to gather community resources by creating a resource map for your office or location of employment. Often a large county map may be obtained by contacting the county commissioner's office, completing a thorough online search, or contacting a commercial sign company. Real estate developers use similar maps, thus this request is not unusual. It is also possible to download a county map and take the file to a local printing company that has the desired paper size. In addition, CHWs begins to collect varied resources of information from sources including individuals, locations, and resources. Personal connections with individuals (e.g., coworkers, community members, neighborhood organizations) are a valuable source of community resource information.

Additionally, driving around the neighborhood, also known as a windshield assessment, provides information through observation about the area's local grocery stores, bus stops, parks, sidewalks, bike lanes, etc. Last, searching the internet provides detailed information about the community, such as locations of hospitals, nursing homes, churches, schools, libraries, and public institutions. By collecting information from diverse people and places, the resource map begins to reveal the community's current resources and deficits. After organizing the collected information, the CHW decides what is the best way to store the information, such as color-coded dots on the map, computer files, paper files in a binder, or other creative ways. Once the collected information is entered into the resource map and resource guide, the CHW is prepared to provide patients, clients, or other individuals with valuable information and referrals to community resources. See **Table 4.3**.

Table 4.3 Examples of a Community Resource Guide

Community Resource Guide
Adult Education: GED = General education development equivalent of high school diploma. ESL = English as a second language
Advocacy
Alcoholic Anonymous
Bail Bonds
Car Seats
Child Behavioral Support
Child Care
Children and Family Services
Consumer Information
Counseling
Day Care for Adults
Department of Motor Vehicles including driver's license and vehicle license plates
Dental Care
Dialysis Centers
Domestic and Family Violence Shelters
Drug and Alcohol Supports
Emergency Shelters for Pending Weather Conditions
Employment
Evacuation Routes for Pending Weather Conditions
Food and Nutrition Programs: SNAP = Supplemental Nutrition Assistance Program, formerly food stamps and WIC = Women, Infant, Children food supplement program
Financial Emergency Assistance
Food Banks
Health Care Clinics (Free or Low Cost) such as Federally Qualified Health Clinics (FQHC)

(continues)

Table 4.3 **Examples of a Community Resource Guide** *(continued)*

Health-Related Service Agencies

Head Start Children's Programs

Home Buying Programs

Hotlines

Home Health Care and Services

Homelessness

Housing and Renter's Assistance

Immigration Legal Services

Legal and Pre-Legal Services

Libraries

Meals-on-Wheels: home delivery service for elderly

Medical Providers

Mental Health Services

Parenting Support and Classes

Parks, Community Gardens, and Green Space

Prescription Drug Assistance

Pre-School Programs (No Cost)

Public Assistance

Recreation and After-School Programs

School Districts

Services for Individuals with Disabilities including lists of physically accessible buildings, large print written materials, services for individuals who are blind, an American Sign Language interpreter, free medical equipment, medical transportation services, prescription costs, etc.

Support Groups

Tax Filing Assistance

Thrift Shops, Goodwill, and Salvation Army Services

Transportation

Unemployment Compensation

Utilities (including assistance with past due payments)

Veteran Services

Veterinary Vaccines and Pet Medical Care

Victim Advocacy

Voter Registration

As a CHW accumulates information for the community resource guide, it is important to collect the necessary information and ensure that the guide is regularly updated to make a successful referral.

Access Community Resources

Now that the community resource map and guide are developed, it is time to think about how the individuals in the community can access the resources and what barriers they may encounter while obtaining access.[23] The community resource is not as simple as referring the individuals and assuming they will receive the needed services. There are four general categories of access to community resources: availability, physical access, information, and effectiveness.[23]

Availability. Availability of service or product is essential for the community, such as adequate supplies, services open for extended hours, translators for individuals with English as a second language, and services and products for individuals with disabilities (e.g., physical, visual, hearing, mental, mobility, post-traumatic stress disorder).[23] CHWs assist in a variety of situations. For example, a family that is moving out of the area may need support or assistance from a CHW to help research services and ensure availability in the new area where the family is moving. Furthermore, the CHW may be the first point of contact for the family moving into the new community. In either situation, the CHW becomes an essential point of contact for the family and helps to connect residents to a variety of available services.

Physical. Ensuring appropriate physical access to a service is an essential community resource.[23] For example, public transportation is vital for anyone with mobility needs due to physical impairment. If a rural community lacks public bus service or medical transport services, it is difficult for elderly individuals requiring kidney dialysis or cancer treatments and individuals who attend weekly mental health counseling. Physical access may involve appropriate and safe entree into a variety of public areas.[23] This can be accomplished with doors that have push-plate automatic door openers, stalls with disability bars, wide doors, access ramps, kneeling busses for individuals that are unable to navigate steps, sloping sidewalk curbs for walkers or wheelchairs, and pedestrian lights with signal flashing lights and beeps for safe street crossings.

Information. Ensuring obtainable access to information is important for community wellness.[23] For example, access to information through educational materials located on the computer or making information available in public locations such as libraries, clinics, or pharmacies where individuals or various professionals search for learning materials.[23] Whether on the computer or on paper, the font must be large enough for the visually impaired individuals and available in Braille for individuals with blindness. The education materials must be written in a low literacy format for ease of understanding. Appropriately, translating the materials into the common language of the possible reader is an additional factor to consider, ensuring educational attainment.[23] Last, television, radio and social media ads provide valuable information with public service announcements (PSA). Keep in mind that there are situations where some corporations, political figures, and local officials do not wish for specific information to be readily available and understandable to the public. For example, the way in which amendments are worded on voter ballots are not always easy to understand.

Effectiveness. Determining how effective a service is to the community is an essential element to access.[23] If a service is available, but not effective, then it is of minimal use to the individual. See **Case Study 4.3**.

Case Study 4.3 The Obesity Epidemic

Debra has been employed for 5 years as a CHW at a high school in a large metropolitan border city in Texas. The high school is composed of 60 percent adolescents from the Black and Brown community, and the majority of the more than 4,000 students are from low-income families living in government-subsidized housing. Most of the parents are immigrants from Mexico, working in the service or construction industries, and speak Spanish as their primary language. Debra speaks Spanish fluently, so she can talk to the families.

Debra is concerned about the number of students who are obese in the high school. She investigated the topic on the Centers for Disease Control and Prevention (CDC) website and found that "obesity is reducing our nation's ability to have a productive workforce as well as the number of young adults able to take part in the armed forces.[24] Obesity can lead to type 2 diabetes, heart disease, and some cancers."[24] She approached the Parent/Teacher Association (PTA) president and the school principal to discuss starting a campaign to make healthy living easier for all students and their families. She suggested the student clubs may wish to embrace this initiative for their annual project. The PTA president and the principal approved Debra's idea if she has a plan to show the effectiveness of this campaign.

Immediately, Debra contacted the leaders of student clubs. The leaders meet once per month, so Debra was added to the upcoming monthly agenda. She made copies of **Figure 4.4** for distribution at the meeting.

Because there are more than 25 student clubs, the club leaders decided that the entire high school would focus on the phrase in the middle of the handout: "Americans don't eat healthy enough or get the right amount of physical activity."[24]

Questions

1. Since Debra is your friend, she asks you for ideas to help the high school students with their new campaign. What advice would you give to her?
2. The PTA president and the principal want Debra to write a quarterly report to show the effectiveness of the student campaign. What should Debra write in the first quarter report?

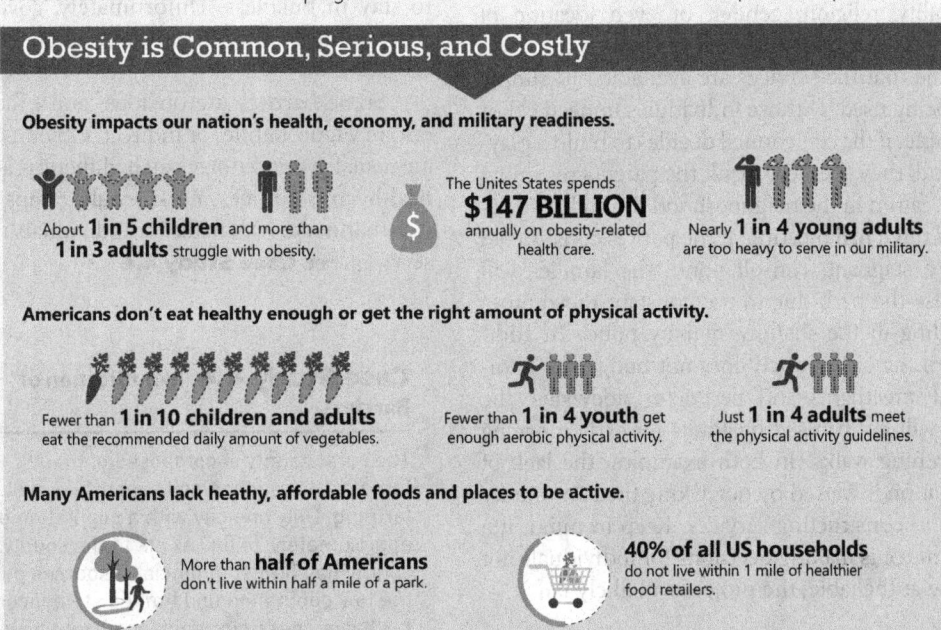

Figure 4.4 Obesity Is Common, Serious, and Costly

Data from Centers for Disease Control and Prevention, CDC Division of Nutrition, Physical Activity, and Obesity. Making Healthy Living Easier. https://www.cdc.gov/nccdphp/dnpao/docs/Obesity-Fact Sheet 508.pdf. Accessed November 24, 2021. Reference to specific commercial products, manufacturers, companies, or trademarks does not constitute its endorsement or recommendation by the U.S. Government, Department of Health and Human Services, or Centers for Disease Control and Prevention.[24]

Barriers to Community Resources

Barriers to community resources include personal, societal, and institutional barriers.[23]

Personal Barriers. Personal barriers are defined as any obstacle that impedes personal basic care needs.[23] The list may include, but is not limited to, adequate food, clothing, shelter, physical and mental health care, safety, medical equipment for disabilities, low literacy, English as a second language, and legal issues.[23]

Societal Barriers. Societal barriers includes the broader domains, such as education and employment inequalities unjustly based on race, ethnicity, sexual orientation, disabilities, or religious or cultural beliefs and practices.[23] Societal barriers are related to decisions that are made for individuals rather than involving people in the decisions, including illegal and unequal treatment of individuals simply because of their ethnicity, disability, religion, gender, or even location of their home address.[23] Too often people in power assume that the services are available but simply not being used by those individuals in need.[23] For example, if the city council decides to build a playground, they should consult the parents regarding the location in the neighborhood through a structured town hall meeting. If the park is constructed near a stagnant, run-off pond, the families will not use the park due to the constant mosquitoes breeding in the shallow, marshy pond. In addition, if the city council does not budget for additional streetlights and perimeter sidewalks, the park will not be used by adults for early morning or evening walks. In both examples, the lack of utilization is caused by not asking the community prior to constructing services. Keep in mind, if a committee is making decisions for individuals not sitting at the table, the project will likely fail.[23]

Institutional Barriers. Institutional barriers include location, physical access, administrative interaction, poor communication, and lack of cultural sensitivity.[23] The institutional barriers are intentional or unintentional barriers often with limited or no awareness. Location barriers assume that if the service is built, that the people in need of the service will come to the location.[23] However, if inadequate public transportation is an issue, the individuals in need of the service, have no way to overcome the lack of transportation.[23] Transportation continues to be a persistent obstacle across many communities. Physical access requires equal access for individuals with disabilities, by engineering the appropriate elevators, ramps, and large, private restroom facilities for families with children, caregivers, and other types of accommodations.[23] Administrative barriers include complex forms that require high literacy to complete and that use a small font, confusing phone systems with long wait times, and overall poor customer service. Since government agencies serve the public and provide needed services, they often do not view customer service as essential.[23] Commercial establishments offer excellent service because they must retain their customers to stay in business. Unfortunately, government services may not view the public customers in the same way.

Some barriers are obvious, and other barriers are vague, subtle, or indirect. Obvious barriers are usually conditions, such difficulty accessing healthcare resources, no sidewalk ramps or policies that make it difficult for individuals to access services. See **Case Study 4.4**.

Case Study 4.4 Identification of Barriers

The rural county is composed of mostly large cattle ranches and expansive soybean farming. Only one city with a population of approximately 78,000 exists in the county. The county has limited financial resources due to the low population and limited state income tax base. These circumstances limit how the county commissioners expand new services across the county. Since the parents are anxious to get educational computer services for the children in the rural areas, the county commissioners made the difficult decision to limit the hours of the county library to 3 days per week to save money on personnel. The saved money was used to purchase computers for rural schools and one computer per teacher to service the rural schools. Since the instructional designer is from this county, she has relatives in the rural areas. She is paid her salary and mileage but stays with relatives during the week to save mileage.

Questions

1. Name two barriers in this case study.
2. Name two barriers that were addressed.

When CHWs identify an issue related to barriers that block access to community services, they investigate current policies, engage in dialogue with administrators, and ask community members to explore ways to reduce the barriers for greater access to needed services.[23] Working in groups improves the chances of success in modifying community policies.[23]

Improving Access by Decreasing Barriers

After the discussion of access and barriers regarding community resources, it is time to think about how to improve access and decrease barriers. CHWs play a role in improving access, so this discussion involves some of the action plans that illustrates how to decrease barriers to improve access.[23] See **Table 4.4**.

Table 4.4 Improving Access by Decreasing Barriers

Decreasing Barriers	Example
Decrease availability of unhealthy food products.	A modest tax for soda and high sugar drinks; install streetlights for safety and build continuous sidewalks to encourage walking.
Expanding opportunities for community members.	Extend hours of operations to meet the needs of the community.
Improve availability of services for individuals with disabilities.	Mandatory installation of family restrooms; visit the Americans with Disabilities website (https://www.ada.gov[25]) to read important details.
Provide outreach services with a mobile health bus to rural areas.	Provide vaccinations for children, adolescents, adults, and elderly populations.
Enhance awareness and knowledge about chronic health conditions by offering health education seminars at local libraries, retirement communities, clinic conference rooms, and within faith-based communities.	Convert confusing health forms into low literacy formats with large fonts and appropriate language for the community. Maintaining cultural sensitivity is a crucial component to enhancing awareness.
Decrease the use of tobacco products.	Prohibit smoking at outside public places and parks.
Increase access to healthy practices, information, and practices.	Offer free yoga classes in the parks, and initiate neighborhood walking clubs to engage the community in exercise and fellowship.
Modify community policies to reflect education and employment equity across all neighborhoods in the county.	Offer adult GED courses in the local libraries and at convenient times for those who work during the day.

Data from Community ToolBox. Chapter 23: Section 1. Overview of Tactics for Modifying Access, Barriers, and Opportunities. https://ctb.ku.edu/en/table-of-contents/implement/access-barriers-opportunities/overview/main. Accessed July 15, 2021.[23]

Changes always begin with a single idea, then taking actionable baby steps, acquiring funding and finally, years later completing the project that began as a simple idea. See **Critical Thinking 4.1** and **Case Study 4.5**.

Critical Thinking 4.1 Examples of Improving Access by Decreasing Barriers

In your lifetime, you have likely witnessed barriers such as social, institutional, physical, familial, psychological, cultural, etc. that were changed to provide greater access to opportunity and increase participation within your community. List three examples.

Case Study 4.5 Betty's Meeting with a CHW

Betty is 56 years old and Black. She was recently diagnosed with an early stage of breast cancer. She has been a widow for the last 26 months after being married 28 years. She has an associate degree from a community college and has been employed for 12 years as an office manager for a real estate company. She has basic health insurance and is concerned about the cost of her cancer treatment. Betty has two sons in high school. Her oldest son has a driver's license and can drive the family's car. Betty is scared and looking for answers to her numerous questions. Her oncologist (cancer physician) referred her to a CHW located at the local American Cancer Society (ACS) office.

Betty called ACS on Monday morning and scheduled an appointment with Marilyn, the CHW. She was thrilled to learn that Marilyn schedules evening appointments on Wednesdays and had an appointment open this week at 7:00 p.m. Marilyn emailed an attachment to Betty containing directions to the ACS office, Marilyn's cell phone number, and a brief questionnaire for Betty to complete and return to Marilyn prior to her appointment on Wednesday. The questionnaire included basic demographic information (age, marital status, living arrangement, employment, date of cancer diagnosis, physician's name, and treatment completed).

Betty liked the next section because she had the opportunity to write her questions so Marilyn would be prepared to provide Betty with specific information and referrals. Betty completed the questionnaire on Monday evening when she got home from work.

Since Betty gets off work at 5:30 p.m., she had time for dinner at her favorite café near the ACS office. She wanted to collect her thoughts and go over the questions that she had submitted on the questionnaire. The directions to the ACS office were easy to follow, and there was ample parking behind the building since it was after usual office hours. Marilyn was waiting in the lobby for Betty since the main door locked at 6:00 p.m. Marilyn and Betty went up the elevator to Marilyn's cozy office filled with brochures, pamphlets, brightly colored posters, and soft quiet background music. Immediately, Betty felt at ease as she sat down in a puffy overstuffed red loveseat with flowered pillows and Kleenex on the side table. Marilyn offered Betty a cup of hot tea as she began by telling Betty that she was a 12-year breast cancer survivor herself and had experience working only with female cancer patients, especially those battling breast cancer. Betty accepted the hot tea as Marilyn opened her laptop. Marilyn began to review Betty's questionnaire and encouraged Betty to add information or questions throughout the process. Betty felt like she was talking to a close friend rather than talking to a stranger. She had no problem asking additional questions as Marilyn took notes.

At the end of the appointment, Marilyn reviewed her notes with Betty and provided a summary of their first appointment. In addition, she gives Betty a pink canvas bag to collect the brochures of interest from the display rack and her notes. Here is the summary:

Question 1: Betty is going to have 8 weeks of chemo prior to her surgery. Where can she obtain wigs or scarves after her hair thins or falls out?

Answer 1: Marilyn explained that ACS has a closet filled with wigs, scarves, camisoles with pockets to hold breast prosthesis if needed after surgery, and many other necessary items. All supplies are free. Women donated to the closet after their treatment is completed. In addition, Marilyn describes the ACS Reach to Recovery support group program for individuals with a breast cancer diagnosis. There are three active groups in their community. Each group meets once per month at various dates, times, and locations. Women are welcome at any group, and they are not limited or obligated to one meeting per month. Marilyn hands Betty the brochure.

Question 2: Betty had questions about her health insurance policy.
Answer 2: Marilyn suggested that Betty bring her health insurance policy to their next meeting. They will read it together. Marilyn will take notes and tell Betty what to ask when she calls the health insurance company.

Question 3: Betty is afraid that she will not be able to drive to her chemotherapy appointments. Even though her son drives, she does not wish to take him out of school. Also, she does not wish to impose on her friends.
Answer 3: Marilyn explained that ACS has a program called "Ride to Recovery." Volunteers at ACS volunteer to drive individuals with cancer to their appointments or treatments. Some drivers wait for the individuals, or another driver arrives for the trip home.

Question 4: Betty has not yet told her two sons about her cancer diagnosis. She is afraid that they will be so afraid that she might die. Her husband did not die of cancer, but a tragic unintentional injury at work.

She cannot bring herself to tell them since they are still grieving the loss of their father. Answer 4: Marilyn understood Betty's situation and offered her a few useful booklets to read. Also, she suggested that Betty schedule a phone appointment with the school counselor at the boys' high school. She thought that the school counselor may have some useful ideas or would a referral to the high school grief counselor for the county. In the meantime, Marilyn would investigate additional resources for Betty related to this question.

Betty nodded after a summary was provided to sensitively answer each question. Marilyn asked Betty if she had any further questions before they scheduled Betty's next appointment. Betty had no further questions and scheduled the next appointment with Marilyn for the following Wednesday. On her drive home, Betty felt a sense of relief. She felt that Marilyn was going to accompany her on this cancer journey.

Questions

1. Describe in detail three things that Marilyn did to make Betty feel comfortable.
2. List three resources that are available at most ACS office in most cities and that Marilyn recommended to Betty.
3. What questions would you add to the first questionnaire that Betty received from Marilyn prior to her first appointment?

Chapter Summary

This chapter focuses on social justice, advocacy, and community-based resources essential to CHWs. Social justice is defined as equal rights, equal opportunities, and equal treatment. There are several types of advocacy categories, two of which include self-advocacy and community advocacy. Self-advocacy is speaking for oneself and effectively communicating with others about your emotional, physical, and mental needs regardless of a known health condition.[2] Community advocacy involves speaking for individuals or identifying an issue or cause to initiate the change of a policy or program to improve conditions for a specific people group or the entire community including age, race, ethnicity, disabilities, and

sexuality. Regardless of the advocacy category, the goal of advocacy is to speak on behalf of marginalized individuals and be a voice for the overlooked and underrepresented.[2] CHWs are trained to teach individuals to advocate for themselves as well as to be an advocate on behalf of the community. The chapter introduces community resources including how to develop a community resource map and create a community resource guide. Once the guides are completed, the CHWs learns to investigate, verify, and make a successful referral to a community service or resource for individuals in need of services and information. Last, the discussion explores the process of improving access by decreasing barriers to community resources.

References

1. Meaning of advocate in English. Lexico Web site. https://www.lexico.com/definition/advocate. Accessed July 6, 2021.
2. Hubinette M, Dobson S, Scott I, Sherbino J. Health advocacy. *Med Teach.* 2017;39(2):128–135.
3. What is social justice? Pachamama Alliance Web site. https://www.pachamama.org/social-justice/what-is-social-justice. Accessed November 22, 2021.
4. What is social justice? The San Diego Foundation Web site. https://www.sdfoundation.org/news-events/sdf-news/what-is-social-justice/. Accessed November 22, 2021.
5. Cirillo A. Fighting ageism in health care. https://www.enlivant.com/blog/fighting-ageism-in-health-care. Accessed November 22, 2021.
6. Racism and health. Centers for Disease Control and Prevention Web site. https://www.cdc.gov/healthequity/racism-disparities/index.html. Accessed November 23, 2021.
7. Disability impacts all of us infographic. Centers for Disease Control and Prevention Web site. https://www.cdc.gov/ncbddd/disabilityandhealth/infographic-disability-impacts-all.html#:~:text=26%20percent%20(one%20in%204)%20of%20adults%20in,South.%20Percentage%20of%20adults%20with%20functional%20disability%20types:. Accessed July 8, 2021.
8. Disability and health information for health care providers. Centers for Disease Control and Prevention Web site. https://www.cdc.gov/ncbddd/disabilityandhealth/hcp.html. Accessed November 23, 2021.
9. Morris M, Cooper RL, Ramesh A, et al. Training to reduce LGBTQ-related bias among medical, nursing, and dental students and providers: A systematic review. *BMC Medical Education.* 2019;19(325).
10. Types of blood pressure medication. American Heart Association Web site. https://www.heart.org/en/health-topics/high-blood-pressure/changes-you-can-make-to-manage-high-blood-pressure/types-of-blood-pressure-medications. Accessed July 6, 2021.
11. What does social justice mean? Human Rights Careers Web site. https://www.humanrightscareers.com/issues/what-does-social-justice-mean/. Accessed November 23, 2021.
12. Human rights. United Nations Web site. https://www.un.org/en/global-issues/human-rights. Accessed November 24, 2021.
13. What is accessibility? SeeWriteHear Web site. https://www.seewritehear.com/learn/what-is-accessibility/. Accessed November 24, 2021.
14. United Nations, Economic and Social Commission for Western Asia (ESCWA). Social justice and participation policy brief. https://yptoolbox.unescapsdd.org/wp-content/uploads/2017/08/ESCWA_Policy-Brief-on-%e2%80%98Social-Justice-and-Participation%e2%80%99.pdf. Accessed November 24, 2021.
15. Federal employment discrimination laws. Find Law Web site. https://www.findlaw.com/civilrights/discrimination/employment-discrimination-federal-laws.html. Accessed November 24, 2021.
16. Age discrimination. U.S. Department of Labor Web site. https://www.dol.gov/general/topic/discrimination/agedisc. Accessed November 24, 2021.
17. LGBTQ rights and gender identity discrimination. Find Law Web site. https://www.findlaw.com/civilrights/discrimination/gay-and-lesbian-rights-sexual-orientation-discrimination.html. Accessed November 24, 2021.
18. Willison K. 12 self-advocacy skills for adults with a disability or chronic illness. The Ability Toolbox Blog. https://theabilitytoolbox.com/self-advocacy-skills-disability-chronic-illness/. Accessed July 8, 2021.
19. Advocacy. The American Heritage Dictionary of the English Language Web site. https://www.ahdictionary.com/word/search.html?q=advocacy. Accessed July 8, 2021.
20. 2-1-1. United Way Web site. https://www.unitedway.org/our-impact/featured-programs/2-1-1#. Accessed July 8, 2021.
21. Blackburn BR, Blackburn R, Williamson R. 8 Characteristics of effective advocates. https://www.edcircuit.com/8-characteristics-of-effective-advocates-education/. Accessed July 12, 2021.
22. Neely CK. Examples of community resources. https://pocketsense.com/examples-community-resources-5677.html. Accessed July 12, 2021.
23. Chapter 23: Section 1. Overview of tactics for modifying access, barriers, and opportunities. Community ToolBox Web site. https://ctb.ku.edu/en/table-of-contents/implement/access-barriers-opportunities/overview/main. Accessed July 15, 2021.
24. Making healthy living easier. Centers for Disease Control and Prevention Web site. https://www.cdc.gov/nccdphp/dnpao/docs/Obesity-Fact-Sheet-508.pdf. Accessed November 24, 2021.
25. Information and technical assistance on the Americans with Disabilities Act. ADA.gov. https://www.ada.gov/. Accessed July 8, 2021.

Appendix

1. What Is Advocacy: https://www.youtube.com/watch?v=NnOk2tTz468
2. Invisible Disabilities: https://www.youtube.com/watch?v=2nI3kSy__OA&t=4s
3. Fighting for Disability Rights: https://www.youtube.com/watch?v=C6c6gZEFQdg
4. Advocacy and Self-Determination: https://www.youtube.com/watch?v=5r-kVhemaAQ
5. How Community Resources Can Help: https://www.youtube.com/watch?v=KEFd6hwqcHk
6. CDC Obesity Epidemic: https://www.youtube.com/watch?v=vCORDl4bqDE

Health and Disease

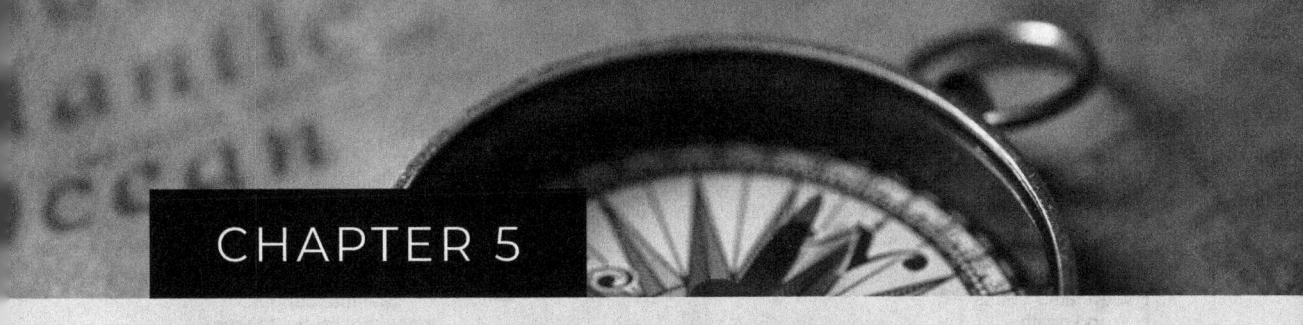

CHAPTER 5

Environmental Impact of Health

LEARNING OBJECTIVES

1. Explain how the health hazards of climate effects, water, air, and noise pollution affect health.
2. Describe the mental health impact and various influence of stress related to climate.
3. Discuss the negative effects of water pollution on human health.
4. Examine three types of air pollution and the consequences on health.
5. Describe how noise pollution causes the deterioration of health.
6. Define risk factors and protective factors in relationship to health.

KEY WORDS

positive stress (eustress)
negative stress (distress)
physical stress
environmental stress

social stress
risk factors
personal risk factors
environmental risk factors

protective factors
personal protective factors
environmental protective factors

Introduction

This chapter explores environmental health as the branch of public health that focuses on the interrelationships between people and their environment, the promotion of health and well-being, and the importance of fostering healthy and safe communities. Environmental health works to advance policies and programs to reduce chemical and other environmental exposures to protect residents and provide communities with healthier environments. For this discussion, we are referring to the health hazards produced by climate, such as water, air, and noise pollution.[1]

Health Hazards of Climate Effects: Water, Air, and Noise Pollution

This section discusses the health hazards related to the climate effects of water, air, and noise pollution and how these elements impact the health of individuals and the communities that are exposed. The adverse exposures are caused by numerous factors. The 2020 data show life expectancy in the United States as an average of 78.7 years: 76.2 years for men and 81.2 years for women.[2] However, the overall longevity across various communities

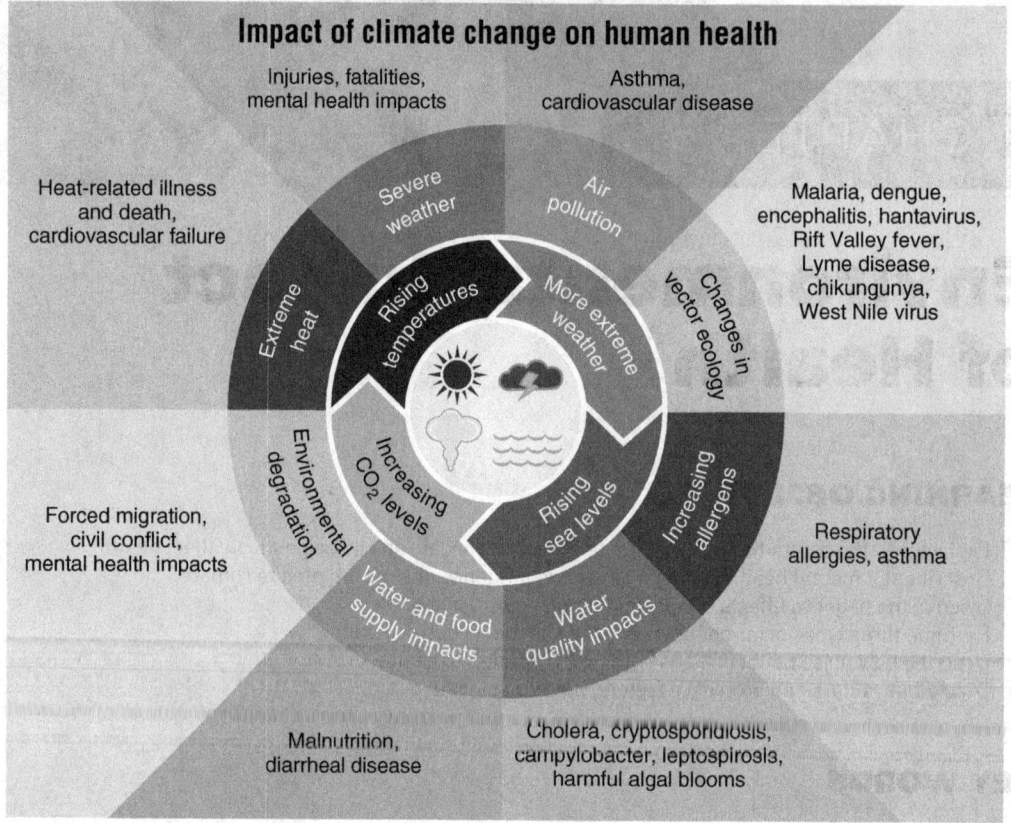

Figure 5.1 Climate Effects on Health

Figure from Centers for Disease Control and Prevention. Climate Effects on Health. https://www.cdc.gov/climateandhealth/effects/default.htm. Accessed November 19, 2021. Reference to specific commercial products, manufacturers, companies, or trademarks does not constitute its endorsement or recommendation by the U.S. Government, Department of Health and Human Services, or Centers for Disease Control and Prevention.[3]

largely depends on the environmental conditions related to climate and adverse exposures throughout a community. It is important to understand how environmental conditions contribute to a community's health. See **Figure 5.1**.

Climate Effects

As described in Figure 5.1, climate impacts many aspects of health. This section explores mental health and stress disorders along with temperature extremes, precipitation extremes, and how the environment influences food security.

Mental Health and Stress

Mental illness is one of the major causes of suffering in the United States, and extreme weather events can affect one's mental health in several ways.[4] Following environmental disasters, mental health problems increase, both among people with no history of mental illness, and those at risk—a phenomenon known as "common reactions to abnormal events."[4] These reactions may be short-lived or, in some cases, long-lasting.[4] For example, hurricanes, floods, heat waves, and wildfires have demonstrated high levels of anxiety and post-traumatic stress disorder among individuals. All these events are increasingly fueled by climate change. Other health consequences of stress exposures include pre-term birth, low birth weight, and maternal complications.[4]

In addition, some individuals with a mental illness, such as depression and schizophrenia, are susceptible to heat. Dementia is a risk factor for hospitalization and death during heat waves.[4]

Other potential mental health impacts, though less understood, include the possible distress associated with environmental displacement, and anxiety and despair linked to climate change.[4]

The topic of stress is complex and involves behavior, lifestyle, biological properties, genetics, and psychological processing.[5] While there are two major categories of stress, such as positive stress (eustress) and negative stress (distress), continued stress overtime has negative impacts on physical, mental, emotional, and spiritual health.[6] The body recognizes stress as tension regardless of if the stress is identified as positive or negative. Therefore, it is crucial to be cognizant of stress levels to prevent chronic disease, immune vulnerability, the development of stress-related disorders, tissue damage, and a suppressed central nervous system.[5] Additionally, prolonged stress is identified as a complicated social determinant of health, which considers how stress can be uniquely rooted within the built environment, throughout the workplace, among marginalized communities, and co-exist with many other identified determinants of health.

Positive Stress. Positive stress, also known as **eustress**, is natural, and biological reaction to a specific demand or event in which the individual faces or chooses to accept.[6] Positive stress helps individuals in the short-term to cope with difficult situations, increase performance, motivate, or achieving a specific goal (e.g., stop smoking, lose weight, or exercise consistently each week).[6]

Negative Stress. Negative stress, also known as **distress**, is a more complex, intricate topic because everyone responds to negative stress differently.[6] An individual's response to a stressor is unique based on their past experiences, genetics, trauma, coping mechanisms, and behavioral patterns. Research has indicated that high levels of stress may cause increased inactivity (e.g., watching television, computer games, sleeping), withdrawing from daily activities, and increased eating and drinking habits.[7] In addition to the two types of stress just discussed, there are three additional categories of stress that impact an individual and their health: physical, environmental, and social and emotional.[7]

Physical Stress: **Physical stress** is short term or long term. In short-term situations, the body has a fight-or-flight response that is a natural, life-saving system that allows the muscles to move quickly and effectively.[5,7] However, long-term physical stress occurs when the body is caught in the fight-or-flight mode.[5] When long-term stress prevents the body from returning to a relaxation mode, the body remains in a constant state of readiness for physical action (i.e., fight-or-flight). When the body has no time to recuperate, the immune system become weak and susceptible to sickness.[5]

Environmental Stress: **Environmental stress** is caused by multiple factors related to climate change, wildfires, air quality, water pollution, extreme weather conditions, noise, traffic, and poor quality of housing.[1,3] Unfortunately, environmental stress is usually not related to a single incident. Additionally, environmental stress is often defined as catalyst that causes additional repercussions to one's quality of life, sense of safety and security, and living conditions. For example, a hurricane destroys a home which leads to lack of utility services, poor housing conditions due to mold, and flooding. Each incident is stressful, but multiple environmental events lead to major stress over a long period of time for entire communities including unemployment, highway damage, loss of transportation, and school closing.[3]

Social and Emotional Stress: **Social stress** is caused by living in neighborhoods with poor quality housing and schools, exposure to institutional racism, low-income employment opportunities, neighborhood violence, lack of law enforcement protection, and discrimination based on ethnicity, religious beliefs, gender, disability, age, and sexual orientation.[5,7] Emotional stress involves relationships, such as divorce, domestic violence, housing eviction, loss of property, loss of family members via child protection removal, foster care, incarceration, mental health conditions, suicide, homicide, and the lack of adequate treatment of disease or delay of diagnosis.[7]

It is normal for everyone to experience some form of stress in their lifetime.[8] However, whether someone is feeling routine stress related to school, housing, financial security, or life-changing stress, such as the death of a loved one, loss of housing due to a fire, or severe storm damage, it is important to practice effective coping skills. Long-term stress that is not controlled becomes overwhelming and leads to a future of chronic health problems.[8]

Temperature Extremes

Extreme heat events are linked to deaths from heat stroke and related conditions, such as cardiovascular disease, respiratory disease, and cerebrovascular disease.[9] Heat waves are associated with increased hospital admissions for cardiovascular, kidney, and respiratory disorders. Extreme heat remains a cause of preventable death nationwide. Urban heat areas are projected to increase the vulnerability of urban and aging populations to heat-related health impacts in the future.[9] Extreme summer heat is increasing, and climate projections indicate that extreme heat will become more frequent and intense in the coming decades. Milder winters resulting from a warming climate can reduce illness, injuries, and deaths associated with cold and snow. While deaths and injuries related to extreme cold events are projected to decline due to climate change, these reductions are not expected to compensate for the increase in heat-related deaths.[9]

Precipitation Extremes: Heavy Rainfall, Flooding, and Droughts

The frequency of heavy precipitation is increasing in all U.S. regions.[10] Floods are the second deadliest of all weather-related hazards in the United States, most due to drowning. Flash floods and flooding associated with tropical storms result in the highest number of deaths.[10]

In addition to the immediate health hazards of flooding, elevated waterborne disease outbreaks can easily occur. Water intrusion into buildings can result in mold contamination leading to compromised indoor air quality. Buildings damaged during hurricanes are especially susceptible to water intrusion. Damp indoor environments lead to an increased prevalence of asthma and other upper respiratory tract symptoms, such as coughing and wheezing, as well as lower respiratory tract infections such as pneumonia.[10]

At the opposite end, drought conditions may increase the environmental exposure to a broad set of health hazards including wildfires, dust storms, extreme heat events, flash flooding, degraded water quality, and reduced water quantity. Dust storms associated with drought conditions contribute to reduced air quality due to harmful particles circulating in the air.[10]

Food Security

Globally, climate change threatens food production and certain aspects of food quality as well as food prices and distribution systems.[11] Many crop yields are predicted to decline because of the combined effects of changes in rainfall, severe weather events, and increasing competition from weeds and pests on crop plants. Livestock and fish production are also projected to decline. Prices are expected to rise in response to declining food production and associated trends such as increasingly expensive petroleum.

In such situations, individuals will likely turn to nutrient-poor, high calorie foods.[11] Thus, the nutritional value of some foods is projected to decline. The nutrient content of crops is also projected to decline if soil nitrogen levels are suboptimal. In addition, farmers are expected to need to use more herbicides and pesticides because of the increase of pests and weeds as well as decreased effectiveness and duration of some chemicals.[11] Farmers, farmworkers, and consumers will be increasingly exposed to these substances, which can be toxic and are often associated with chronic diseases. The impacts of climate change on the nutritional value of food exist within a larger context. Therefore, it is necessary to prevent food insecurity by protecting the environment and acknowledge the importance of early interventions to prevent health consequences.[11]

Water

Humans, animals, and plants depend on water for survival. Without water, death occurs within a few days. When water is polluted, consumption may lead to disease and death. Although this dire situation is observed in impoverished countries, access to abundant clean water is a global concern.[12] This section discusses the effects of water pollution and hazards of lead exposure in drinking water.

Water Pollution

Water pollution is mostly caused by urban development, such as building houses, roads, and factories.[12] Reports indicate that 75 percent to 80 percent of water pollution is caused by the domestic sewage, and 25 percent of pollution is caused by industries, which produce more pollution than urban development.[12] In homes, individuals contribute to water pollution by pouring chemicals down toilets and applying weed killers and chemical fertilizers on lawns. Factories and industries discharge radioactive wastes, marine waste dumping, oil leaks and spills, plastics and other waste into rivers, lakes, oceans. The health of ecosystems, plants, animals, fish, and humans are adversely affected by water pollution.[12] See **Table 5.1**.

For example, water pollutants cause death and contamination of fish, impacting the entire food chain and other forms of aquatic life.[12] These events are linked to the destruction of coastal waters (e.g., red, green, and blue algae). Overall, some types of fish are no longer safe for human consumption.[12] See **Figure 5.2**.

Table 5.1 Negative Effects of Water Pollution on Human Health

Disease	Symptoms
Traveler's Diarrhea	Bacteria causes by contaminate water or food. Symptoms include abdominal cramps and loose stools.[13]
Salmonella	Bacteria causes an infection including fever, abdominal cramps, diarrhea, headache, and vomiting lasting 4 to 7 days.[14]
Cholera	Bacteria causes mild to severe symptoms: vomiting, leg cramps, and profuse watery diarrhea.[15]
Dysentery	Bacteria, virus, or parasite causes inflammation of intestines, stomach pain, cramping, and bloody diarrhea.[16]
Escherichia Coli (E. Coli)	Bacteria found in intestines of humans. Bad strains found in drinking water polluted with human or animal feces causes severe diarrhea, vomiting, and cramps.[17]
Hepatitis A	Highly contagious liver infection is transferred through the consumption of contaminated food or water. Symptoms include fatigue, stomach pain, low appetite, nausea, and jaundice.[18]
Hepatitis E	Type of liver disease associated with contaminated water in areas with poor sanitation. Symptoms include fever, fatigue, nausea, jaundice, vomiting, and joint pain.[19]
Parasitic Infections	Harmful parasites found in contaminated water. Symptoms include diarrhea, stomach pain, dehydration, weight loss, and flu-like symptoms.[20]
Botulism	Rare poisoning by toxin. If untreated, paralysis occurs with death from respiratory failure. This disease is particularly dangerous for infants.[21]
Typhoid Fever	Spread by contaminated food or water. Symptoms include high fever, stomach pain, weakness, loss of appetite, and headache.[22]

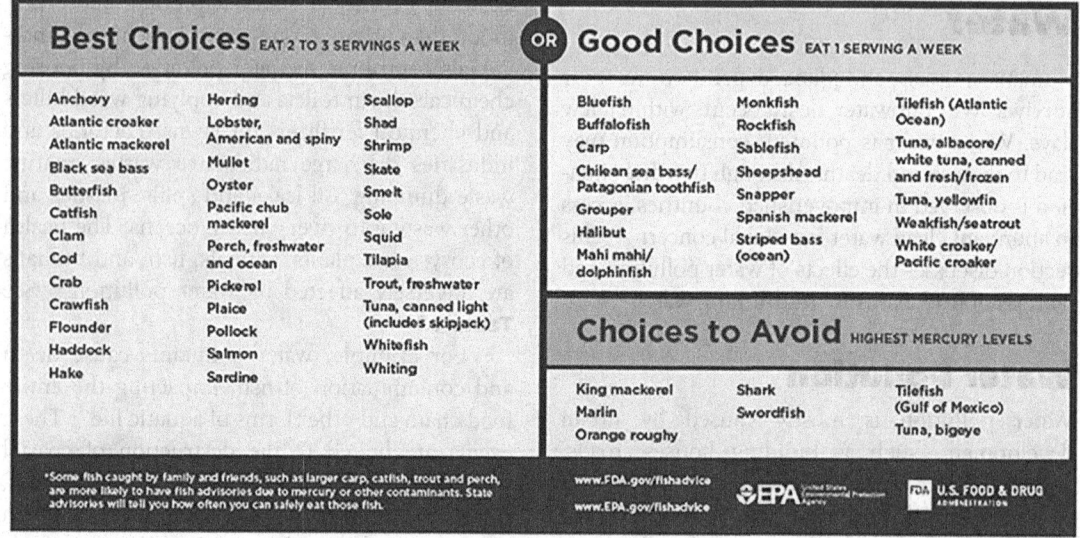

Figure 5.2 Advice on Fish Consumption

Figure from Environmental Protection Agency. Fish Advice. https://www.epa.gov/system/files/images/2021-09/fish-chart.jpg. Accessed November 19, 2021.[23]

Lead Exposure in Drinking Water

The most common sources of lead found in drinking water are from lead pipes, faucets, and plumbing fixtures.[24] Certain pipes that carry drinking water from the water source to the home may contain lead. Household plumbing fixtures, welding solder, and pipe fittings made prior to 1986 may also contain lead. Steps taken during the last few decades have reduced exposures to lead in sources of tap water. Even so, lead in water can come from homes with lead service lines that connect the home to the main water line. Homes without lead service lines may still have brass or chrome-plated brass faucets, galvanized iron pipes, or other plumbing soldered with lead.[24]

Some drinking water fountains with lead-lined tanks and other plumbing fixtures not intended for drinking water (e.g., lab faucets, hoses, spigots, hand washing sinks) may also have lead in the water.[24] Lead exposure occurs when a child touches, swallows, or breathes in lead or lead dust particles. Because no safe blood level has been identified for young children, all sources of lead exposure for children should be controlled or eliminated to prevent adverse health

consequences. For example, infants who drink formula prepared with lead-contaminated tap water may be at a higher risk of exposure because of the large volume of water they consume relative to their body size. Protecting children from exposure to lead is important to lifelong good health.[24]

The U.S. Environmental Protection Agency (EPA) has set the maximum contaminant level for lead in drinking water at zero because lead can be harmful to human health even at low exposure levels.[24] Lead is a toxic metal that is persistent in the environment and can accumulate in the body over time. Risks vary depending on the individual, the chemical conditions of the water, and the amount consumed. Bathing and showering should be safe because human skin does not absorb lead if found within the water source. If individuals are concerned about lead in water or know that their plumbing contains lead, they can take the following actions to reduce the amount of lead in their drinking water and minimize their potential for exposure.[24]

- Reduce or eliminate the exposure to lead in tap water by drinking or using only tap water that has been run through a "point-of-use" certified filter by a licensed independent testing organization to reduce or eliminate lead.[25] Only used the water that passes through the filter for drinking or cooking.[25-26]

- Reduce potential exposure from household lead plumbing by running the tap, taking a shower, doing laundry, or doing a load of dishes. These actions flush the pipes and is especially important when the water has been off and sitting in the pipes for more than 6 hours.[25-26] Drink or cook only with water that comes out of the tap cold. Water that comes out of the tap warm or hot can have higher levels of lead. Boiling this water will not reduce the amount of lead in the water.[25-27]
- Eliminate exposure to lead in water by drinking or using *only* bottled water that has been certified by a licensed independent testing organization.[25-27] For more information, visit: https://info.nsf.org/certified/bwpi/[27] to search for products that have undergone strict filtering, adhere to safety standards, maintain certification, and oversee product development from start to finish to ensure public health protection when consuming water.[25-27] See **Box 5.1**.

Box 5.1 Commercial Bottled Water

In the United States, individuals spend billions of dollars every year on commercially bottled water.[28] People choose bottled water for a variety of reasons including taste, convenience, consume as a substitute for other beverages, or because of perceived health benefits. The Food and Drug Administration (FDA) regulates the safety of bottled water and bases its standards on the EPA standards for tap water.[28] If these standards are met, water is considered safe for most healthy individuals. The bottled water industry must also follow the FDA's good manufacturing practices for processing and bottling drinking water.[28]

While there is currently no standardized label for bottled water, labels may discuss how the water was treated, filtered, or produced.[28] Check the label for a toll-free number or webpage address of the company that manufactured the bottled water to learn more.[28]

Commercially bottled water. Centers for Disease Control and Preventionhttps://info.nsf.org/certified/bwpi/. https://www.cdc.gov/healthywater/drinking/bottled/index.html. Accessed November 19, 2021. Reference to specific commercial products, manufacturers, companies, or trademarks does not constitute its endorsement or recommendation by the U.S. Government, Department of Health and Human Services, or Centers for Disease Control and Prevention

Last, a tragic example of water pollution occurred in 2014, when the residents of Flint, Michigan, experienced lead contamination due to inadequate testing and treatment of their water supply.[29] The water contaminated with lead caused rashes, hair loss, and itchy skin. Lead levels in the bloodstream of children who drank the water increased, causing major health concerns.[29]

Air Pollution

When examining the topic of air pollution, it is easy to recognize common air pollutants and their daily sources. For individuals living in cities, air pollution is caused by vehicle emissions, factories, fires, construction sites, heating/cooling equipment, and various other environmental contaminants.[30] Due to daily air pollution exposure, the pollutants accumulate over time within the body, which causes organ damage, lung disease, eye and skin irritation, memory impairment, various disabilities, and chronic illness.[30] While air pollution comes in many forms, the Clean Air Act mandates the EPA to set quality standards to inform the public about the six most common air pollutants that are harmful to human health.[31]

For example, climate change is projected to harm human health by increasing the particulate matter causing air pollution in many locations. Particulate matter concentrations are affected by wildfire emissions and air stagnation episodes, among other factors. By increasing these different factors, climate change is projected to lead to increased concentrations of ozone and increased particulate matter in some regions. Increases in global temperatures could cause associated increases in premature deaths related to particle pollution.[32] Outdoor air quality has improved since the 1990s; however, many challenges remain in protecting Americans from air quality problems. This section explores several types of air pollution (e.g., wildfires, cigarette smoke, radon, and carbon monoxide) that threaten air quality and public health in the United States.[32]

Wildfires

Climate change is increasing the vulnerability and frequency of wildfires in many forests across certain regions of the United States.[33] Long periods of record high temperatures are associated with droughts that contribute to dry conditions and causing wildfires. The smoke produced from wildfires contains particulate matter, and various volatile organic compounds can significantly reduce air quality in the areas near the fires.[33]

Wildfire smoke exposure increases respiratory and cardiovascular hospitalizations and medical visits for lung illnesses.[33] It has also been associated with hundreds of thousands of deaths annually from landscape fire smoke. Climate change is projected to increase wildfire risks and associated emissions, with harmful impacts on health.[33] See **Figure 5.3**.

Cigarette Smoking

It is important to acknowledge how human behavior and lifestyle factors can instigate air pollution. According to the Centers for Disease Control and Prevention (CDC), although air pollution is generally blamed on environmental hazards, cigarette smoking is the leading preventable cause of death in the United States.[35] Cigarette smoking harms nearly every organ of the body, causes many diseases, and causes poor health outcomes for those who smoke or use tobacco products.[36] For example, in the United States, cigarette smoking causes nearly one in five deaths.[37] If no one smoked, one of every three cancer deaths in the United States would not occur.[35] See **Figure 5.4**.

Last, it is important to recognize the risks related to exposure to secondhand smoke. Secondhand smoke includes a combination of

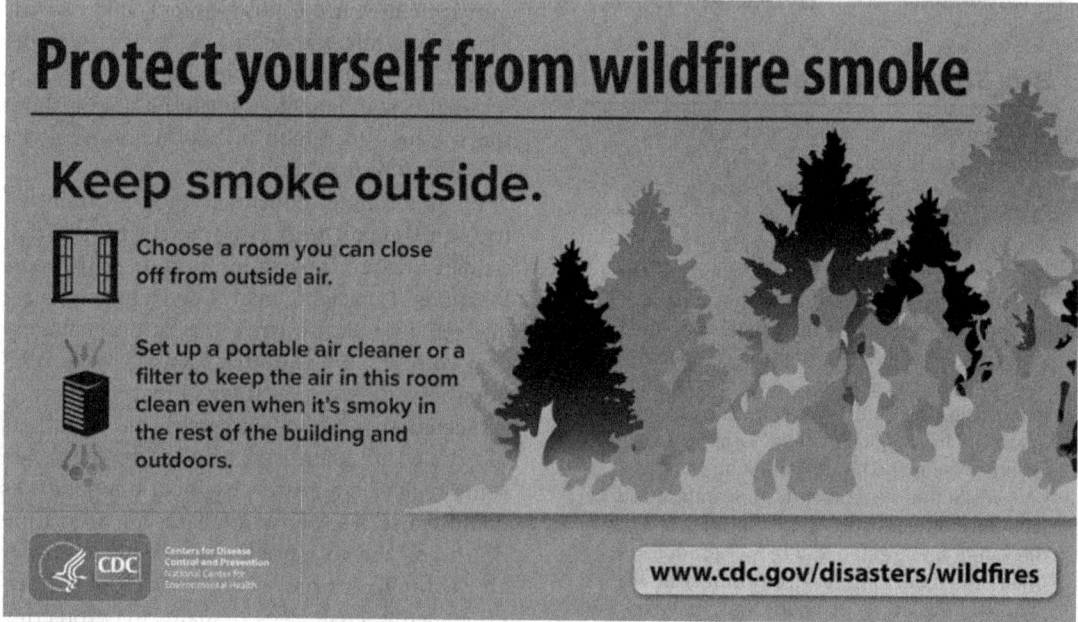

Figure 5.3 Protect Yourself from Wildfire Smoke

Figure from Centers for Disease Control and Prevention. Protect Yourself from Wildfire Smoke. https://www.cdc.gov/nceh/features/wildfires/index.html#:~:text=%20Who%20is%20at%20greatest%20risk%20from%20 wildfire,health%20threats%20from%20smoke.%20Children%E2%80%99s%20airways...%20More%20. Accessed November 20, 2021. Reference to specific commercial products, manufacturers, companies, or trademarks does not constitute its endorsement or recommendation by the U.S. Government, Department of Health and Human Services, or Centers for Disease Control and Prevention.[34]

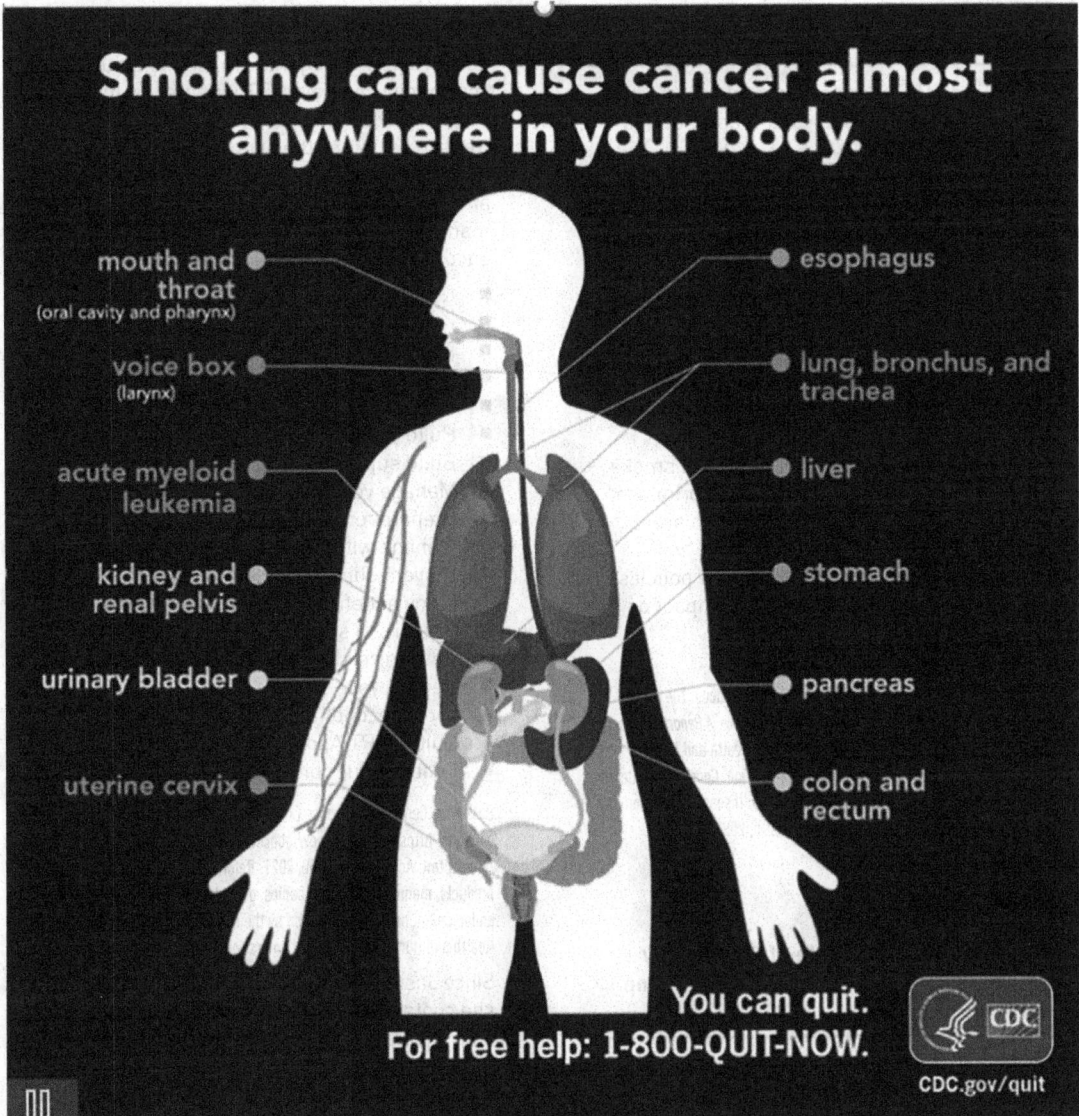

Figure 5.4 Cancer Linked to Smoking

Figure from Centers for Disease Control and Prevention. Health effects of cigarette smoking. https://www.cdc.gov/tobacco/data_statistics/fact_sheets/health_effects/effects_cig_smoking/index.htm. Accessed June 30, 2021. Reference to specific commercial products, manufacturers, companies, or trademarks does not constitute its endorsement or recommendation by the U.S. Government, Department of Health and Human Services, or Centers for Disease Control and Prevention.[35]

smoke from the burning end of a cigarette and the smoke breathed out by smokers.[38] Secondhand smoke contains hundreds of toxic chemicals and approximately 70 of those chemicals can cause cancer.[38] Additionally, secondhand smoke causes numerous health problems in infants and children including asthma attacks, respiratory infections, ear infections, and sudden infant death syndrome. For adults, the health conditions caused by secondhand smoke include coronary heart disease, stroke, and lung cancer.[39] See **Box 5.2** and **Case Study 5.1**.

Box 5.2 Secondhand Smoke Exposure

In 2006, the U.S. Surgeon General reported the following conclusions to control secondhand smoke exposure:

- Studies show that there is a no level of risk-free exposure to secondhand smoke.
- Eliminating smoking in indoor spaces is the only way to fully protect nonsmokers from secondhand smoke exposure.
- Workplace smoking restrictions reduce secondhand smoke exposure and leads to an increase in the number of workers who reduce or quit smoking.
- Establishing smoke-free workplaces is the only way to ensure secondhand smoke exposure does not occur in the workplace.
- Most workers in the United States are covered by smoke-free policies.
- Research shows that smoke-free policies do not have an adverse economic impact on the hospitality industry.

Data from U.S. Department of Health and Human Services. *The Health Consequences of Involuntary Exposure to Tobacco Smoke: A Report of the Surgeon General.* Atlanta, GA: U.S. Department of Health and Human Services, Centers for Disease Control and Prevention, Coordinating Center for Health Promotion, National Center for Chronic Disease Prevention and Health Promotion, Office on Smoking and Health, 2006.[38]

Case Study 5.1 Role of Community Health Worker (CHW) in Community Stop Smoking Campaign

Since Jasmyn was raised in rural east Tennessee, she was hired as the first CHW for the Mountain City Health Clinic. Recently, she graduated from Nashville Community State College with an associate degree. She was anxious to return to her hometown of Mountain City, Tennessee, and start her new position. On the first day, Martha McKinney, Jasmyn's supervisor, said that the leading cause of death for Mountain City was lung cancer. The clinic leadership wanted Jasmyn to focus on starting a stop smoking campaign in the community. Jasmyn was thrilled to initiate this community project because her grandfather died of lung cancer a few years previous. Jasmyn learned in her health education courses about the CDC website Guide for Quitting Smoking, but she was not sure how to begin to prepare for a successful community campaign.[40] Therefore, Jasmyn began by exploring the topics on the CDC website list, since the agency offers a variety of lessons based on evidence-based research and practice. The following list showcases the many offerings to build a successful campaign to encourage smoking cessation:

- Quitline
- Know your reasons for quitting
- Plan to quit
- Take steps to quit
- Learn about nicotine replacement therapy
- Build your quit plan
- Build support to stay quit
- Manage your quit day
- Prepare for cravings
- Manage withdrawal
- Prevent slips
- Enjoy benefits of being smoke-free
- Prepare to stay smoke-free
- Recognize signs of depression
- Reduce your stress
- Avoid secondhand smoke
- Quit START App
- Learn about quit smoking medicines

Data from Centers for Disease Control and Prevention. Guide for quitting smoking. https://www.cdc.gov/tobacco/campaign/tips/quit-smoking/guide/index.html. Accessed June 30, 2021. Reference to specific commercial products, manufacturers, companies, or trademarks does not constitute its endorsement or recommendation by the U.S. Government, Department of Health and Human Services, or Centers for Disease Control and Prevention

Since Jasmyn could not decide where to begin, she contacted five of her friends from the health education course to obtain their opinions. Pretend that you are one of Jasmyn's friends and answer the following questions as if she were asking you.

Questions

1. After reviewing the list of topics above, what are your top three topics to suggest to Jasmyn for a successful plan to support the Stop Smoking campaign? Explain why you selected those three topics.
2. How should Jasmyn discover which topics would gain most interest for the patients who do smoke and receive their health care at the Mountain City Health Clinic?
3. What are some ways to get the clinic healthcare providers involved in the stop smoking campaign?

Radon Gas

Radon is an odorless and invisible radioactive gas released when some naturally occurring radioactive materials break down in rocks, soil, and water and can build up to dangerous levels inside homes or buildings.[41–42] Any home can have a radon problem; whether the home is drafty or well sealed, radon can still build up and get trapped inside. Radon can enter the home through several ways, including cracks in solid floors and walls, construction joints, gaps in suspended floors and service pipes, cavities inside walls, and water supplies.[41–42] When an individual breathes in radon, radioactive particles from the decay of radon gas becomes trapped in the lungs. Over time, these radioactive particles increase the risk of lung cancer. It may take years before health problems appear.[41–42] See **Figure 5.5**.

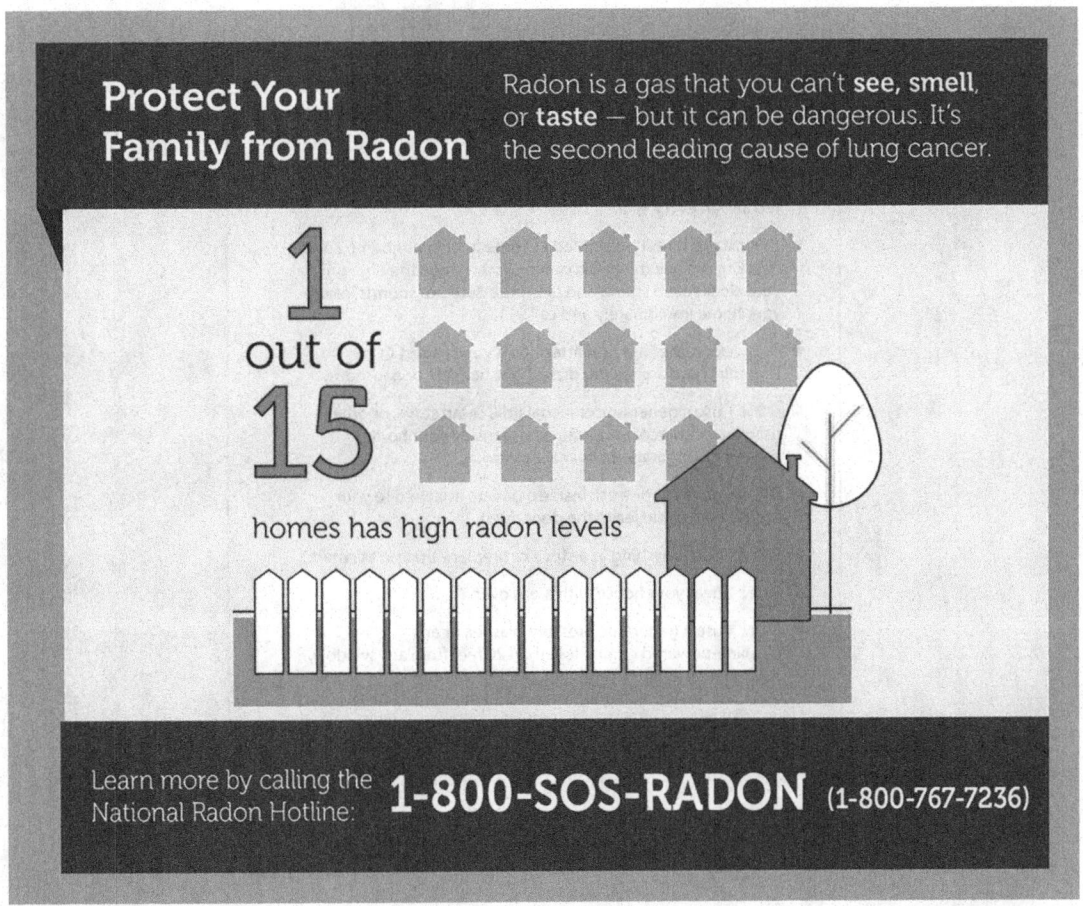

Figure 5.5 Facts About Radon

Carbon Monoxide Exposure

Carbon monoxide (CO) is a colorless, odorless, and tasteless gas that can cause sudden illness and death. CO is produced any time a fossil fuel is burned in a furnace, vehicle, generator, grill, or elsewhere.[43] CO from these sources can build up in enclosed or semi-enclosed spaces and can poison the people and animals in them. The most common symptoms of carbon monoxide poisoning are headaches, dizziness, and nausea.[43] See **Figure 5.6**.

Mold

Mold is located within a variety of settings, including indoors and outdoors. Mold can enter homes through open doorways, windows, vents, and heating and air conditioning systems.[45] Mold in the air outside can also attach itself to clothing, shoes, and pets and be carried indoors. When mold spores drop on places where there is excessive moisture, such as where leakage may have occurred in roofs, pipes, walls, plant pots,

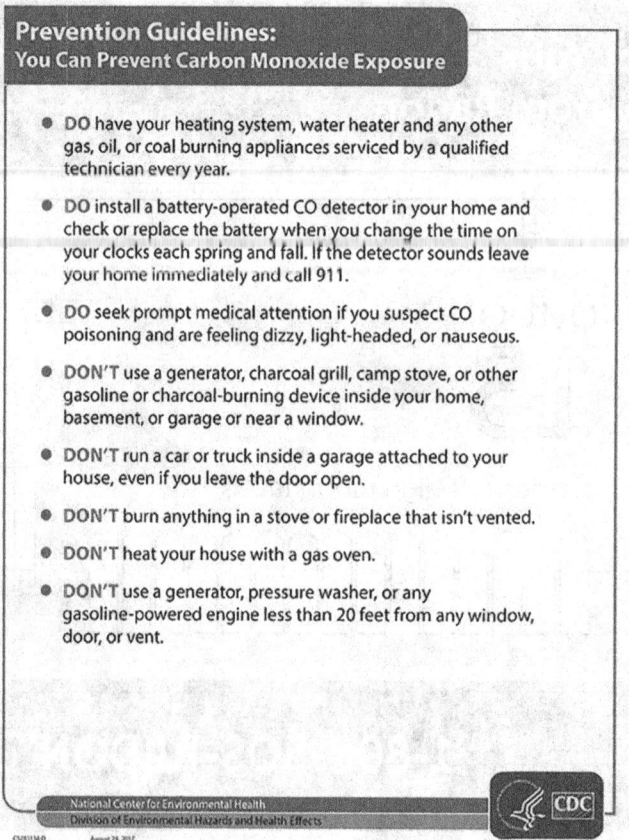

Figure 5.6 Prevention of Carbon Monoxide Exposure

Figure from Centers for Disease Control and Prevention. Carbon Monoxide Prevention Guidance. https://www.cdc.gov/co/guidelines.htm. Accessed November 20, 2021. Reference to specific commercial products, manufacturers, companies, or trademarks does not constitute its endorsement or recommendation by the U.S. Government, Department of Health and Human Services, or Centers for Disease Control and Prevention.[44]

or where there has been flooding, the spores will grow. Many building materials provide suitable nutrients that encourage mold to grow.[45] Wet cellulose materials, including paper and paper products, cardboard, ceiling tiles, wood, and wood products, are particularly conducive for the growth of some molds. Other materials such as dust, paints, wallpaper, insulation materials, drywall, carpet, fabric, and upholstery, commonly support mold growth.[45]

Large mold infestations can usually be seen or smelled.[45] Exposure to damp and moldy environments may cause a variety of health effects, especially to individuals sensitive to mold. For these people, exposure to molds can lead to symptoms such as stuffy nose, wheezing, and red or itchy eyes or skin. Other individuals have more intense reactions. Severe reactions, such as fever and shortness of breath, may occur among workers exposed to large amounts of molds in occupational settings.[45] Currently, there are no definitive blood tests for mold. However, some physicians can do allergy testing for possible allergies to mold, but no clinically proven tests can pinpoint when or where a particular mold exposure took place.[45]

After a hurricane or major flood, some individuals may have to live in a home that is affected by mold.[45] This circumstance could last for weeks, if the families have nowhere else to go, or even months, if the whole community was affected. As a CHW, it is important to know how to guide individuals in these situations.[45] See **Table 5.2**.

Table 5.2 **Steps to Reduce Exposure to Mold**

- If the individuals have asthma, chronic obstructive pulmonary disease (COPD), or are immunocompromised, they must avoid mold within the home completely until it is cleaned, removed, or dried.

- Spend less time in the home. Stay with friends or relatives until the home is dried and cleaned thoroughly. If the weather is good, spend more time outdoors. During the day, visit libraries, malls, and other public places.

- Seal off the mold. Use plastic tarps to seal off moldy rooms in the house until the rooms are cleaned.

- Create a separate sleeping area. If the family must sleep in a home with mold, seal off the cleanest room for sleeping with plastic tarps and always leave shoes outside the room. Shower and wash your hair before you go to bed. Avoid wearing moldy clothes in the room designated for sleep. Do not carry items from other parts of the house into the room. Open a window to let fresh air into this room if possible.

- Use air conditioners and fans wisely. If the home has a whole-house heating, ventilation, and air conditioning system, do not turn it on until it has been inspected—it could spread mold.

- Clean, throw away, or seal moldy items. Wash and dry or throw away moldy bedding, towels, clothing, and draperies. If there are moldy papers that cannot be destroyed, the papers should be dried and sealed in a bag until the papers can be properly cleaned.

Centers for Disease Control and Prevention. Reduce Your Exposure to Mold in Your Home. https://www.cdc.gov/mold/reduce-your-exposure-to-mold.html. Accessed November 20, 2021. Reference to specific commercial products, manufacturers, companies, or trademarks does not constitute its endorsement or recommendation by the U.S. Government, Department of Health and Human Services, or Centers for Disease Control and Prevention.[46]

Noise Pollution

This section investigates the effects of noise on health. While experiencing loud noise for a short period of time is annoying, long-term noise pollution can cause a variety of health issues, such as irritability, sleep disturbance, cardiovascular diseases, disruption to the metabolic system, and cognitive impairment. See **Figure 5.7**.

Noise pollution causes the deterioration of health as noted in the following list:

Hearing Loss. Exposure to high levels of noise of above 85 decibels (dB) can cause hearing loss. When the noise is loud and prolonged, the hearing loss occurs faster. Once the inner ear is damaged by noise, it is not possible to reverse the hearing loss.[48] Sensorineural hearing loss is caused by the malfunction of the inner ear (the cochlea).[49] The inner ear cells are called hair cells, which look like hairs under a microscope. When sounds are too loud for too long, these bundles are damaged. Damaged hair cells cannot respond to sound, causing noise-induced hearing loss.[50]

Sleep Disorder. Noise as low as 30 dB disturbs sleep, causes amnesia, and contributes to behavior disorders and aggression. For example, living close to an active railroad crossing causes repeated disturbed sleep.[48]

Memory Loss and Lack of Concentration. Constant noise affects the ability to focus and concentrate, slows down performance, lowers productivity, and decreases ability to learn new information. For example, if an office is located near a noisy loading dock of the building, individuals assigned to this office experience a decrease in their ability to concentrate and focus on assigned projects.[48]

Tinnitus. An auditory disorder often associated with hearing loss, depending on the noise exposure, can be temporary or permanent.[48]

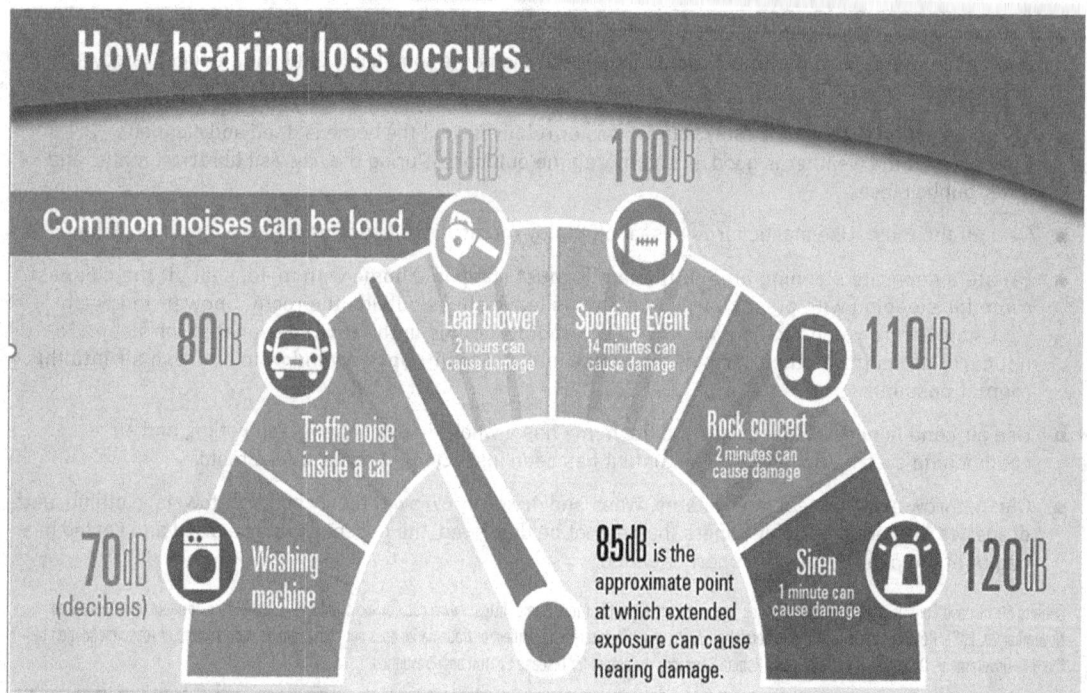

Figure 5.7 How Hearing Loss Occurs

Cardiovascular Diseases. Noise levels greater than 50 dB may increase the risk of myocardial infarction, coronary artery disease, hypertension (high blood pressure), constriction of blood flow in arteries and veins, and increased reaction to stress.[48] For example, if a man works outside on construction sites for his entire career, he was exposed to constant, loud noise for years. It is likely that he will develop deafness and coronary artery disease. The CHW would note the connection when assisting the gentleman with completing the health history form at the clinic.[48]

In conclusion, while sound is a valuable part of life, noise has a negative impact on physical and mental health.[48] It is important to recognize the noise pollution as a serious health concern for not only workers, but among communities who experience long periods of sustained noise. Here are two examples to showcase how noise can be harmful. First, noise affects individuals living in poverty. The thin walls of inexpensive apartments do not block the sounds of crime, domestic violence, or other late-night disturbances. These cumulative instances of prolonged noise can cause psychological stress, which then impacts physical health and well-being.[48,51] Second, neighborhoods and workers benefit from changing the city's trash pick-up schedule from a 2:00 a.m. pick-up to a 6:00 a.m. scheduled pick-up. Early morning trash pick-up is considered an environmental noise source. Therefore, it is paramount to reduce noise as an environmental disturbance because research has thoroughly shown how constant noise increases the risk of tinnitus, cognitive impairment, and cardiovascular issues. Additionally, the workers would benefit from more daylight working hours, and the neighbors would likely have improved sleep without the additional noise.[48,51]

Risks Factors and Protective Factors

This section introduces the topic of risk factors and protective factors relative to the environment.[52] The definitions presented illustrate these simple, yet important terms. Keep in mind that individuals, families, and communities are a combined mixture of risk and protective factors. Also, a CHW never assigns blame if an individual develops a chronic disease based on their multiple risk factors and limited protective factors. Life is complex; therefore, the individual may have been exposed to environmental risk factors, such as poor air and water quality in childhood.[52] Additionally, the individual may have protective factors, such as moving to a healthier neighborhood later in life. It is critical to acknowledge that every individual is unique with a blend of risk factors and protective factors. Individuals should strive to focus on protective environmental factors and attempt to minimize the harm from risk factors with healthy behaviors, such as never smoking.[52]

Risk Factors. Risk factors are viewed as negative, personal, or environmental indicators.[52] **Personal risk factors** are linked to an individual's knowledge, skills, experience, personal behavior, and lifestyle.[52] The greater number of risk factors in an individual's life, the greater chance of developing an illness, disease, or injury. **Environmental risk factors** include the social environment and physical environment (e.g., poor air and water quality and noise pollution). If a geographical location has numerous environmental risk factors, the community members are more likely to be at-risk of developing chronic health conditions.[52] See **Case Study 5.2**.

Case Study 5.2 Risk and Protective Factors

As a CHW, it is important to evaluate the community, the families, and individuals when exploring the risk factors and the protective factors. Drive around the community to assess which types of factors exist. What types of factors currently exist within the community and where can positive change occur?

Questions

1. Make a table and list five risk factors and five protective factors.
2. Write a brief scenario that links two factors from each list.

Protective Factors. Protective factors are defined as positive assets.[52] There are two kinds of protective factors: personal and environmental. **Personal protective factors** are linked to an individual's knowledge, skills, experience, personal behavior, and lifestyle.[52] When individuals have a greater number of protective factors (e.g., healthy weight, nutritious food, never smoking, and routine exercise), there is a decreased likelihood of developing a chronic illness or disease. **Environmental protective factors** include social support and physical (e.g., clean air and water, safe outdoor space, access to resources and health care). Whether it is an individual, a family, or a community, more protective factors lead to improved health outcomes and decreased development of chronic disease.[52]

It is important to know that risk factors and protective factors are flexible and fluctuate in environmental settings. Individuals or communities can change their ratio of risk and protective factors. It is possible for individuals to positively alter their life by engaging in more protective factors and disengaging from risk factors.[52] For example, an individual joins Alcoholic Anonymous (AA) to stop drinking and find new nondrinking friends who will support their journey toward sobriety. AA members attend support meetings daily or weekly. Some AA members add other protective factors through the years, such as exercising or practicing smoking cessation through the motivation of the other AA members. Communities achieve improvement by organizing change from within the community. For example, community organizations may obtain funding to achieve urban renewal from grants and tax incentives for the development of new businesses, school improvement, expansion of neighborhood sidewalks, lighting, and parks, and to increase access to health care, improve safety, and create more resources. These community revitalization efforts take years of dedicated hard work, but each successful program begins with an idea.[52] See **Case Study 5.3**.

Case Study 5.3 Role of CHW Related to Public Environmental Factors

After Jamal graduated from high school, he attended the local community college, worked part-time, and lived at home to reduce his tuition debt. His advisor suggested that because Jamal had always been involved in community activities throughout high school that he might wish to explore the CHW associate degree. Since Jamal had lived in Carter County his entire life, he assumed that he knew the community well. After he registered for his first course for the CHW degree, he bought the textbook and started reading before the semester started. When he read Chapter 4, he realized that Carter County has serious pollution issues. He was surprised to learn the link between pollution and chronic health conditions. Throughout his life, he noticed that members of his family worked hard, developed chronic health conditions, and died around 70 years of age. It never occurred to him that their health could be related to the environment and present working conditions. This knowledge motivated Jamal to explore the information and further investigate Carter County conditions.

Questions

1. If you were Jamal's friend, where would you tell him to look to gain more information about the adverse environmental factors affecting the health of community members?
2. Who would you recommend that Jamal should contact to gather further information about the environmental health concerns?

Chapter Summary

This chapter covers the health effects of environmental conditions present in numerous communities. The information covers the topics of environmental impact on climate, water, air, and noise pollution. Each topic covers the reason for the pollution and the adverse health effects. First, climate change effects the stress (e.g., mental, physical, environmental, and social), extreme temperature and precipitation extremes, and food security. Second, it discusses the negative effects on health due to water pollution, including bacteria, viruses, and lead exposure. Third, there is a discussion about how noise pollution causes the deterioration of health. Last, risk factors and protective factors are defined in relationship to environmental health.

References

1. Definitions of environmental health. National Environmental Health Association Web site. https://www.neha.org/about-neha/definitions-environmental-health. Accessed November 19, 2021.
2. Mortality in the United States, 2018. Centers for Disease Control and Prevention Web site. https://www.cdc.gov/nchs/products/databriefs/db355.htm. Accessed May 8, 2021.
3. Climate effects on health. Centers for Disease Control and Prevention Web site. https://www.cdc.gov/climateandhealth/effects/default.htm. Accessed November 19, 2021.
4. Mental health and stress-related disorders. Centers for Disease Control and Prevention Web site. https://www.cdc.gov/climateandhealth/effects/mental_health_disorders.htm. Accessed November 19, 2021.
5. Schneiderman N, Ironson G, Siegel SD. Stress and health: Psychological, behavioral, and biological determinants. *Annu Rev Clin Psychol*. 2005;1:607–628.
6. Types of stressors (eustress vs. distress). Mentalhelp.net. https://www.mentalhelp.net/stress/types-of-stressors-eustress-vs-distress/. Accessed July 2, 2021.
7. Post-core: stress and time management. Centers for Disease Control and Prevention Web site. https://www.cdc.gov/diabetes/prevention/pdf/posthandout_session12.pdf. Accessed July 2, 2021.
8. What are the long-term effects of stress? (17 symptoms to know). Mellowed Web site. https://mellowed.com/long-term-effects-stress/. Accessed July 8, 2021.
9. Temperature extremes. Centers for Disease Control and Prevention Web site. https://www.cdc.gov/climateandhealth/effects/temperature_extremes.htm. Accessed November 19, 2021.
10. Precipitation extremes: heavy rainfall, flooding, and droughts. Centers for Disease Control and Prevention Web site. https://www.cdc.gov/climateandhealth/effects/precipitation_extremes.htm. Accessed November 19, 2021.
11. Food security. Centers for Disease Control and Prevention Web site. https://www.cdc.gov/climateandhealth/effects/food_security.htm. Accessed November 19, 2021.
12. Smith A. What effects does water pollution have on human health? Medical News Today Web site. https://www.medicalnewstoday.com/articles/water-pollution-and-human-health#combatting-water-pollution. Accessed June 4, 2021.
13. Cunha JA. Traveler's diarrhea: treatment and prevention. Medicinenet Web site. https://www.medicinenet.com/travelers_diarrhea/article.htm. Accessed June 9, 2021.
14. Salmonella (*salmonellosis*). WebMD. https://www.webmd.com/food-recipes/food-poisoning/what-is-salmonella. Accessed June 9, 2021.
15. Cholera—*vibrio cholerae* infection. Centers for Disease Control and Prevention Web site. https://www.cdc.gov/cholera/general/index.html. Accessed June 23, 2021.
16. Dysentery. WebMD. https://www.webmd.com/digestive-disorders/what-is-dysentery. Accessed June 23, 2021.
17. E. coli. Mayo Clinic Web site. https://www.mayoclinic.org/diseases-conditions/e-coli/symptoms-causes/syc-20372058. Accessed June 23, 2021.
18. Hepatitis A. Centers for Disease Control and Prevention Web site. https://www.cdc.gov/hepatitis/hav/index.htm. Accessed June 23, 2021.
19. Hepatitis E. Centers for Disease Control and Prevention Web site. https://www.cdc.gov/hepatitis/hev/index.htm#:~:text=Hepatitis%20E%20is%20a%20liver,virus%20%E2%80%93%20even%20in%20microscopic%20amounts. Accessed June 23, 2021.
20. Transmission of parasitic diseases. Centers for Disease Control and Prevention Web site. https://www.cdc.gov/parasites/transmission/index.html. Accessed June 23, 2021.
21. Botulism. Centers for Disease Control and Prevention Web site. https://www.cdc.gov/botulism/index.html. Accessed June 23, 2021.
22. Typhoid fever. Mayo Clinic Web site. https://www.mayoclinic.org/diseases-conditions/typhoid-fever/symptoms-causes/syc-20378661#:~:text=Typhoid%20fever%20is%20caused%20by,infected%20person%20cause%20typhoid%20fever. Accessed June 23, 2021.
23. Fish advice. Environmental Protection Agency Web site. https://www.epa.gov/system/files/images/2021-09/fish-chart.jpg. Accessed November 19, 2021.
24. Health effects of lead exposure. Centers for Disease Control and Prevention Web site. https://www.cdc.gov/nceh/lead/prevention/health-effects.htm. Accessed November 19, 2021.
25. Certified product listings for lead reduction. NSF. https://info.nsf.org/Certified/DWTU/listings_leadreduction.asp. Accessed November 19, 2021.
26. Lead in drinking water. Centers for Disease Control and Prevention Web site. https://www.cdc.gov/nceh/lead/prevention/sources/water.htm. Accessed November 19, 2021.
27. Search for NSF certified bottled waters and beverages. NSF. https://info.nsf.org/certified/bwpi/. Accessed November 19, 2021.
28. Commercially bottled water. Centers for Disease Control and Preventionhttps://info.nsf.org/certified/bwpi/. https://www.cdc.gov/healthywater/drinking/bottled/index.html. Accessed November 19, 2021.
29. Denchak M. Flint water crisis: Everything you need to know. NRDC Web site. https://www.nrdc.org/stories/flint

-water-crisis-everything-you-need-know. Accessed June 23, 2021.

30. Ghorani-Azam A, Riahi-Zanjani B, Balali-Mood M. Effects of air pollution on human health and practical measures for prevention in Iran. *Journal of Research in Medical Sciences.* 2016;21:65.

31. Criteria air pollutants. Environmental Protection Agency Web site. https://www.epa.gov/criteria-air-pollutants. Accessed July 20, 2021.

32. Air pollution. Centers for Disease Control and Prevention Web site. https://www.cdc.gov/climateandhealth/effects /air_pollution.htm. Accessed November 19, 2021.

33. Wildfires. Centers for Disease Control and Prevention Web site. https://www.cdc.gov/climateandhealth/effects /wildfires.htm. Accessed November 20, 2021.

34. Protect yourself from wildfire smoke. Centers for Disease Control and Prevention Web site. https://www.cdc.gov/nceh /features/wildfires/index.html#:~:text=%20Who% 20is%20at%20greatest%20risk%20from%20wildfire, health%20threats%20from%20smoke.%20 ChildrenE2%80%99s%20airways...%20More%20. Accessed November 20, 2021.

35. Health effects of cigarette smoking. Centers for Disease Control and Prevention Web site. https://www.cdc.gov /tobacco/data_statistics/fact_sheets/health_effects/effects _cig_smoking/index.htm. Accessed June 30, 2021.

36. National Center for Chronic Disease Prevention and Health Promotion (US) Office on Smoking and Health. *The Health Consequences of Smoking—50 Years of Progress: A Report of the Surgeon General.* Atlanta, GA: Centers for Disease Control and Prevention; 2014.

37. Murphy SL, Xu J, Kochanek KD. Deaths: final data for 2010. *Natl Vital Stat Rep.* 2013;61(4):1–117.

38. U.S. Department of Health and Human Services. *The Health Consequences of Involuntary Exposure to Tobacco Smoke: A Report of the Surgeon General.* Atlanta, GA: U.S. Department of Health and Human Services, Centers for Disease Control and Prevention, Coordinating Center for Health Promotion, National Center for Chronic Disease Prevention and Health Promotion, Office on Smoking and Health, 2006.

39. Health effects of secondhand smoke. Centers for Disease Control and Prevention Web site. https://www.cdc.gov /tobacco/data_statistics/fact_sheets/secondhand_smoke /health_effects/index.htm. Accessed June 30, 2021.

40. Guide for quitting smoking. Centers for Disease Control and Prevention Web site. https://www.cdc.gov/tobacco /campaign/tips/quit-smoking/guide/index.html. Accessed June 30, 2021.

41. Protect yourself and your family from radon. Centers for Disease Control and Prevention Web site. https://

www.cdc.gov/radon/index.html?CDC_AA_refVal =https%3A%2F%2Fwww.cdc.gov%2Fradon%2Fradon -health.html. Accessed November 20, 2021.

42. Get the facts on radon. Center for Disease Control and Prevention Web site. https://www.cdc.gov/radon/radon -facts.html. Accessed November 20, 2021.

43. Poison control center. The University of Kansas Health System Web site. https://www.kansashealthsystem.com /care/centers/poison-control-center/common-poisons /carbon-monoxide#:~:text=Carbon%20Monoxide% 20Carbon%20monoxide%20%28CO%29%20 is%20a%20colorless%2C,can%20poison%20the% 20people%20and%20animals%20in%20them. Accessed November 20, 2021.

44. Carbon monoxide prevention guidance. Centers for Disease Control and Prevention Web site. https://www. cdc.gov/co/guidelines.htm. Accessed November 20, 2021.

45. Basic facts about mold and dampness. Centers for Disease Control and Prevention Web site. https://www.cdc.gov /mold/faqs.htm. Accessed November 20, 2021.

46. Reduce your exposure to mold in your home. Centers for Disease Control and Prevention Web site. https:// www.cdc.gov/mold/reduce-your-exposure-to-mold.html. Accessed November 20, 2021.

47. Too loud! For too long! Centers for Disease Control and Prevention Web site. https://www.cdc.gov/vitalsigns /hearingloss/index.html. Accessed June 25, 2021.

48. Noise pollution affecting human health. Nature Talkies Web site. https://www.naturetalkies.com/30/11/2020/pollution /noise-pollution-affecting-human-health/. Accessed June 28, 2021.

49. Venail F, Camilleri M, Lorenzi A. What's a hearing impairment? A tinnitus? http://www.cochlea.org/en /impairment. Accessed November 22, 2021.

50. It's a noisy planet protect their hearing. Line up! To reverse hearing loss, new hair cells need to stand in formation. U.S. Department of Health and Human Services Web site. https://www.noisyplanet.nidcd.nih.gov/have-you-heard /new-hair-cells-need-to-stand-in-formation-to-reverse -hearing-loss. Accessed November 22, 2021.

51. It's just noise... right? Australian Academy of Science Website. https://www.science.org.au/curious/earth-environ ment/health-effects-environmental-noise-pollution. Accessed June 28, 2021.

52. Risk and protective factors. Substance Abuse and Mental Health Services Administration Web site. https://www .samhsa.gov/sites/default/files/20190718-samhsa-risk -protective-factors.pdf. Accessed July 24, 2021.

Appendix

1. Your Zip Code Can Determine How Long You Live: https://www.rwjf.org/en/library/interactiveswhereyou liveaffectshowlongyoulive.html

2. Flint, Michigan Water Crisis: https://www.youtube.com /watch?v=I-KaqTyuVJY

3. Stress Management Test: https://www.thecalculator.co /personality/Stress-Management-Test-626.html

CHAPTER 6

Body Systems

LEARNING OBJECTIVES

1. Explain the major body systems with examples to specific diseases.
2. List common prefixes and suffixes from medical terminology with examples.
3. Define leading causes of death in the United States.
4. Explain behaviors for chronic disease prevention.

KEY TERMS

nervous system
urinary system
cardiovascular system
reproductive system
endocrine system
lymphatic system

immune system
muscular system
skeletal system
morbidity
morbidity rate
mortality

mortality rate
suicide
suicide attempt
alcohol use disorder
obesity

Introduction

This chapter begins with an overview of major body systems and describes basic anatomical and physiological principles. Increased risk factors and disabilities occur when body systems become compromised, leading to injury and disease. It is important to acknowledge the complexity of risk factors, such as genetic links, and disabilities that are not always visible including post-traumatic stress syndrome (PTSD), arthritis, autoimmune conditions, high blood pressure, or mental health issues. The important definitions of morbidity (disease) and mortality (death) are linked to various medical conditions. After

an overview of major body systems and related conditions, the discussion shifts to the leading causes of death in the United States. Each of the causes are described in-depth for greater understanding and comprehension. With the previous knowledge of major body systems, one will better understand the delicate balance of the body and how it affects other systems. Next this chapter includes many of the prefixes and suffixes used in basic medical terminology. Although it is not extensive, the reader learns common terminology used in health care. Last, the chapter ends with an overview of the aging process, a summary of the top five healthy behaviors, and finishes with a robust case study.

Major Body Systems

This section reviews the human body organs and systems. Keep in mind that each system has unique functions but work in conjunction with all body systems. In this section, the function of each organ is explained after each description of the system.

Digestion. Organs involved include the mouth and teeth, esophagus, stomach, liver, pancreas, small intestine, and large intestine.[1] The rectum and anus are the excretion portion of the digestive system. The primary function of digestion includes the physical and chemical breakdown of food to allow absorption of nutrients.[1] Think of the digestive system as a tube in which food and fluids are consumed, and then digested and converted into energy for use by the body. After food and fluids are converted into energy, fiber and nondigested food is then excreted.

Mouth: Entry into the digestive system.

Teeth: Teeth helps to form words for speech; tear, cut, and grind food in preparation for swallowing.

Esophagus: The esophagus is straight muscular tube through which food passes from the pharynx to the stomach. The esophagus can contract or expand to allow for the passage of food. Anatomically, it lies behind the trachea and heart and in front of the spinal column.[2]

Stomach: The stomach is located between the esophagus and the small intestine. It secretes digestive enzymes and gastric acid to aid in food digestion.

Liver: The liver detoxifies various metabolites, synthesizes proteins, and produces biochemicals necessary for digestion. It is also the largest internal organ in the body.

Pancreas: The pancreas is a glandular organ in the digestive system and endocrine system located in the abdominal cavity behind the stomach. It is an endocrine gland producing several important hormones, including insulin.

Small intestine: The small intestine, the part of the gastrointestinal tract between the stomach and the large intestine, is where most of the end absorption of food takes place. The small intestine has three distinct regions: the duodenum, jejunum, and ileum.

Large intestine: The large intestine is the last part of the gastrointestinal tract and of the digestive system. Water is absorbed here, and the remaining waste material is stored as feces before being excreted through the rectum and anus.

Rectum: The rectum is the final straight portion of the large intestine.

Anus: The anus is the opening at the base of the rectum.

Respiration. Organs involved include nose, mouth, trachea, bronchi, and lungs.[1] Each time individuals inhale a breath through their nose and/or mouth, the oxygenated air travels down the tube (trachea) that connects to the back of the throat to the tube-like branches into the top of the lungs.[1] In the lungs, bronchi form tiny branches to the alveoli. The alveoli are the tiny sacs at the end of the bronchi. In the tiny alveoli sacs, the oxygenated air is exchanged with the carbon dioxide in the blood. When the individual exhales, the carbon dioxide is exhaled, and the process begins with the next inhalation breath.[1]

Nervous System. Organs involved include the brain, spinal cord, and central nervous system. The function of the **nervous system** is described as the processing center for sensory input and using the input to produce appropriate body responses.[1] The brain fills the skull and controls many complex body functions, such as emotions, vision, hearing, thought, memory, speech, and movement. The spinal cord runs through the vertebrae of the spine (back bone) and connects the brain to the nerves of the body.[3] The spinal cord allows the brain to send messages throughout the body. The network of the brain and spinal cord is called the central nervous system (CNS). The brain is divided down the middle from front to back into

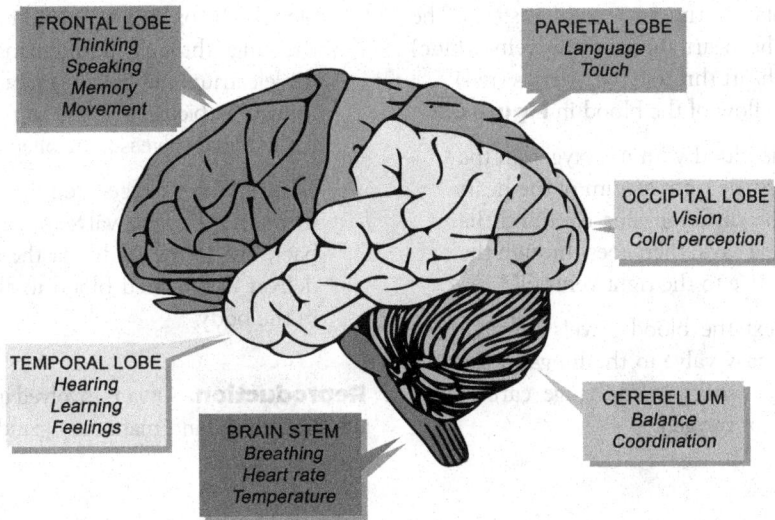

FRONTAL LOBE
Thinking
Speaking
Memory
Movement

PARIETAL LOBE
Language
Touch

OCCIPITAL LOBE
Vision
Color perception

TEMPORAL LOBE
Hearing
Learning
Feelings

BRAIN STEM
Breathing
Heart rate
Temperature

CEREBELLUM
Balance
Coordination

Figure 6.1 Lobes of the Brain
© Noiel/Shutterstock

two halves called the cerebral hemispheres. Each hemisphere is divided into four lobes: frontal, parietal, occipital, and temporal.[3] See **Figure 6.1**.

Urinary System. Organs involved include kidneys, urinary bladder, and urethra. The primary function of the **urinary system** is the filtration of blood and excretion of wastes from the body.[1] As individuals drink fluids, the fluid goes down the esophagus to the stomach and into the small intestine.[1] In the small intestine, villi are the finger-like folds that increase the surface area of the membrane and assist in the movement of fluid passage. The small intestine, with the help of villi increases the absorption of the fluid and nutrients into the blood.[1]

Kidneys. The blood is constantly passing through the kidneys on its way back to the heart to gain more oxygen. The circulation of blood within the kidneys allows the kidneys to filter and remove any impurities, toxins, or excess nutrients and fluids that the body no longer needs (e.g., sodium, potassium, nitrites). The two kidneys act like miniature sophisticated chemistry laboratories that work in unison and help maintain proper electrolyte balance. If the individual is

thirsty, the kidneys send a signal to the brain, so the individual increases their fluid intake.[1] It is possible for an individual to live a full life with only one kidney. As a result, a healthy individual may donate one kidney to an individual in need, due to kidney failure.[1] Also, the individual receiving the donated kidney can resume a full life if the donated kidney is not rejected by the recipient's body. The recipient must consume anti-rejection medication for the rest of their life to maintain the donated kidney.

Urinary Bladder. If the body has excess fluid, the kidneys remove the extra fluid where it is stored in the bladder. Once the bladder reaches capacity, the individual feels the need to urinate. The urine travels from the bladder to the urethra out of the body.

Urethra. The duct by which urine is conveyed out of the body from the bladder and in males the semen travels out of the body through the urethra.

Cardiovascular System. Organs involved include heart, blood, arteries, and veins. The primary function of the **cardiovascular system** includes the circulation of blood, which transports gases, nutrients, hormones, and wastes.[1] The blood enters the heart through the veins (blue) and leaves the heart through the arteries (red).

Follow the flow of the blood in **Figure 6.2**.[5]

Step 1: The blood with no oxygen in the veins enters the right atrium of the heart through the superior vena cava and the inferior vena cava, then goes through the tricuspid valve to the right ventricle.

Step 2: Next the blood travels through the pulmonary valve to the lungs in the pulmonary artery to exchange carbon monoxide for oxygen.

Step 3: The oxygenated blood returns from the lungs through the pulmonary vein to the left atrium through the mitral valve (also known as bicuspid valve) to the left ventricle. Mitral valve is more often replaced.

Step 4: The oxygenated blood travels through the mitral valve to the aorta and back out to the body via the arteries to deliver oxygenated blood to all the cells in the body.

Reproduction. Organs involved include (female) uterus, ovaries, and mammary glands (breasts) and

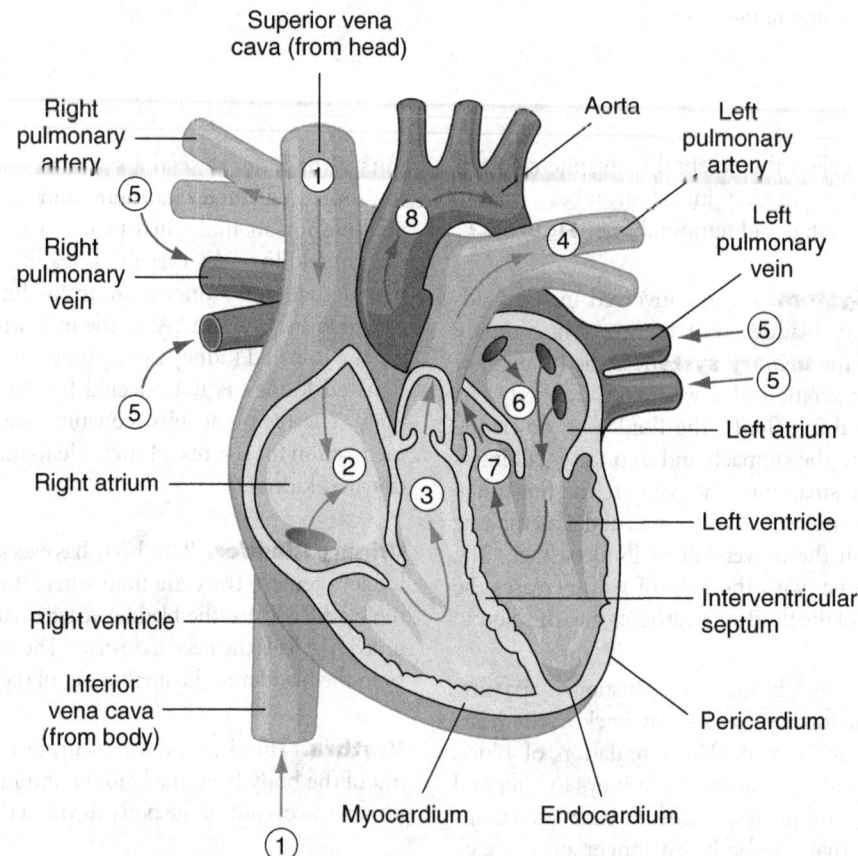

Figure 6.2 Diagram of the Heart

Figure from Anchoradvocates.com. Your heart health. https://www.anchoradvocates.com/blog. Accessed July 16, 2021.[5]

(male) testes, scrotum, prostate gland, and penis. The function of the **reproductive system** is to produce reproductive cells that generate offspring.[1] For the males, the reproductive organs include the testes, scrotum, prostate gland, and penis.

Endocrine System. Organs involve pituitary gland, adrenal, thyroid, pancreas, parathyroid, prostate glands.[1] The function of the **endocrine system** is to ensure the regulation of body processes through hormone production.[6] The endocrine system is composed of glands located throughout the body.[6] Hormones are made by the glands and released into the blood or the fluid surrounding cells. Receptors in various organs and tissues recognize and respond to the hormones.[1] Hormones act as chemical messengers to control or regulate processes within the body. The hormone-receptor complex switches on or switches off specific biological processes in cells, tissues, and organs. For example, insulin controls blood sugar levels, while growth hormones and thyroid hormones control body growth and energy production.[6] See **Figure 6.3**.

Hypothalamus: Hypothalamus drives the endocrine system and links the endocrine system to the nervous system.[6]

Pituitary gland: Pituitary gland receives signals from the hypothalamus.

Thyroid gland: Thyroid gland is important for healthy development, energy production and metabolism regulation.[6]

Adrenal glands: Adrenal glands are located on top of the kidneys and produce hormones in response to stress and regulate blood pressure, glucose metabolism, and help the kidneys regulate the salt and water balance in the body.[6]

Pancreas: The pancreas is responsible for producing the hormones that regulate the concentration of glucose (sugar) in the blood.[6]

Testes and ovaries: Male reproductive gonads (testes) and female reproductive gonads (ovaries) produce steroids that affect growth and development and regulate reproductive cycles and behaviors.[6]

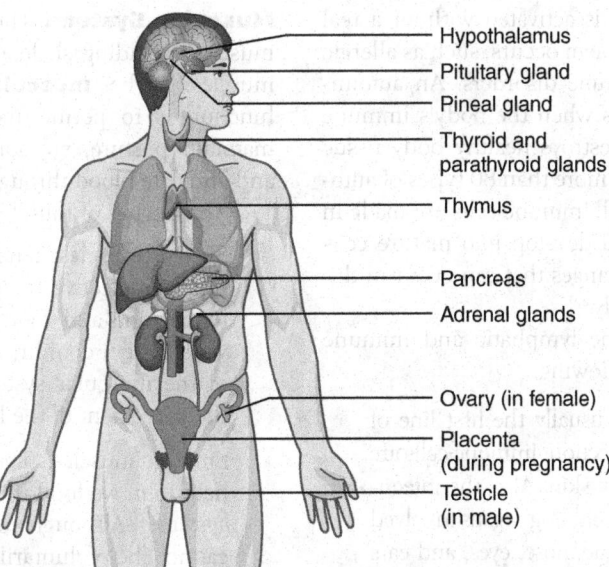

- Hypothalamus
- Pituitary gland
- Pineal gland
- Thyroid and parathyroid glands
- Thymus
- Pancreas
- Adrenal glands
- Ovary (in female)
- Placenta (during pregnancy)
- Testicle (in male)

Figure 6.3 Endocrine Glands in the Body

Figure from United States Environmental Protection Agency. What Is the Endocrine System? https://www.epa.gov/endocrine-disruption/what-endocrine-system. Accessed July 28, 2021.[4]

Lymphatic and Immune System. Organs involve the skin, bone marrow, tonsils and adenoid, appendix, blood, thymus, spleen, and mucosal tissue.[7] The **lymphatic system** is a network of vessels and tissues composed of extracellular fluid and lymph nodes. The primary function of this complex system is to collect the excess fluid from tissues, vessels, and cells and return it to the blood stream to be recirculated.[7] Additionally, the lymphatic system is a channel for the blood and immune cells to communicate about possible problems. Immune cells are carried through the lymphatic system and converge in lymph nodes, which are found throughout the body. Swollen lymph nodes may indicate an active immune response, such as an infection.[7]

A strengthened immune system response prevents or limits infection. The **immune system** recognizes normal, healthy cells and unhealthy cells.[8] Cells are unhealthy due to infection or damage, such as sunburn, cancer, or congenital immune deficiency. The immune system recognizes a problem and responds.[8] If the response is not sufficient, the infection spreads throughout the body unless treatment or medication is provided to stop the infection. In contrast, when an immune response is activated without a real threat, a different problem occurs, such as allergic reactions or autoimmune disorders. An autoimmune disorder occurs when the body's immune system attacks and destroys healthy body tissue by mistake. There are more than 80 types of autoimmune disorders.[9] All immune cells are made in the bone marrow and develop into mature cells through a series of changes that can occur in different parts of the body.[8,9]

The organs of the lymphatic and immune system include the following:

Skin: The skin is usually the first line of defense against infection. Immune cells are in specific layers of skin. Also, the integumentary system, including organs involved include skin, tongue, nose, eyes, and ears are the organs involved with the senses. The function of the skin is to provide protection against the external environment and regulation of the temperature.[8]

Bone marrow: The bone marrow contains stems cells that can develop into a variety of cell types that are important first-line responders to infection.[7-8]

Blood: Immune cells constantly circulate throughout the bloodstream, patrolling for problems. Blood tests are used to monitor white blood cells (WBCs). When there are too many or too few WBCs in the blood, the problem needs further investigation.[7-8]

Thymus: A small organ located in the upper chest, it produces a specific type of immune cells called T cells.[7-8]

Spleen: The spleen is an organ located behind the stomach. The spleen filters and creates WBCs, which are a vital component for adequate immune defense.[7-9]

Mucosal tissue: Mucosal surfaces are prime entry points for pathogens in the respiratory tract (mouth, nose, trachea, and lungs) and the gastrointestinal tract (mouth, esophagus, stomach, small intestines, and large intestines).[8]

Muscular System. There are three types of muscles including skeletal, smooth, and cardiac muscles.[10] The **muscular system**'s primary function is to permit movement of the body, maintain posture, support the skeletal system, and circulate blood throughout the body.[10]

Three types of muscles:

Skeletal muscles: Tendons, cartilage, and other connective tissues secure muscles to the joints and skeleton bones. The nervous system coordinates the contraction of the muscular system to synchronize the movement of the limbs.[10]

Smooth muscles: The smooth muscles help to move food through the digestive system.[10] Although the digestive organs cannot be voluntarily contracted like skeletal muscles, it is controlled subconsciously and automatically. When food needs to be moved through the gut, the muscles produce a contraction in a synchronized, wave-like motion called peristalsis.[10]

Cardiac muscles: The cardiac muscle refers to the heart. The heart is the main circulatory support and blood supply required for healthy organ function.[10] Unlike other muscles, the heart never stops. The average heart beats 72 times per minute. With an average lifespan of 75 years, the heart beats 4,320 times per hour, 103,680 times a day, 37,843,200 times a year, and 2,838,240,000 times during an average lifespan.[11]

Skeletal System. The **skeletal system** is the underlying structure of the body and includes the bones, joints, ligaments, tendons, and cartilage. There are a total of 206 bones in the adult human body. Vitamin D and calcium are important in the diet to maintain a strong and healthy skeletal system. It is important to maintain a healthy weight, because extra weight places extra pressure on the joints and cartilage that causes damage and pain. In addition, weight bearing exercise (e.g., walking) is essential to keep bones and joints strong. When exercising, wear proper footwear to avoid falls and injuries. If biking, wear a bike helmet and follow rules of the road to stay safe.

Bones: The function of the bones is to support and protect the body. The support allows movement to stand, sit, squat, walking, and all other activities. The skull protects the brain, the ribs protect the heart and lungs, and the spine protects the spinal cord. Lastly, bone marrow is in the interior of the bone produces red blood cells and white blood cells and stores Vitamin D and calcium.

Joints: Joints are located at the end of bones and allow movement. There are three different types of bones: immovable (skull), partly movable (ribs), and moveable (fingers, toes, elbows, ankles, knees, hips, shoulders, and jaw.

Ligaments: Ligaments are the connective tissue that hold the bones together.

Tendons: Tissue bands connect the ends of the muscle to the bones.

Cartilage: Cartilage is a smooth gel-like substance that covers the ends of the bones, so movement is possible without friction. Arthritis occurs when the cartilage wears away and causes painful movement and limits mobility.

Basic Medical Terminology

Medical terminology is composed of prefixes, word root, and suffixes. The list in **Table 6.1** introduces some of the commonly used prefixes and suffixes. It is highly recommended that all CHWs purchase a medical dictionary. Each time that an unfamiliar medical term is found, it is important to search for the meaning in the medical dictionary.

Leading Causes of Death in the United States

Before discussing the leading causes of death in the United States, it is important to define the terms: morbidity and mortality.

Morbidity. Morbidity (sickness) is references as having a specific illness, disease, or condition. Morbidity is calculated by carefully considering the number of cases of disease occurring in approximately 100,000 persons of the population.[12] In addition, the **morbidity rate** is the frequency or proportion with which a disease appears in a population. For example, during the COVID-19 pandemic, the number of people testing positive was stated as a percent. The Center for Disease Control and Prevention (CDC) wanted that percentage to be under 5% for two consecutive weeks to declare that the spread of the virus was under control. Morbidity rates are used in a variety of professions, such as health insurance, life insurance, and long-term care insurance to determine the premiums to charge to customers, public health, chronic disease management, and research.[13]

Mortality. Mortality is defined as the cause and number of deaths in a specific population during a set period of time. **Mortality rate** is typically expressed in units of deaths per 1,000 individuals per

Table 6.1 Basic Prefixes and Suffixes in Medical Terminology

Prefixes and Suffixes	Definition
a-, an-	denotes an absence of
ab-	away from
abdomin(o)-	of or relating to the abdomen
-ac, -acal	pertaining to
ad-	near, forward
aesthesio-	sensation
-al	pertaining to
alb-	denoting a white or pale color
alge(si)-	pain
-algia	pain
an-	not, without
ana-	back, again, up
angi(o)-	blood vessel
anti-	describing something as "against" or "opposed to" another
arthr(o)-	of or pertaining to the joints, limbs
arteri(o)-	of or pertaining to an artery
articul(o)-	joint
-ary	pertaining to
-ase	enzyme
aut(o)-	self
aux(o)-	increase, growth
axill-	of or pertaining to the armpit
-blast	immature cell
brachi(o)-	of or relating to the arm
brachy-	indicating short
brady-	slow
bronch(i)-	bronchus
burs(o)-	bursa (fluid sac between the bones)
carcin(o)-	cancer
cardi(o)-	of or pertaining to the heart
carp(o)-	of or pertaining to the wrist
cata-	down, under

(continues)

Table 6.1 Basic Prefixes and Suffixes in Medical Terminology *(continued)*

Prefixes and Suffixes	Definition
-cele	pouching, hernia
cerebell(o)-	of or pertaining to the cerebellum
cerebr(o)-	of or pertaining to the brain
cervic(o)-, cervix	of or pertaining to the neck (cervical spine) or pertaining to the neck of the uterus
chol(e)-	of or pertaining to bile
cholecyst(o)-	of or pertaining to the gallbladder
chondr(i)o-	cartilage, gristle, granule, granular
-cidal, -cide	killing, destroying
-cision	process of cutting
co-	with, together, in association
col-, colo-, colono-	colon
colp(o)-	of or pertaining to the vagina
contra	against
cost(o)-	of or pertaining to the ribs
-crine	to secrete
cyst (o, i)-	of or pertaining to the urinary bladder
cyt(o)-	cell
-cyte	cell
de-	away from, cessation
dent-	of or pertaining to teeth
dermat(o)-	pertaining to the skin
di-	two
dia-	across
digit-	of or pertaining to the finger or the toe
dis-	separation, taking apart
dors(o, i)-	of or pertaining to the back
ecto-	outside of, without
-ectomy	excision
end-	within, inside
epi-	above, upon
hyper-	excessive

(continues)

Table 6.1 Basic Prefixes and Suffixes in Medical Terminology *(continued)*

Prefixes and Suffixes	Definition
hypo-	insufficient
inter-	between
intra-	middle
-itis	inflammation
-lysis	decline, disintegration, or destruction
-oid	resembling
-ology	study of
-oma	tumor, swelling
-pathy	disease or a system for training disease
per-	through
peri-	surrounding, around, outer
-phasia	pertaining to speech
-phobia	fear
-pnea	pertaining to breathing
poly-	many
pro-	before, for, in front of
-ptosis	dropping
re-	back, again
retro-	behind, back
-rrhea	flow or discharge
-scope	instrument for viewing
-scopy	visual examination
-sis	state of, process, or condition
sub-	under, below
sym-, syn-	union, association, or joined
tachy-	fast
-therapy	treatment
trans-	across, through
-version	to turn
ultra-	excess
-uria	pertaining to a substance in the urine

year. Thus, a mortality rate of 9.5 (out of 1,000) in a population of 1,000 persons would mean 9.5 deaths occurred per year within that entire population.[14]

Now that body systems have been reviewed, the discussion moves to the leading causes of death in the United States and includes a brief description of each condition. Because these conditions are the top leading causes of death in the United States, it is likely that CHWs will regularly encounter these diseases. **Box 6.1** showcases the leading causes of death.

1. Heart Disease

There are numerous types and causes of heart disease.

Heart Attack (MI). Myocardial (myo = muscle; cardi = heart) infarction (blockage) is defined by the symptoms and conditions caused by coronary heart disease.[16] When a blood vessel is blocked with a blood clot or atherosclerotic plaque, there is an insufficient supply of oxygen and nutrition to the muscle causing a heart attack or MI.[16]

Coronary Artery Disease (CAD). A disease of the artery caused by the accumulation of atherosclerotic plague within the walls of the artery.[17]

Cardiovascular (Cardio = heart; vascular = veins and arteries) Disease. Any number of specific diseases affecting the heart and blood vessels (veins and arteries) leading to and from the heart including:

a. atherosclerosis (a disease of the arteries characterized by the deposition of plaques of fatty material on their inner walls)
b. ischemic heart disease (when blood flow to the heart is reduced, preventing the heart muscle from receiving enough oxygen, and heart failure).[18–20]

Hypertensive. Heart disease is caused by chronic high blood pressure.[18]

Arrhythmias. Arrhythmias (abnormal heart beats) occur when the electrical impulses that coordinate the heartbeats fail to work properly. Arrhythmia occurs when the heartbeats are too slow, too rapid, too irregular, or too early.[18–19] Tachycardia (tachy = fast; cardi = heart) are defined as rapid arrhythmias greater than 100 beats per minute. Bradycardia (brady = slow; cardi = heart) refers to a heart that has arrhythmias slower than 60 beats per minute.[18–19]

Valvular Heart Disease. Valvular heart disease is when any valve in the heart has damage or is diseased.[20] When any of the heart valves are diseased, the heart is unable to pump blood throughout the body and must work harder to pump. The heart valve conditions can lead to heart failure, sudden cardiac arrest, and death.[20]

Congestive Heart Failure (CHF) or Heart Failure (HF). Heart failure occurs when the heart muscle is not pumping blood as well as it should.[21–22] Certain conditions, such as narrowed arteries in the heart (coronary artery disease) or high blood pressure, gradually leave the heart too weak or stiff to fill and pump efficiently. Not all conditions that lead to heart failure can be reversed, but treatments can improve the signs and symptoms.[21–22] See **Box 6.2**.

Although these signs and symptoms may be due to heart failure, there are many other possible causes, including other life-threatening heart and lung conditions with symptoms that overlap.[22] Do not try to diagnose. Call 911 or

---

Box 6.1 The Top 10 Leading Causes of Death in 2019

1. Heart disease
2. Cancer
3. Accidents (unintentional injuries)
4. Chronic lower respiratory diseases
5. Stroke (cerebrovascular diseases)
6. Alzheimer's disease
7. Diabetes
8. Nephritis, nephrotic syndrome, and nephrosis
9. Influenza and pneumonia
10. Intentional self-harm (suicide)

Data from Kochanek KD, Xu J, Arias E. Mortality in the United States, 2019. https://www.cdc.gov/nchs/data/databriefs/db395-H.pdf. Accessed July 21, 2021.[15]

Box 6.2 Heart Failure (HF)

Signs and symptoms of heart failure:
- Shortness of breath (dyspnea)
- Fatigue and weakness
- Swelling (edema) in the legs, ankles, and feet
- Rapid or irregular heartbeat
- Reduced ability to exercise
- Persistent cough or wheezing
- Increased need to urinate at night
- Swelling of your abdomen (ascites)
- Persistent cough or wheezing
- Very rapid weight gain from fluid retention
- Lack of appetite and nausea
- Difficulty concentrating or decreased alertness
- Sudden, severe shortness of breath and coughing up pink, foamy mucus
- Chest pain if heart failure is caused by a heart attack

Data from Mayo Clinic. Heart Failure. https://www.mayoclinic.org /diseases-conditions/heart-failure/symptoms-causes/syc-20373142. Accessed July 21, 2021.[16]

your local emergency number for immediate help Emergency room doctors will stabilize the individual's condition and determine if the symptoms are due to heart failure or something else.[22]

2. Cancer

Cancer can develop anywhere in the body, and there are many types of cancer.[23] It starts when cells grow out of control and invade normal cells.[23] Cancers are alike in some ways and different in the ways that cells grow, multiply, and spread. Most cancers form a lump called a tumor or a growth; however, not all tumors are cancerous. Healthcare providers remove a piece of the tumor to perform a biopsy to determine if it is not cancer (benign) or is cancer (malignant).[23] Cancer of the blood, known as leukemia, grows within the blood cells or within other cells of the body rather than forming tumors.[23] Cancer is a complex group of diseases and can be associated with or caused by a variety of genetic components, lifestyle habits, the environment, and exposure to carcinogens. Many times, it is difficult to find the exact cause of this complicated disease.[23]

A. Four Types of Cancer

The four common types of cancer are: carcinoma, sarcoma, leukemia, and lymphoma.

Carcinoma. Cancer that is found in the internal organs (e.g., lungs, breast, colon, and uterus) and skin.

Sarcoma. Cancer that is found in connective tissues and bones, such as muscles, nerves, joints and tendons.

Leukemia. Cancer of the blood that spreads throughout the body.

Lymphoma. Cancer of the lymphatic system that is a complex system of vessels and glands that fight infections.

B. Stages of Cancer

The stages of cancer range from 0 to 4.

Stage 0: This stage is called "in situ" and means that the cancer has not spread to nearby tissue. Most likely curable when surgery removes the entire tumor.

Stage 1: This early-stage cancer is a small tumor that has not grown into nearby tissue or lymph nodes.

Stage 2 and 3: These two stages of cancer have spread to nearby tissues or lymph nodes.

Stage 4: This advanced (metastatic) stage of cancer has spread to other organs or other parts of the body.

C. Common Cancer Treatments

Cancer treatment options vary by diagnosis, stage, and type of cancer.[24] Treatments include surgery, chemotherapy, radiation therapy, bone marrow transplant, immunotherapy, hormone therapy, targeted drug therapy, cryoablation, radiofrequency ablation, and clinical trials. This list is not meant to be comprehensive because new cancer treatments become available through current clinical trials.[24] This list is a reference guide for understanding types of cancer treatments:

Surgery: Remove the cancer or as much of the cancer as possible.[24]

Chemotherapy: Uses drugs to kill cancer cells.

Radiation therapy: Uses high-powered energy beams to kill cancer cells, such as X-rays or protons.[24]

Bone marrow transplant: Also called stem cell transplant.[24] The stem cells are used from the patient or a donor. A bone marrow transplant allows the physician to use higher doses of chemotherapy to treat the cancer. It may also be used to replace diseased bone marrow.[24]

Immunotherapy: Also known as biological therapy. This type of treatment uses the body's immune system to fight cancer.[24] Cancer can survive unchecked in the body because if the immune system fails to recognize the cancer as an intruder. Immunotherapies assist the body's immune system to "see" the cancer and attack it.[24]

Hormone therapy: Used for some types of cancer are fueled by the body's hormones, such as breast cancer and prostate cancer.[24] If the effects of the hormones are blocked, the cancer cells stop growing.

Targeted drug therapy: Focuses on specific abnormalities within cancer cells that allow them to survive.[24]

Cryoablation: Cryoablation (cryo = cold; ablation = remove or destroy material) treatment kills cancer cells with cold.[24] During cryoablation, a thin, wand-like needle (cryoprobe) is inserted through the skin into the cancerous tumor. A gas is pumped into the cryoprobe to freeze the tissue. A freezing and thawing process is repeated several times during the same treatment session to kill the cancer cells.[24]

Radiofrequency ablation: A treatment that uses electrical energy to heat cancer cells.[24] The physician guides a thin needle through the skin into the cancer tissue. High-frequency energy passes through the needle and causes the surrounding tissue to heat up and kill the cancer cells.[24]

Clinical trials:Studies that investigate new ways of treating cancer.[24]

3. Accidents and Unintentional Injuries

Data for accidents and unintentional injuries in the United States account for 39.5 million physician office visits, 24.5 million emergency department visits, and 173,040 unintentional injury deaths (52.7 deaths per 100,000 population).[25] Without including COVID-19 deaths, accidents and unintentional injuries remain the third leading cause of death. Other unintentional deaths include falls (39,433 deaths), motor vehicle traffic deaths (37,595 deaths), and poisoning deaths (65,773 deaths).[25]

4. Chronic Lower Respiratory Disease

There are two types of chronic lower respiratory diseases.[26–27]

A. Asthma

Asthma affects the lungs and causes repeated episodes of wheezing, breathlessness, chest tightness, and nighttime or early morning coughing. Asthma can be controlled by taking medicine and avoiding the triggers that can cause an attack. Specifically, it is important to remove the environmental triggers to avoid asthma attacks.[26]

B. Chronic Obstructive Pulmonary Disease (COPD)

COPD is a chronic inflammatory lung disease that causes obstructed airflow from the lungs.[27] Symptoms include difficulty breathing, cough, mucus (sputum) production, frequent respiratory infections, lack of energy, swelling in ankles, feet or legs, and wheezing.[27] It is typically caused by long-term exposure to cigarette smoke. COPD increases the risk of developing heart disease and lung cancer. Symptoms appear after significant lung damage has occurred and worsen over time if individual continues to smoke.[27]

There are two kinds of COPD lung diseases: emphysema and chronic bronchitis.[28]

Emphysema. Emphysema develops over time, involves gradual damage of lung tissue, and is strongly linked to smoking. Signs and symptoms of emphysema take years to develop and include shortness of breath, coughing with mucus, wheezing and chest tightness. There is no cure, but treatments are available to help manage symptoms.[28-29]

Chronic Bronchitis. Chronic bronchitis is one of the lung diseases that encompasses COPD. Many treatments are available to help control symptoms and ease breathing problems. Cigarette smoking is a major cause of chronic bronchitis. Other factors that increase the risk of developing this disease include exposure to air pollution as well as dust or toxic gases in the workplace or environment.[28,30]

5. Stroke

A stroke occurs when blood flow to a specific part of the brain is suddenly stopped by a blood clot, and oxygen flow is significantly decreased to that part of the brain.[31] The lack of oxygen may damage or kill the brain cells. Death to a portion of the brain may lead to the loss of certain body functions controlled by that affected part.[31] A stroke is also referred to as a cerebrovascular accident (CVA).[31] Signs of a stroke include sudden numbness or weakness in the face, arm, or leg, especially on one side of the body, sudden confusion, trouble speaking, or difficulty understanding speech, sudden trouble seeing in one or both eyes, trouble walking, dizziness, loss of balance, or lack of coordination and the onset of a severe headache with no known cause.[31] Call 9-1-1 right away if an individual has any of these symptoms. See **Box 6.3**.

Box 6.3 Acting F.A.S.T Is Key for Stroke

Acting F.A.S.T. can help stroke patients get the treatments they desperately need.[31] The stroke treatments that work best are available only if the stroke is recognized and diagnosed within 3 hours of when the first symptoms appear.[31] Stroke patients may not be eligible for these treatments if they do not arrive at the hospital in time.

If you think someone may be having a stroke, act F.A.S.T. and do the following simple test:

F—Face: Ask the person to smile. Does one side of the face droop?
A—Arms: Ask the person to raise both arms. Does one arm drift downward?
S—Speech: Ask the person to repeat a simple phrase. Is the speech slurred or strange?
T—Time: If you see any of these signs, call 9-1-1 right away.

Be sure to make a note of the exact time when any symptoms first appear. This information helps health care providers determine the best treatment for each person. Do not drive to the hospital or let someone else drive you. Call an ambulance so that medical personnel can begin life-saving treatment on the way to the emergency room.

Data from Centers for Disease Control and Prevention. *Stroke*. https://www.cdc.gov/stroke/index.htm. Accessed July 25, 2021.[31]

---

6. Alzheimer's Disease

Alzheimer's disease is a form of dementia that is defined as a chronic disorder of the mental processes caused by brain disease or injury and is marked by memory disorders, personality changes, and impaired reasoning.[32] Alzheimer's disease is the most common type of dementia. Alzheimer's is described as a progressive disease that involves parts of the brain that control thought, memory, and language. It is important to consult a healthcare provider when someone has concerns about memory loss, thinking skills, or behavioral changes.[32] Twice as many Americans fear the loss of mental capabilities as the loss of physical ability.

Due to longer life spans and the growing prevalence of conditions like Alzheimer's, the need for caregivers, both informal (i.e., family and friends) and formal (i.e., paid professionals), will likely increase significantly as the U.S. population ages.[33]

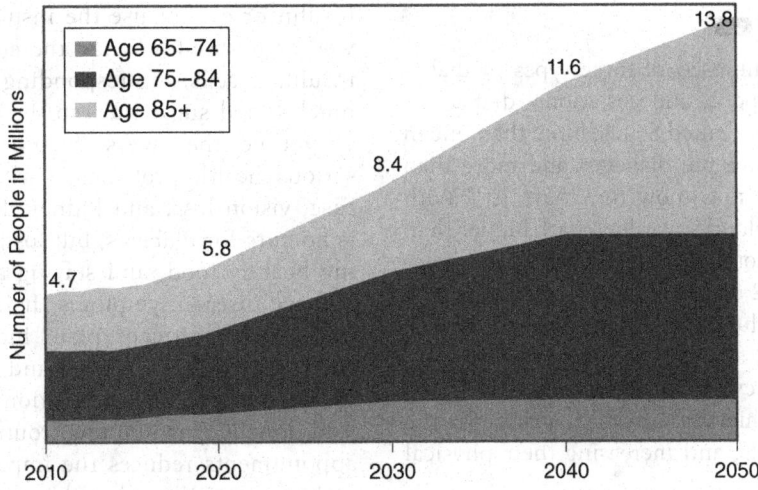

Figure 6.4 Projected Number of People Aged 65 or Older with Alzheimer's Disease, by Age Group, United States, 2010–2050

Data from Hebert LE, Weuve J, Scherr PA, Evans DA. Alzheimer's disease in the United States (2010–2050) estimated using the 2010 Census. *Neurology.* 2013;80(19):1778–1783.[34]

Although caregiving may be rewarding, caregivers are at an increased risk of increased stress, depression, unhealthy behaviors, and poor attention to their own health. Caregivers of people with dementias are at even higher risk of these problems, and they may delay their own health needs. Informal or unpaid caregivers are the backbone of long-term care provided in people's homes.[33] See **Figure 6.4**.

The CDC has create the Healthy Brain Initiative as a uniform national public health program to address dementia and promote implementation of the CDC Healthy Brain Initiative (HBI).[35] It is a series of practical steps for state and local public health officials and for Indian Country, or tribal agencies, to promote brain health, better care for people with cognitive impairment, and increase attention to caregivers. The goal is to improve understanding of brain health as a central part of public health practice.[35] See **Case Study 6.1**.

related to the growing number of seniors who are being diagnosed with Alzheimer's and related dementias. She was conducting a literature search and came across this publication: *Role of Community Health Workers in Addressing Dementia: A Scoping Review and Global Perspective*, PubMed (nih.gov).[36] The 2021 publication stated that limited access to health care and a shortage of healthcare workers are significant shortcomings and how utilizing CHWs could be a promising way to improve dementia care through cost-effective approaches. The five potential roles of CHWs include educational and community awareness, screening for dementia, screening for HIV-associated dementia, utilization of healthcare systems and other dementia-related resources by patients, and services to dementia caregivers. This review publication sheds light on important contributions of CHWs in addressing dementia among vulnerable communities.[36] Amanda was so excited to discover this current publication that she made an appointment with the director of her clinic.

Figure 6.4 shows geriatric care will expand and continue to be relevant in the future.

Case Study 6.1 CHW Role in Alzheimer's and Related Dementias

Amanda is a CHW at a large outpatient clinic linked to a university hospital. She has been working in the Department of Geriatric Care in the outpatient clinic for about 6 years. Although she loves her career, she has a desire to do more

Questions

1. As a CHW, which of the five potential roles related to Alzheimer's and related dementia appeals to you? Why?
2. As a CHW, would you apply for a position in a geriatric clinic? Why or why not?

7. Diabetes

Diabetes is composed of three types of diabetes: type 1, type 2, and gestational diabetes.[37] However, in the United States, more than one in three adults have pre-diabetes, and more than 84 percent do not know they have it.[37] With pre-diabetes, blood sugar levels are higher than normal, but not high enough yet to be diagnosed as type 2 diabetes. Pre-diabetes raises the risk for individuals to develop type 2 diabetes, heart disease, and stroke. Adults with pre-diabetes can reverse their risk of developing diabetes by achieving a healthy weight, eating nutritious foods, and increasing their physical activity.[37]

A. Type 1 Diabetes

Type 1 diabetes is thought to be caused by an autoimmune reaction. An autoimmune reaction occurs when the body attacks itself by mistake. As a result, the body stops making insulin. Individuals with type 1 diabetes need to take insulin every day to survive. Currently, no one knows how to prevent type 1 diabetes, though research continues.[37]

B. Gestational Diabetes

Gestational diabetes develops in pregnant women who have never had diabetes.[37] After the baby is born, gestational diabetes usually goes away but increases the woman's risk and the child's risk for type 2 diabetes later in life.[37]

C. Type 2 Diabetes

Type 2 diabetes is a chronic (long-lasting) health condition that affects how the body uses food to make energy.[37] When food is consumed, the body breaks the food down into sugar (glucose). The glucose is released into the bloodstream.[37] When the blood glucose increases, it signals the pancreas to release the insulin. Insulin acts like a key to let the blood sugar into the body's cells for use as energy.[37] If the individual has diabetes, their body either does not make enough

insulin or cannot use the insulin it makes as well as it should. When there is not enough insulin or cells stop responding to insulin, too much blood sugar stays in the bloodstream.[37] Over time, the excess glucose (sugar) causes serious health problems, such as heart disease, vision loss, and kidney disease.[37] There is no cure for diabetes, but losing weight, eating healthy food, and staying active helps to manage disease symptoms. It is important to follow the treatment plan, including taking the prescribed medication and getting diabetes self-management education and support. Additionally, maintaining routine healthcare appointments reduces the impact of diabetes and promotes better health outcomes.[37]

8. Kidney Disease

Kidney disease includes the following medical terms:

Nephritis = neph (kidney) I (inflammation)[38]

Nephrotic syndrome = a kidney disorder that causes the body to excrete too much protein in your urine[38]

Nephrosis = nephr (kidney) osis (noninflammatory process).[38]

The kidneys are two bean-shaped organs located on each side of the spine and slightly above the waist.[39] Each kidney is about the size of a fist. The kidneys filter extra water and wastes out of the blood and produce urine. Kidney disease is diagnosed when the kidneys are damaged and are unable to filter blood effectively. Individuals are at greatest risk for kidney disease if they have diabetes or high blood pressure.[39] Approximately, one out of three adults with diabetes has kidney disease.[40] Some people live with kidney disease for years and maintain kidney function, while others progress quickly to kidney failure. End-stage renal disease (ESRD) is kidney failure that is treated by dialysis or kidney transplant.[40] Other kidney problems include acute kidney injury, kidney cysts, kidney stones, and kidney infections.[40]

9. Influenza and Pneumonia

Influenza (flu) is a highly contagious viral infection that is one of the most severe illnesses of the winter season.[41] Influenza is spread easily from person to person, usually when an infected person coughs or sneezes. Influenza is a common cause of pneumonia (pneum = breath; onia = abnormal), especially among younger children, the elderly, pregnant women, or those with certain chronic health conditions.[41] Influenza spreads easily across confined areas like nursing homes, college dorms, and among members of the military. While most cases of flu never lead to pneumonia, when a person does contract the flu and it leads to pneumonia, the case can be severe and even deadly. In fact, flu and pneumonia were the eighth leading cause of death in the United States in 2016.[41] For both influenza and some types of pneumonia, there are protective vaccines, although none are 100 percent protective. As flu strains change each year, it is necessary to get a flu vaccination each season to be protected against the most current strains.[41] Pneumonia vaccinations are usually only necessary once, although a booster vaccination may be recommended for some individuals. Healthcare providers determine when to update vaccinations and to determine if any additional vaccinations are needed.[41]

10. Intentional Self-Harm

Suicide is a form of intentional self-harm and is defined as death caused by severely injuring oneself with the intent to die.[42] A **suicide attempt** is when someone harms themselves with any intent to end their life, but they do not die because of their actions.[42] Examples of self-directed harm is action that intentionally cause injury to self, including cutting and death.

If you or anyone that you know needs mental health services, contact the National Suicide Prevention Lifeline. They can connect you to a variety of resources.

- Call 1-800-273-TALK (1-800-273-8255)
- Use the online Lifeline Crisis Chat: https://suicidepreventionlifeline.org/chat/[43]

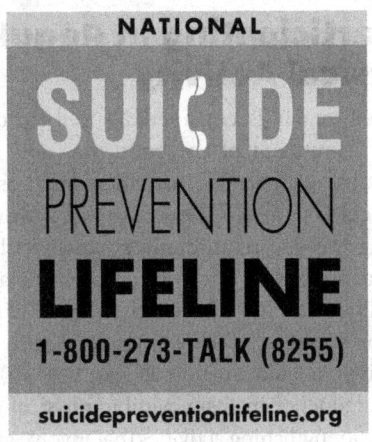

Figure 6.5 National Suicide Prevention
Reproduced from 988 Suicide & Crisis Lifeline.

Both are free and confidential. All callers are connected to a skilled, trained counselor in their area.[44]

Other forms of self-injury behaviors may be unintentional in nature. They are often repetitive, such as head banging, self-biting, cutting, and self-scratching. It is important to try to understand the cause(s) of the behavior so that treatment will be more effective.[44] See **Figure 6.5**.

Behaviors for Chronic Disease Prevention

There are five key health-related behaviors for chronic disease prevention: never smoking, participating in regular physical activity, refraining from consuming alcohol or drinking only moderate amounts, maintaining a healthy body weight, and obtaining daily sufficient nutrition.[45]

1. Never Smoking

This behavior is defined as no use of tobacco or vaping products including chewing tobacco, smoking cigarettes, cigars, and pipes, and vaping.[45]

2. Participating in Regular Physical Activity

Physical activity is considered any form of exercise or movement of the body that uses energy. Some of your daily life activities, such as doing active chores around the house, yard work, and walking the dog require energy and satisfy daily physical activity.[45–46] Activity can include aerobic, flexibility, and muscle-strengthening activities.

For adults aged 18–64 years: Weekly physical activity should include at least 150–300 minutes of moderate-intensity aerobic physical activity, muscle-strengthening activities that involve all major muscle groups on two or more days a week and limit the amount of time spent being sedentary.[46]

For adults 65 years and above: Weekly physical activity should include the same activities as for younger adults. However, older adults should do varied multicomponent physical activity that emphasizes functional balance and strength training at moderate or greater intensity, on three or more days a week, to enhance functional capacity and to prevent falls.[46]

3. Consuming No Alcohol or Only Moderate Amounts

According to the CDC, moderate alcohol consumption is defined as having up to one drink per day for women and up to two drinks per day for men.[47] One drink equals 12 ounces of regular beer, 8 ounces of malt liquor, 5 ounces of table wine, or 1.5 ounce shot of distilled spirits (e.g., gin, rum, tequila, vodka, whiskey, etc.).[47]

Alcohol use disorder involves a pattern of problems controlling consumption of alcohol, preoccupation with alcohol, continued use of alcohol even when it causes problems, consuming more to get the same effect, or experiencing withdrawal symptoms without alcohol consumption.[48] Unhealthy alcohol consumption includes any alcohol use that puts health and safety at risk, such as binge drinking. Binge drinking is defined as a pattern of drinking where a male consumes five or more drinks within 2 hours or a female consumes at least four drinks within 2 hours.[48] Alcohol use disorder is when a pattern of drinking results in repeated significant distress and consistent problems with functioning in daily life ranging from mild to severe. Even a mild alcohol use disorder can escalate and lead to serious problems, so early treatment is important.[48] Alcohol use disorder has been associated with genetics, behavior, lifestyle, and social contacts. See **Figure 6.6**.

4. Maintaining a Normal Body Weight

When a normal body weight is not maintained, underweight or overweight occur. There are three levels of gaining weight outside of the normal body weight limits: overweight, obese, and extreme obesity.[45,50] **Obesity** is a medical condition in which excess body fat may have a negative effect on health. The symptoms of obesity include above average body weight, trouble sleeping or sleep apnea, enlarged veins in the legs, skin problems as moisture accumulates in skin folds, gallstones, and osteoarthritis in hip and knee joints.[50] Obesity increases the likelihood of various diseases and conditions, particularly cardiovascular diseases, type 2 diabetes, obstructive sleep apnea, certain types of cancer, osteoarthritis, and depression.[50] In the past, people were considered overweight when their body mass index (BMI) was over 25.0, while individuals with a BMI of 30 or higher are considered obese.[50] While the use of the body mass index metric has clinical utility, it is largely dependent on height and did not take into account age, gender, genetic, fitness, pre-existing diseases, and distribution of fat on the body.[50-51] Therefore, in some cases where individuals are shorter or taller in height, their BMI may not be accurate or a reliable metric to determine respective normal body weight.

More recently, studies have shown that the measurement of weight circumference as an indicator for normal body weight and as a screening tool to determine the risk of type 2

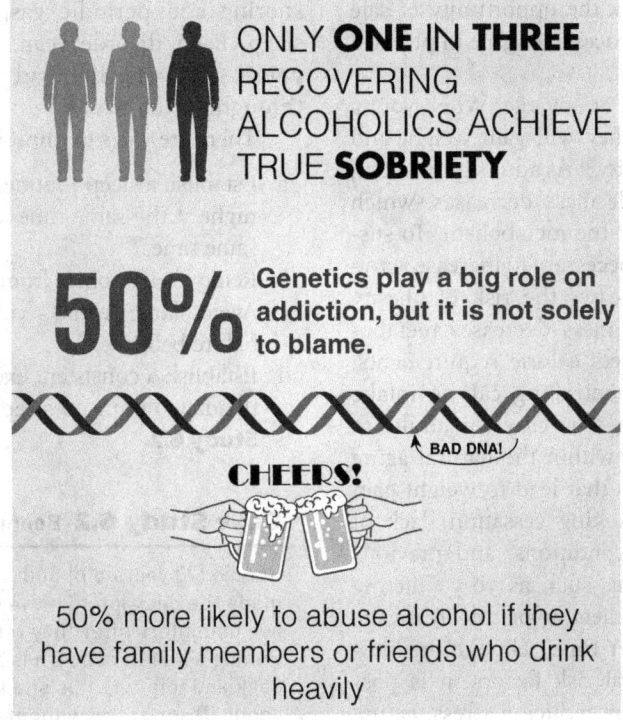

Figure 6.6 Alcoholism

Courtesy of CDC. Reference to specific commercial products, manufacturers, companies, or trademarks does not constitute its endorsement or recommendation by the U.S. Government, Department of Health and Human Services, or Centers for Disease Control and Prevention.

diabetes and other weight associated conditions.[51] In simple terms, the individual's waist circumference should be less than half of the individual's height. For example, a 6-foot (72 inches) man should have a waist circumference less than 36 inches (half of 72 inches). A 5-foot 4-inch (64 inches) woman should have a waist circumference less than 32 inches.[52] The abdominal fat at the waist, abdomen, and hips indicates the heart, liver and kidneys are affected by the excess fat in the waist circumference measurement.[52]

The risk factors associated with obesity have been linked to a combination of causes. Obesity is influenced by genetic factors, such as the amount of fat stored in the body and where the fat is located on the body.[51] For example, it is not uncommon for obesity to run in families due to shared eating, activity habits, and cultural norms. Lifestyle choices influence an individual's risk of becoming overweight or obese due to consistently consuming an unhealthy diet of high-calorie beverages, consuming oversized portions, processed foods, rather than consuming nutritious foods like whole grains, seeds, nuts, fruits, vegetables, and lean proteins.[51]

Additionally, some medications, such as antidepressants, steroids, and hypertension drugs, may lead to weight gain if the individuals do not alter their diet and activities. In addition, social and economic factors are associated with obesity.[51] For example, if the individual's neighborhood is not safe for walking, biking, or exercising or if the individual grew up in a family that did not focus on physical activity or nutritious eating, one may lack the education on the importance of physical activity or lack the opportunity of safe areas and open green spaces to engage in physical activity.

Obesity may occur at any age. When young children are overfed, they will gain weight and become at risk for obesity.[51] As adults grow older, their amount of muscle mass decreases, which reduces the function of the metabolism. To sustain muscle mass, it is necessary to increase activity.[51] Less activity increases the risk of obesity because lower muscle mass decreases metabolism function and lowers calorie requirements. Without consciously controlling calorie intake and increasing activity, it is easy for adults to gain weight, especially within the natural aging process.[51] Other factors that lead to weight gain include pregnancy, smoking cessation, lack of sleep, stress, medical conditions, and previous attempts to lose weight, such as yo-yo dieting or participating in fad diets, which decrease the metabolic function over time. Though an individual may have several risk factors, it is possible to avoid obesity by reducing stress, eating nutritiously, increasing activity, and practicing healthy habits.[51]

5. Obtaining Daily Sufficient Sleep

In the United States, about 30 percent of adults report getting less than 7 hours of sleep each night despite the 7 or more hours of sleep recommended for adults ages 18–60.[53] A lack of sleep is associated with many chronic diseases, including type 2 diabetes, heart disease, obesity, and depression.[54] Sleep is crucial to the health and well-being of individuals, and without the proper amount of sleep, work-related injuries and motor vehicle accidents occur, leading to death or disability.[53] The major sleep disorders include insomnia, which is defined as the inability to go to sleep or stay asleep; narcolepsy, which includes irresistible sleepiness and sudden muscle weakness; restless legs syndrome, which causes aches and pains in the lower legs; and sleep apnea, which causes snoring and periodic gasping for air during sleep. Each disorder can significantly impair one's quality of life and ability to function throughout the day.[55]

There are ways to improve sleep habits:

a. Establish a sleep routine of going to bed each night at the same time and getting up at the same time.[56]
b. Remove electronics from the bedroom.[56]
c. Avoid large meals, caffeine, and alcohol before bedtime.[56]
d. Establish a consistent exercise routine during the day to improve sleep at night.[56] See **Case Study 6.2.**

Case Study 6.2 Bonnie's Decisions

Bonnie (72 years old) and Ron (76 years old) made the decision to move closer to their two daughters after they retired. Currently, Bonnie's health concern is arthritis in her back and left hip, plus she had breast cancer about 20 years ago without any recurrence. Ron is starting to experience some symptoms of congestive heart failure (CHF) due to high cholesterol and hypertension. Since Ron's and Bonnie's waist circumference measurements are more than half of their individual heights, they realize that they should both lose about 15 pounds. Since they knew that they would be moving, they failed to schedule routine prevention screenings as recommended, such as a colonoscopy, an annual dermatology skin screening, bone density scan, several vaccines (e.g., flu, pneumonia, shingles, and pertussis) and routine dental check-ups.

Ann, their older daughter, is a chiropractor, and her husband owns a general contracting business. They have three children ranging from ages 6 to 14 years old. Bonnie and Ron purchased a condo about 7 miles away. They are available to assist driving the grandchildren, which also helps them learn their way around the city. Also, their younger daughter, Beth, lives in the same city, is single, and attends law school. As soon as Bonnie and Ron moved, they established their healthcare team with a primary care physician, cardiologist, dentist, and ophthalmologist. They joined the YMCA, because their health insurance covers the membership cost, but they have not attended any exercise classes yet.

As they got settled into their new community, Bonnie and Ron started volunteering at the local food bank plus other activities of interest. On the first day at the food bank, Bonnie tripped over the curb in the parking lot while carrying a box of fruit. She was more embarrassed than hurt, so she and Ron completed their 4-hour shift. However, by the time they left, Bonnie's ankle was aching and beginning to swell. Since they had not yet had an appointment with their primary care physician, Ron suggested stopping at the urgent care clinic near their condo. Bonnie agreed that her ankle hurt enough to get an X-ray.

Ron drove up to the door and went in the clinic to request a wheelchair for Bonnie. He was pleasantly surprised to be greeted promptly by the clerk at the front desk. When he parked the car, he realized that the urgent care clinic was part of a larger medical building. Coincidentally, it was the same location of their new primary care physician's office.

Bonnie had been taken to an exam room, while he parked the car. The clerk took Ron to Bonnie's exam room. Jasmine, medical assistant (MA) was taking Bonnie's blood pressure when Ron entered the room. Since Ron had not had blood pressure checked for a few months, he asked if she would mind taking his blood pressure also. The MA took his blood pressure also. Bonnie's blood pressure was elevated, probably due to her ankle pain, but

Ron's was elevated also. The MA told Ron that he needed to get it rechecked soon. Bonnie explained that they had their first appointments with Dr. Williamsburg, the primary care physician, next week. The MA pushed Bonnie in the wheelchair back to the technician so she could get her ankle x-rayed. Bonnie returned to the exam room.

Dr. Brighton, the urgent care physician, told Bonnie that she had several hairline fractures in her ankle and one in the arch of her foot. She explained that Bonnie needed to see the orthopedic physician in the next few days for further treatment. The MA had told Dr. Brighton that Ron's blood pressure had been elevated, so she told Ron to get it rechecked soon. Dr. Brighton told Jasmine to take Bonnie to the CHW's office to get her orthopedic appointment scheduled. Jasmine introduced them to Debra, CHW for the urgent care clinic. She reviewed Dr. Brighton's notes and asked Bonnie when she would prefer the appointment. After the appointment was scheduled, Jasmine asked Bonnie and Ron if they had any other questions. After thoroughly reading this case study, answer the following questions below.

Questions

1. What else should Ron be concerned about regarding his BMI since he has high cholesterol, hypertension, and some symptoms of congestive heart failure?
2. What else should the orthopedic physician suggest for Bonnie to have checked given that her ankle fractured in several locations?

Chapter Summary

This chapter describes the major body systems with disease examples followed by common prefixes and suffixes from medical terminology. Next the leading causes of death in the United States are explained in detail. Last, the five key health-related behaviors

for chronic disease prevention are explained, which include never smoking, participating in regular physical activity, refraining from consuming alcohol or drinking only moderate amounts, maintaining a healthy body weight, and obtaining daily sufficient.

References

1. The human body and different organ systems. Office of Science and Technology Web site. https://www.ostc-was .org/2013/04/23/the-human-body-and-different-organ -systems/. Accessed July 16, 2021.

2. Esophagus. *Britannica Encyclopedia*. https://www.britannica .com/science/esophagus. Accessed November 22, 2021.

3. Brain and spine tumor anatomy and functions. National Cancer Institute, Center for Cancer Research Web site. https://www.cancer.gov/rare-brain-spine-tumor/tumors /anatomy#:~:text=The%20brain%20controls%20 many%20important%20body%20functions,%20 such,the%20brain%20to%20send%20messages%20 throughout%20the%20body. Accessed July 6, 2021.

4. Human brain lobes. Bing Images Web site. https://www .bing.com/images/search?view=detailV2&ccid=%2B4awu F9k&id=5E4060D4653A0B4369598069611F70B51513 CA2E&thid=OIP.-4awuF9kKZMNkfPDRWti5AHaD3&ex ph=0&expw=0&q=Human+Brain+Lobes&simid=60804 1888098684411&ck=012EE7B281747954F48E28BB88 81C068&selectedindex=9&form=IRPRST&ajaxhist=0&v t=0&sim=11. Accessed July 16, 2021.

5. Heart organ diagram. Bing Images Web site. https://www .bing.com/images/search?view=detailV2&ccid=7kO4m apB&id=3DC7D57BE726E78C74F89EC037207D723E C96915&thid=OIP.7kO4mapBE192sQIfA8uuyQHaHa &mediaurl=https%3A%2F%2Fi.pinimg.com%2Forigin als%2F06%2F0d%2F48%2F060d48aa995e2da30405e 7cef07679f8.png&exph=1000&expw=1000&q=Heart+ Organ+Diagram&ck=F69F8ED58CA2047545D0A6B2 040FFA5F&selectedindex=0&form=IRPRST&ajaxhist= 0&pivotparams=insightsToken%3Dccid_jpa9zWFx*cp _2D1AD4350EBEC79B5DBC7CC894E626EC*mid_A8 A0C10F3DB9EC3B426E7D53B89FDEB2AA2DED28*s imid_607987745670696167*thid_OIP.jpa9zWFxfvuM cGdLhySH0wHaHa&vt=0&sim=11&iss=VSI. Accessed July 16, 2021.

6. What is the endocrine system? U.S. Environmental Protection Agency Web site. https://www.epa.gov/endocrine -disruption/what-endocrine-system. Accessed July 16, 2021.

7. Lymphatic system. Cleveland Clinic Web site. https:// my.clevelandclinic.org/health/articles/21199-lymphatic -system. Accessed July 16, 2021.

8. Overview of the immune system. National Institute of Allergy and Infectious Diseases, National Institutes of Health Web site. https://www.niaid.nih.gov/research /immune-system-overview. Accessed July 16, 2021.

9. Autoimmune disorders. MedlinePlus Web site. https:// medlineplus.gov/ency/article/000816.htm#:~:text=An%20 autoimmune%20disorder%20occurs%20when%20 the%20body's%20immune,body's%20immune%20 system%20help%20protect%20against%20harmful%20su- bstances. Accessed July 16, 2021.

10. Buckley G. Muscular system. https://biologydictionary.net /muscular-system/. Accessed July 18, 2021.

11. How many times does your heart beat a day? New Health Advisor Web site. https://www.newhealthadvisor.org /How-Many-Times-Does-Your-Heart-Beat-a-Day.html. Accessed July 18, 2021.

12. Morbidity rate. The Free Dictionary Web site. https:// medical-dictionary.thefreedictionary.com/morbidity+rate. Accessed July 18, 2021.

13. Kenton W. Morbidity rate. Investopedia Web site. https:// www.investopedia.com/terms/m/morbidity-rate.asp. Accessed July 18, 2021.

14. Mortality rate. Merriam-Webster Web site. https://www .merriam-webster.com/dictionary/mortality%20rate. Accessed July 21, 2021.

15. Kochanek KD, Xu J, Arias E. Mortality in the United States, 2019. Centers for Disease Control and Prevention Web site https://www.cdc.gov/nchs/data/databriefs/db395-H.pdf. Accessed July 21, 2021.

16. Heart attack symptoms, risk, and recovery. Centers for Disease Control and Prevention Web site. https://www. cdc.gov/heartdisease/heart_attack.htm. Accessed July 21, 2021.

17. Coronary heart disease (CHD). Centers for Disease Control and Prevention Web site. https://www.cdc.gov /heartdisease/coronary_ad.htm. Accessed July 21, 2021.

18. About heart disease. Centers for Disease Control and Prevention Web site. https://www.cdc.gov/heartdisease /about.htm. Accessed July 21, 2021.

19. Other conditions related to heart disease. Centers for Disease Control and Prevention Web site. https://www.cdc.gov/heart disease/other_conditions.htm. Accessed July 21, 2021.

20. Valvular heart disease. Centers for Disease Control and Prevention Web site. https://www.cdc.gov/heartdisease /valvular_disease.htm. Accessed July 21, 2021.

21. Heart failure. Centers for Disease Control and Prevention Web site. https://www.cdc.gov/heartdisease/heart_failure .htm. Accessed July 21, 2021.

22. Heart failure. Mayo Clinic Web site. https://www.mayoclinic .org/diseases-conditions/heart-failure/symptoms-causes/syc -20373142. Accessed July 21, 2021.

23. What is cancer? American Cancer Society Web site. https:// www.cancer.org/cancer/cancer-basics/what-is-cancer.html. Accessed July 21, 2021.

24. Cancer treatment. Mayo Clinic Web site. https://www .mayoclinic.org/tests-procedures/cancer-treatment/about /pac-20393344. Accessed July 21, 2021.

25. Accidents or unintentional injuries. Centers for Disease Control and Prevention Web site. https://www.cdc.gov /nchs/fastats/accidental-injury.htm. Accessed July 21, 2021.

26. Asthma. Centers for Disease Control and Prevention Web site. https://www.cdc.gov/asthma/default.htm. Accessed July 21, 2021.

27. COPD. Mayo Clinic Web site. https://www.mayoclinic .org/diseases-conditions/copd/symptoms-causes/syc -20353679. Accessed July 21, 2021.

28. Chronic obstructive pulmonary disease COPD includes: Chronic bronchitis and emphysema. Centers for Disease Control and Prevention Web site. https://www.cdc.gov/nchs/fastats/copd.htm. Accessed July 21, 2021.

29. Emphysema. American Lung Association Web site. https://www.lung.org/lung-health-diseases/lung-disease-lookup/emphysema. Accessed July 21, 2021.

30. Chronic bronchitis. American Lung Association Web site. https://www.lung.org/lung-health-diseases/lung-disease-lookup/chronic-bronchitis. Accessed July 25, 2021.

31. Stroke. Centers for Disease Control and Prevention Web site. https://www.cdc.gov/stroke/index.htm. Accessed July 25, 2021.

32. Alzheimer's disease and related dementias. Centers for Disease Control and Prevention Web site. https://www.cdc.gov/aging/aginginfo/alzheimers.htm#AlzheimersDisease. Accessed July 25, 2021.

33. At a glance: Alzheimer's disease. Centers for Disease Control and Prevention Web site. https://www.cdc.gov/aging/publications/aag/alzheimers.html. Accessed November 22, 2021.

34. Hebert LE, Weuve J, Scherr PA, Evans DA. Alzheimer's disease in the United States (2010–2050) estimated using the 2010 Census. *Neurology.*2013;*80*(19):1778–1783.

35. Resources for community health and public health professionals: Alzheimer's and related dementias. U.S. Department of Health and Human Services, National Institutes of Health, Alzheimers.gov. https://www.alzheimers.gov/professionals/community-public-health-resources. Accessed November 22, 2021.

36. Alam RB, Ashrafi SA, Pionke JJ, Schwingel A. Role of community health workers in addressing dementia: A scoping review and global perspective. *J Appl Gerontol.* 2021.

37. What is diabetes? Centers for Disease Control and Prevention Web site. https://www.cdc.gov/diabetes/basics/diabetes.html. Accessed July 25, 2021.

38. Nephrotic syndrome. Mayo Clinic Web site. https://www.mayoclinic.org/diseases-conditions/nephrotic-syndrome/symptoms-causes/syc-20375608. Accessed July 25, 2021.

39. Kidney disease. National Institute of Diabetes and Digestive and Kidney Diseases Web site. https://www.niddk.nih.gov/health-information/kidney-disease. Accessed July 25, 2021.

40. Diabetic kidney disease. National Institute of Diabetes and Digestive and Kidney Diseases Web site. https://www.niddk.nih.gov/health-information/diabetes/overview/preventing-problems/diabetic-kidney-disease. Accessed July 25, 2021.

41. What is the connection between influenza and pneumonia? American Lung Association Web site. https://www.lung.org/lung-health-diseases/lung-disease-lookup/pneumonia/what-is-the-connection. Accessed July 25, 2021.

42. Self-directed violence and other forms of self-injury. Centers for Disease Control and Prevention Web site. https://www.cdc.gov/ncbddd/disabilityandsafety/self-injury.html. Accessed July 27, 2021.

43. Lifeline chat. National Suicide Prevention Lifeline Web site. https://suicidepreventionlifeline.org/chat/. Accessed July 27, 2021.

44. Fast facts. Centers for Disease Control and Prevention Web site. https://www.cdc.gov/suicide/facts/index.html. Accessed July 27, 2021.

45. Liu Y, Croft JB, Wheaton AG, et al. Clustering of five health-related behaviors for chronic disease prevention among adults, United States, 2013. *Prev Chronic Dis*, 2016;*13*:160054. https://www.cdc.gov/pcd/issues/2016/16_0054.htm.

46. Physical activity. World Health Organization Website. https://www.who.int/news-room/fact-sheets/detail/physical-activity. Accessed June 27, 2021.

47. Frequently asked questions. Centers for Disease Control and Prevention Web site. https://www.cdc.gov/alcohol/faqs.htm. Accessed June 27, 2021.

48. Alcohol use disorder. Mayo Clinic Web site. https://www.mayoclinic.org/diseases-conditions/alcohol-use-disorder/symptoms-causes/syc-20369243. Accessed June 27, 2021.

49. Alcoholism. North Point Recovery Web site. https://www.northpointrecovery.com/blog/why-is-alcohol-addiction-so-hard-to-beat/. Accessed June 27, 2021.

50. Obesity. Mayo Clinic Web site. https://www.mayoclinic.org/diseases-conditions/obesity/symptoms-causes/syc-20375742. Accessed July 30, 2021.

51. Why BMI is inaccurate and misleading. Medical News Today Web site. https://www.medicalnewstoday.com/articles/265215. Accessed July 30, 2021.

52. What to know about obesity discrimination in health-care. Medical News Today Web site. https://www.medicalnewstoday.com/articles/obesity-discrimination-in-healthcare#negative-effects. Accessed August 1, 2021.

53. Data and statistics. Centers for Disease Control and Prevention Web site. https://www.cdc.gov/sleep/data_statistics.html. Accessed July 30, 2021.

54. Sleep and chronic disease. Centers for Disease Control and Prevention Web site. https://www.cdc.gov/sleep/about_sleep/chronic_disease.html. Accessed July 30, 2021.

55. Key sleep disorders. Centers for Disease Control and Prevention Web site. https://www.cdc.gov/sleep/about_sleep/key_disorders.html. Accessed July 30, 2021.

56. Healthy sleep habits. AASM Web site. https://sleepeducation.org/healthy-sleep/healthy-sleep-habits/. Accessed July 30, 2021.

Appendix

1. Women's Reproductive Health: https://www.youtube.com/watch?v=4e1hVHrf4sw
2. Men's Reproductive Health: https://www.youtube.com/watch?v=RhBS9ANCVL8
3. Immune System Explained: https://www.youtube.com/watch?v=pnFJGqORj74
4. Muscular System: https://www.youtube.com/watch?v=VVL-8zr2hk4
5. Type 2 Diabetes: https://www.youtube.com/watch?v=4SZGM_E5cLI&t=63s

CHAPTER 7

Infectious Diseases

LEARNING OBJECTIVES

1. Identify and define the four categories of infectious diseases.
2. Explain why antibiotics resistance is so challenging and important.
3. Explain the risk factors and transmission of acquiring infectious diseases.
4. Describe the four steps of food safety.
5. Demonstrate how to properly use personal protective equipment.
6. Explain herd immunity and how it is achieved.

KEY WORDS

personal protective equipment (PPE)
bacteria
antibiotic
antibiotic resistance
sepsis
viruses
vaccination
fungus
systemic infections
parasites
direct contact
indirect contact
herd immunity

Introduction

This chapter introduces infectious diseases, including the categories of disease, risk of transmission, symptoms, and prevention. Infectious diseases do not move without help from humans, animals, and the environment. Unlike noncommunicable diseases (i.e., diabetes, obesity, Alzheimer's, and hypertension), it is possible to acquire human-to-human infectious diseases through the respiratory system by inhaling the virus, such as the cold, flu, and COVID-19 virus. Additionally, viruses can be acquired by consuming contaminated food, water, or being exposed to organisms in the environment. Most infectious diseases cause mild symptoms, such as fever, fatigue, diarrhea, muscle aches, and coughing; however, some infectious diseases are serious and require treatment or hospitalization to prevent death or long-term effects. Precautions and prevention of infectious diseases include food safety, the use of **personal protective equipment (PPE)**, and vaccinations.[1] In 2020, due to the spread of the COVID-19 virus, public health prevention was promoted to reduce the virus through frequent and thorough hand-washing, using hand sanitizer, wearing a face mask, social distancing, practicing isolation after exposure, and obtaining the vaccine.

Categories of Infectious Diseases

Infectious diseases are categorized by bacteria, viruses, fungi, and parasites. Each disease operates uniquely and affects body systems differently. Researchers and scientists use certain characteristics to properly define these four categories.[2] For example, to determine an infectious agent scientists may observe the size of the infectious agent, its' biochemical attributes, the method of interaction with the human or animal host, and the treatment options available.[2] While the full details regarding infectious agents are beyond the scope of this text, it is important to know the basic characteristics of bacteria, viruses, fungi, and parasites. As a community health worker (CHW), this basic information enhances knowledge and understanding to assist in important field work.[3]

Bacterial Infections

Bacteria are an inevitable part of life.[2] Bacteria can live in almost any type of environment, from extreme heat to intense cold, and some can even survive in radioactive waste. Some "good" bacteria attack "bad" bacteria and prevent them from causing sickness.[2]

Bacteria enter the body through droplets into the mouth, genitals, open wounds, nose, and eyes and can be transmitted via bodily fluids, skin-to-skin contact, contaminated items, or airborne particles or droplets.[2] After the bacteria enter, they begins to multiply, causing an infection. For treatment options, antibiotics are the standard of care for bacterial infections. The best way to prevent infection is through vaccination efforts.[2]

Common Bacterial Infections

Severe diseases
- Bubonic plague: extremely rare, transmitted by infected fleas[2]
- Cholera: often fatal, contracted from infected water supplies
- Diphtheria: infection in nose and throat; preventable by vaccine
- Dysentery: infection of intestines[3,12]
- Tuberculosis: serious lung infection when left untreated
- Typhoid: contaminated food and water; vaccine advised in some areas[2]
- Typhus: spread with infected insects due to poor basic sanitation[2,3]

Less severe diseases
- Bacterial meningitis: serious inflammation of brain and spinal cord
- Conjunctivitis (pink eye): eye infection[2,12]
- Food poisoning: bacteria contamination of food; see **Figure 7.1**.
- Gastritis: inflammation of stomach
- Helicobacter pylori (H pylori): linked to stomach cancer and peptic ulcers[2]
- Methicillin-resistant staphylococcus aureus (MRSA): a type of staph bacteria resistant to antibiotics used to treat staph infections[2,3,12]
- Otitis media: ear infection
- Pneumonia: lung infection[3,12]
- Skin infections: lacerations (cuts)
- Sexually transmitted infections (STIs): chlamydia, gonorrhea, and syphilis
- Tuberculosis: lung infection[3,12]
- Urinary tract infections: bladder infection[12]

Antibiotic Resistance

The first commercialized **antibiotic** was discovered by Alexander Fleming in 1928.[5] Since the introduction of antibiotics, there has been a reoccurring discovery of new antibiotics to treat various bacterial infections. However, as new antibiotics come to market, germs find ways to survive and resist these new drugs, thus making it harder for research to keep up and treat ongoing bacterial infections successfully.[5] Currently, antibiotic resistance is one of the largest public health concerns. Each year in the United States, at least 2.8 million people get an antibiotic-resistant infection, and more than 35,000 people die.[5] Fighting this threat is a public health priority that requires a collaborative global approach across sectors.[5]

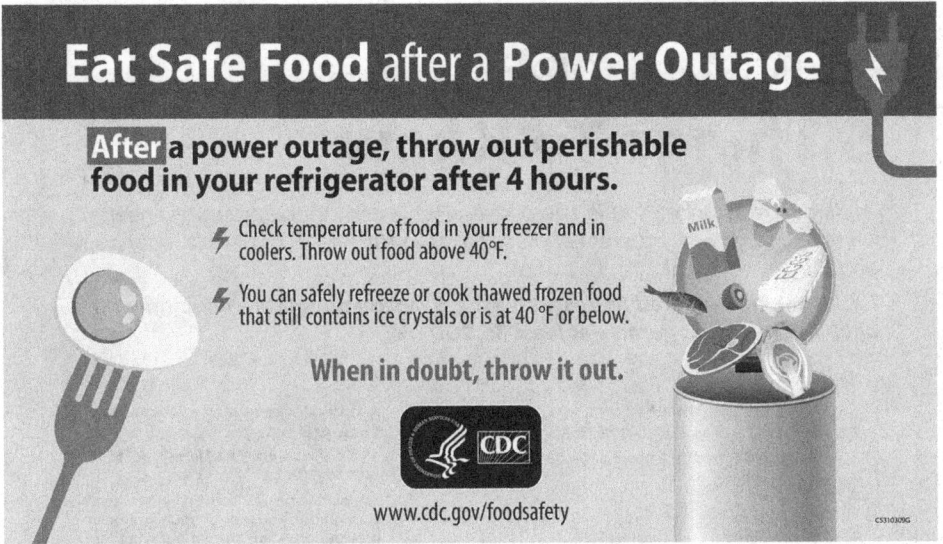

Figure 7.1 Eat Safe Food After a Power Outage

Figure from Centers for Disease Control and Prevention. Food Safety for Power Outages. Available at https://www.cdc.gov/foodsafety/food-safety-during-a-power-outage.html. Accessed September 1, 2021. Reference to specific commercial products, manufacturers, companies, or trademarks does not constitute its endorsement or recommendation by the U.S. Government, Department of Health and Human Services, or Centers for Disease Control and Prevention.[4]

Antibiotic resistance happens when bacteria and fungi develop the ability to defeat the drugs that were initially designed to kill them. When bacteria and fungi are not killed, they continue to rapidly multiply. Infections caused by antibiotic-resistant germs are difficult, and sometimes impossible, to treat. In most cases, antibiotic-resistant infections require extended hospital stays and additional follow-up visits with clinicians, which contributes to the cost of health care. Antibiotic resistance does not mean the body has become resistant to antibiotics. Rather, it means that bacteria have become resistant to the antibiotics designed to kill them.[5]

Avoiding unnecessary use of antibiotics helps slow the spread of antibiotic resistance. For example, most of the time, people should not take antibiotics to treat foodborne illnesses. However, antibiotics can be lifesaving for more severe infections. Additionally, individuals at risk for severe infections include young children, pregnant women, older adults, and people with other chronic health conditions.[5]

The U.S. food supply is among the safest in the world, but people can still get sick from foodborne infections or from contact with animals and their environments. These infections can be caused by antibiotic-resistant bacteria.[5] Animals and humans have bacteria in their gut, including antibiotic-resistant bacteria. Bacteria can spread between animals and throughout their environments (such as on farms, in animal markets, and during transportation). When animals are slaughtered and processed for food, these bacteria can contaminate meat or other animal products. Animal waste can also carry antibiotic-resistant bacteria. Fruits, vegetables, and other produce can become contaminated through contact with soil or water containing waste from animals.[5]

What CHWs Need to Know About Antibiotic Resistance

Antibiotic resistance happens when bacteria develop the ability to defeat the drugs designed to kill them. Simply, the bacteria are not killed and continue to grow. Antibiotic resistance has the potential to affect people at any stage of life, as well as the healthcare, veterinary, and agriculture industries. Antibiotic resistance is one of the world's most urgent public health problems.[6-7] see **Figure 7.2**.

Antibiotic Resistance:
5 Things To Know

Antibiotic resistance (AR) is one of the most urgent threats to public health. AR is a "one health" problem and connects to the health of people, animals, and the environment.

Each year in the United States, at least 2.8 million people are infected with antibiotic-resistant germs—at least 35,000 die.

1 **Antibiotic resistance occurs when germs defeat the drugs designed to kill them.**

It does **NOT** mean the body is resistant to antibiotics.

2 **Antibiotic resistance can affect people at any stage of life.**

Infections caused by resistant germs are difficult—sometimes impossible—to treat. In many cases, these infections require extended hospital stays, additional follow-up doctor visits, and the use of treatments that may be costly and potentially toxic to the patient.

3 **Healthy habits can protect you from infections and help stop germs from spreading.**

Get recommended vaccines, keep hands and wounds clean, and take good care of chronic conditions, like diabetes.

4 **Antibiotics save human and animal lives. Any time antibiotics are used, they can lead to side effects and resistance.**

Antibiotics do not work on viruses, such as colds and the flu. Talk to your healthcare provider or veterinarian about whether antibiotics are needed.

5 **Antibiotic resistance has been found in all regions of the world.**

Modern trade and travel mean AR can move easily across borders. It can spread in places like hospitals, farms, the community, and the environment. Tell your healthcare provider if you recently traveled to or received care in another country.

Your actions can help combat antibiotic resistance.
Learn more at **www.cdc.gov/DrugResistance**

COMMIT TO ACTION
DELIVER RESULTS
COMBAT AMR

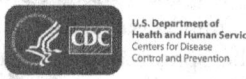

CDC — U.S. Department of Health and Human Services, Centers for Disease Control and Prevention

Figure 7.2 Antibiotic Resistance: Five Things to Know

Figure from Centers for Disease Control and Prevention. 5 Things to Know. Available at https://www.cdc.gov/drugresistance/about/5-things-to-know.html. Accessed February 1, 2022. Reference to specific commercial products, manufacturers, companies, or trademarks does not constitute its endorsement or recommendation by the U.S. Government, Department of Health and Human Services, or Centers for Disease Control and Prevention.[6]

Resistance to even one antibiotic may equal serious problems:

- Antibiotic-resistant infections may require the use of other drug treatments that may harm patients by causing serious side effects,

such as organ failure, and prolong care and recovery for months.[6–7]

- Many medical advances depend on the ability to fight infections using antibiotics, including joint replacements, organ transplants, cancer therapy, and the treatment of chronic diseases, such as diabetes, asthma, and rheumatoid arthritis.[6–7]

- In some cases, antibiotic-resistant infections have no treatment options.[6–7]

If antibiotics lose their effectiveness, health care is no longer able to treat infections and control these public health threats. See **Figure 7.3**.

Antibiotic resistance increases when a combination of germs is exposed to antibiotics, and

How Antibiotic Resistance Spreads

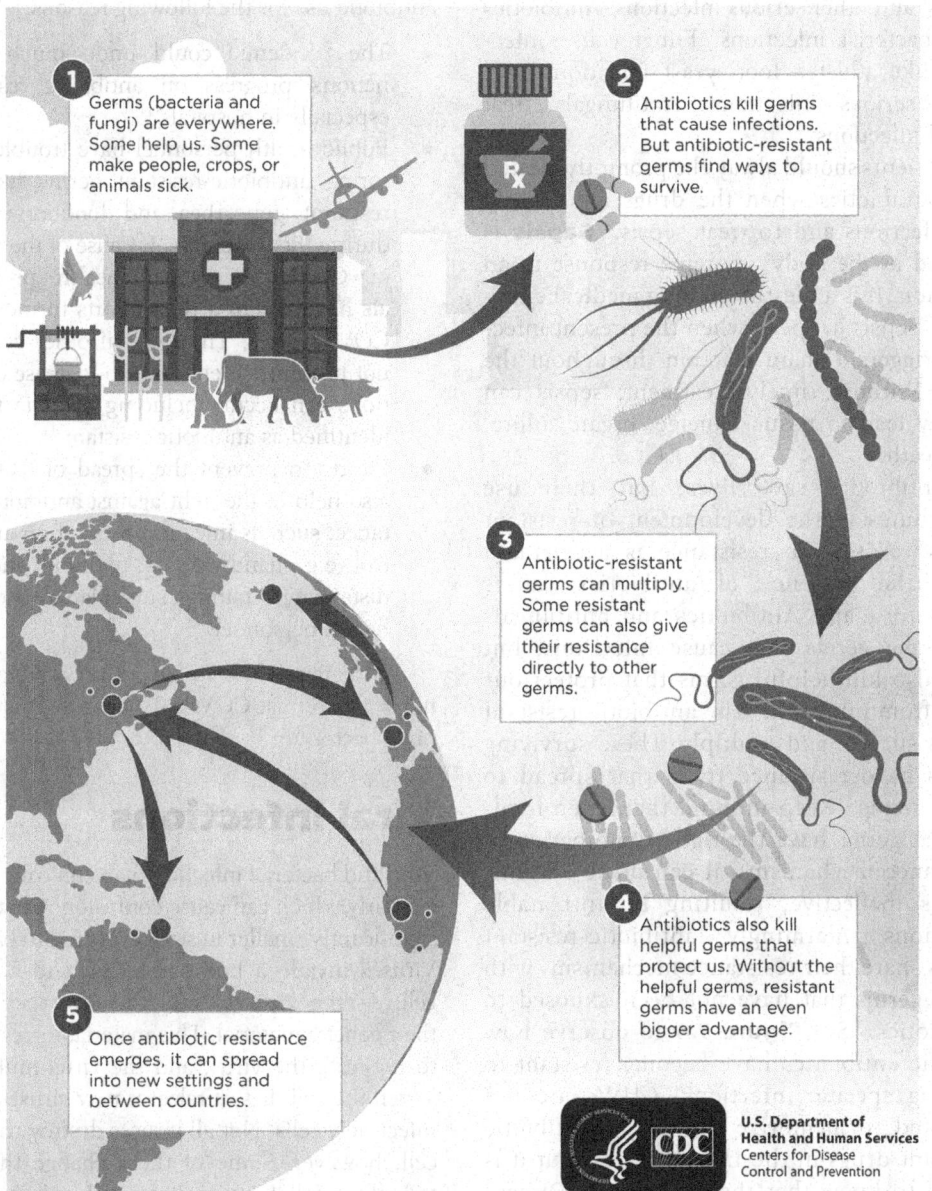

1. Germs (bacteria and fungi) are everywhere. Some help us. Some make people, crops, or animals sick.

2. Antibiotics kill germs that cause infections. But antibiotic-resistant germs find ways to survive.

3. Antibiotic-resistant germs can multiply. Some resistant germs can also give their resistance directly to other germs.

4. Antibiotics also kill helpful germs that protect us. Without the helpful germs, resistant germs have an even bigger advantage.

5. Once antibiotic resistance emerges, it can spread into new settings and between countries.

U.S. Department of Health and Human Services
Centers for Disease Control and Prevention

Figure 7.3 How Antibiotic Resistance Spreads

Figure from Centers for Disease Control and Prevention. How Antibiotic Resistance Happens. Available at https://www.cdc.gov/drugresistance/pdf/threats-report/How-AR-Spreads.pdf. Accessed February 1, 2022. Reference to specific commercial products, manufacturers, companies, or trademarks does not constitute its endorsement or recommendation by the U.S. Government, Department of Health and Human Services, or Centers for Disease Control and Prevention.[8]

those germs and their resistance mechanisms spread.[6-7] Antibiotic resistance does not necessarily mean our body is resistant to antibiotics. However, it does mean the bacteria or fungi causing the infection are resistant to the antibiotic treatment. For example, bacteria cause infections such as strep throat, foodborne illnesses, and other serious infections. Antibiotics treat bacterial infections. Fungi cause infections like athlete's foot, yeast infections, and other serious infections. Antifungals treat fungal infections.[6-7]

Patients should always be promptly treated with antibiotics when the drugs are needed for infections and to treat sepsis.[9] **Sepsis** is defined as the body's extreme response to an infection. It is a life-threatening medical emergency. Sepsis happens when the present infection triggers a chain reaction throughout the body. Without timely treatment, sepsis can rapidly lead to tissue damage, organ failure, and death.[9]

Antibiotics save lives, but their use contributes to the development of resistant germs.[7] Antibiotic resistance is accelerated when the presence of antibiotics causes germs to adapt. Antibiotics and antifungals kill some germs that cause infections, but they also kill helpful germs that protect our body from infection.[7] The antibiotic-resistant germs survive and multiply. These surviving germs have resistance traits that spread to other germs.[7] Keep in mind that when hard-to-treat germs have the right combination of resistance mechanisms, it can make all antibiotics ineffective, resulting in untreatable infections. Alarmingly, antibiotic-resistant germs share their resistance mechanisms with other germs that have not been exposed to antibiotics.[7] See **Figure 7.4** to observe how specific antibiotics have become resistant to treating specific infections. CHWs are not expected to memorize the list of antibiotic resistant drugs in the United States, but it is useful to know that the Centers for Disease Control and Prevention (CDC) list is available and updated regularly.

COVID-19 and Antibiotic Resistance

Antibiotic resistance is still a public health threat during the COVID-19 pandemic. CDC experts closely monitor the possible effects of COVID-19 on the national state of antibiotic resistance and antibiotic use for the following reasons:

- The pandemic could undo much of the nation's progress on antibiotic resistance, especially in hospitals.[11]
- Public health personnel have trouble monitoring antibiotic-resistant germs like drug resistant gonorrhea and foodborne germs during the pandemic. Because of the urgency of COVID-19, public health professionals have diverted their efforts to monitoring COVID cases. Therefore, if other germs are not promptly identified, an increase of infections can occur, including bacteria that are identified as antibiotic resistant.[11]
- Efforts to prevent the spread of COVID-19 also help in the fight against antibiotic resistance, such as infection prevention and control (e.g., handwashing, masking, and social distancing), training, surveillance, and public health personnel.[11]

It is important to note that antibiotics do not work to treat COVID-19 because it is a virus, not a bacterium.[11]

Viral Infections

Viral and bacterial infections can clinically present similarly which can cause confusion. **Viruses** are significantly smaller in size compared to bacteria.[2] Viruses invade a body and attach to a healthy cell. As the viruses enter the cell, they release their genetic material. This material forces the cell to replicate the virus, and the virus multiplies.[2] When the cell dies, it releases new viruses, which infect new cells. Not all viruses destroy their host cell, however. Some of them change the function of the cell. Some viruses, such as human papillomavirus (HPV) and Epstein-Barr virus (EBV), can lead to cancer by forcing cells to replicate in

Germs Develop Antibiotic Resistance

Select Germs Showing Resistance Over Time

Since the discovery of penicillin more than 90 years ago, germs have continued to develop new types of resistance against even our most powerful drugs. While antibiotic development has slowed, antibiotic resistance has not. This table demonstrates how rapidly important types of resistance developed after approval and release of new antibiotics, including antifungals.

Antibiotic Approved or Released	Year Released	Resistant Germ Identified	Year Identified
Penicillin	1941	Penicillin-resistant *Staphylococcus aureus*[20, 21]	1942
		Penicillin-resistant *Streptococcus pneumoniae*[9,10]	1967
		Penicillinase-producing *Neisseria gonorrhoeae*[11]	1976
Vancomycin	1958	Plasmid-mediated vancomycin-resistant *Enterococcus faecium*[12,13]	1988
		Vancomycin-resistant *Staphylococcus aureus*[14]	2002
Amphotericin B	1959	Amphotericin B-resistant *Candida auris*[15]	2016
Methicillin	1960	Methicillin-resistant *Staphylococcus aureus*[16]	1960
Extended-spectrum cephalosporins	1980 (Cefotaxime)	Extended-spectrum beta-lactamase- producing *Escherichia coli*[17]	1983
Azithromycin	1980	Azithromycin-resistant *Neisseria gonorrhoeae*[18]	2011
Imipenem	1985	*Klebsiella pneumoniae* carbapenemase (KPC)-producing *Klebsiella pneumoniae*[19]	1996
Ciprofloxacin	1987	Ciprofloxacin-resistant *Neisseria gonorrhoeae*[20]	2007
Fluconazole	1990 (FDA approved)	Fluconazole-resistant *Candida*[21]	1988
Caspofungin	2001	Caspofungin-resistant *Candida*[22]	2004
Daptomycin	2003	Daptomycin-resistant methicillin-resistant *Staphylococcus aureus*[23]	2004
Ceftazidime-avibactam	2015	Ceftazidime-avibactam-resistant KPC-producing *Klebsiella pneumoniae*[24]	2015

Revised Dec. 2019

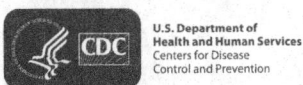

U.S. Department of
Health and Human Services
Centers for Disease
Control and Prevention

Figure 7.4 Antibiotic Resistance Threat in the United States

an uncontrolled way.[3,12] It well known that viruses are more difficult to treat than bacteria. Thus, the use of antibiotics will not work to treat a virus. The symptoms of most viruses are treated with over-the-counter (OTC) medications and are available at the local pharmacy. These medications will help with symptom management while the immune system works to naturally fight the virus.[2] Antiviral medications can help relieve the symptoms of some viruses while the disease passes. They can either prevent the virus from reproducing or boost the host's immune system to counter the effects of the virus.[3,6] These drugs will not stop the virus, and their use only increases the risk of antibiotic resistance.[6] See **Figure 7.5**.

One of the best ways to prevent viral infections is through **vaccination**. For example, influenza or the flu is one of the most common viruses that circulates yearly and replicates quickly.[2]

Common Viral Infections

Chickenpox: linked to shingles later in life
Common cold: respiratory and sinus infection[2,3,12]
COVID-19: serious lung infection

Dengue fever: mosquito-borne viral disease in tropical areas[12]
Ebola: spread through contact with bodily fluids; severe bleeding
Encephalitis: inflammation of the brain due to an infection
Hepatitis B and C have been linked to liver cancer[2,3,12]
Herpes simplex virus (HSV): produce viral infections in humans
Human immunodeficiency virus (HIV): links to acquired immunodeficiency virus (AIDS)
HPV: linked to cervical and throat cancer
Influenza: highly contagious respiratory infection including H1N1 and swine flu[3,12]
Middle East Respiratory Syndrome (MERS-CoV): respiratory infection
Norovirus: infection in the intestinal tract; gastroenteritis[2]
Polio: causes paralysis; transmitted through water, food, and others infected[12]
Pneumonia: lung infection
Meningitis: inflammation of brain and spinal cord[3,12]

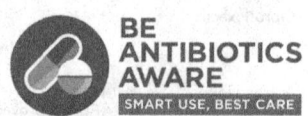

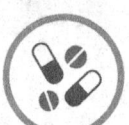
SAY YES TO ANTIBIOTICS
when needed for certain infections caused by **bacteria**.

SAY NO TO ANTIBIOTICS
for **viruses**, such as colds and flu, or runny noses, even if the mucus is thick, yellow or green. Antibiotics also won't help for some common bacterial infections including most cases of bronchitis, many sinus infections, and some ear infections.

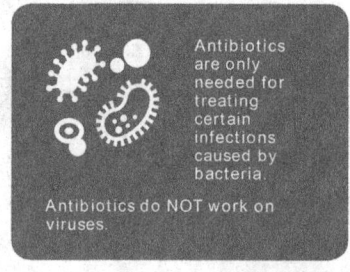
Antibiotics are only needed for treating certain infections caused by bacteria.

Antibiotics do NOT work on viruses.

To learn more about antibiotic prescribing and use, visit www.cdc.gov/antibiotic-use

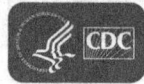

Figure 7.5 Do I Really Need Antibiotics?

Figure from Centers for Disease Control and Prevention. Do I really need antibiotics? Available at https://www.cdc.gov/antibiotic-use/graphics.html. Accessed September 1, 2021. Reference to specific commercial products, manufacturers, companies, or trademarks does not constitute its endorsement or recommendation by the U.S. Government, Department of Health and Human Services, or Centers for Disease Control and Prevention.[13]

Rabies: deadly virus spread to people from saliva of infected animals

Warts: caused by various strains of HPV; person-to-person contact[3,12]

West Nile virus: transmitted by mosquitoes

Zika virus: transmitted by mosquitoes[3,12]

In addition to the brief list above, CHWs benefit from the current information about HIV/AIDS. HIV is a virus that attacks the immune system.[14] When left untreated, HIV can lead to AIDS. While there is no current cure, HIV/AIDs can be controlled with effective treatment and medical care.[14] HIV/AIDS is transmitted through unprotected sexual contact, sharing needles, or through bodily fluids such as breast milk.[15] The CDC estimates that, as of 2019, about 1.2 million people in the United States have HIV.[16] New HIV infections have declined in recent years, after a period of general stability due to advanced treatment options and public health preventative efforts. Overall, new infections fell 8 percent from 37,800 in 2015 to 34,800 in 2019.[16]

However, despite overall progress, some groups remain more affected than others:

- Gay and bisexual men continue to account for most new HIV infections (66 percent).[16]
- Black individuals face infection rates that are eight times as high as White individuals.[16]
- Hispanic/Latino individuals face infection rates that are almost four times as high as White individuals. However, Hispanic/Latino people can be of any race.[16]
- Geographically, the South is disproportionately affected. The region accounted for more than half (53 percent) of new HIV infections in 2019, even though it only represented 38 percent of the U.S. population.[16]

The CDC has accelerated efforts to reduce health disparities among transgender women, MSM (men who have sex with men), homeless youth, Black individuals, and Hispanic/Latino people. These are key populations for the CDC's major HIV prevention funding programs, including funding to state and local health departments and community-based organizations.[16] See **Figure 7.6**.

Fungal Infections

Fungi are significantly different compared to bacteria and viruses.[2,12] A **fungus** can decompose and absorb organic matter using an enzyme. Fungi almost always reproduce by spreading single celled spores.[2] Many human-to-human fungal infections develop in the upper layers of the skin, and some progress to the deeper layers, such as the intestines, mouth, vagina, and other parts of the body. Inhaled yeast or mold spores can sometimes lead to fungal infections, such as pneumonia, or infections throughout the body, which are also known as **systemic infections**. Those with a higher risk of developing a fungal infection include people who are required to use antibiotics for a long time, aging population, and those with a weakened immune system, such as individuals living with HIV or diabetes, receiving chemotherapy treatment, or have undergone a transplant because they take medications to prevent their body from rejecting the new organ. Antibiotics and antifungal medications are used in combination to treat the infected individual.[2,12]

Common Fungal Infections

Athlete's foot: fungal infection; begins between the toes[12]

Candidiasis: lung infection from inhaling spores

Coccidioidomycosis: fungus found in soil; inhaled

Histoplasmosis: lung infections[2,3,12]

Rash: temporary outbreak of red, bumpy, scaly, or itchy patches of skin[12]

Ringworm: highly contagious, fungal infection; spread by skin-to-skin contact[12]

Parasites

Parasites are living organisms that are capable of laying eggs in the host while undetected. Parasites attach to the host, lay eggs, and then symptoms occur once the eggs hatch and infection has taken place.[2] Most medications to treat parasites are not approved or licensed by the federal U.S. Food and Drug Administration (FDA).[2] In the United States, parasite treatment options are not in demand compared

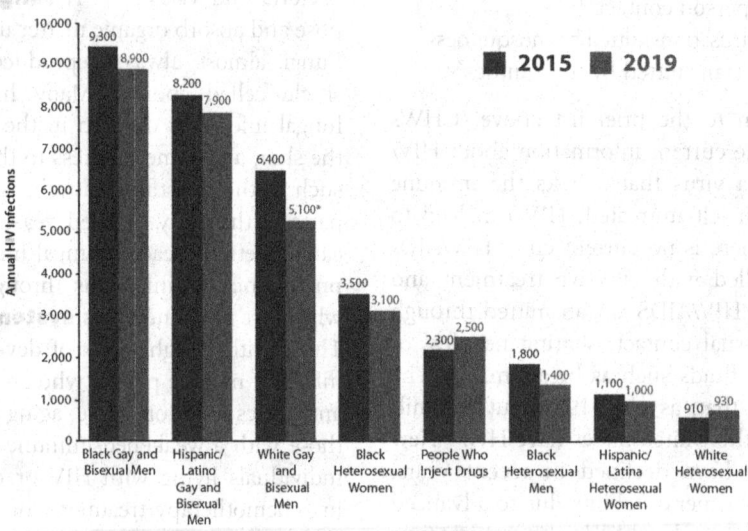

New HIV Infections by Race and Transmission Group, U.S., 2015 vs. 2019

*Indicates that difference from 2015 estimate was deemed statistically significant

For more information, visit
cdc.gov/nchhstp/newsroom

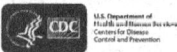

U.S. Department of
Health and Human Services
Centers for Disease
Control and Prevention

Figure 7.6 New HIV Infections by Race and Transmission Groups, United States, 2015 Versus 2019

Figure from Centers for Disease Control and Prevention. The State of the HIV Epidemic in the U.S. Available at https://www.cdc.gov/nchhstp/newsroom/fact-sheets/hiv/state-of-the-hiv-epidemic-factsheet.html. Accessed February 4, 2022. Reference to specific commercial products, manufacturers, companies, or trademarks does not constitute its endorsement or recommendation by the U.S. Government, Department of Health and Human Services, or Centers for Disease Control and Prevention.[16]

to other countries where infections such as malaria (a mosquito-borne disease) and giardia (a parasite causing diarrheal diseases) are more common.[12,17] Some anti-parasitic medications can be prescribed by physicians in the United States, though not officially approved by the FDA. The best way to prevent parasitic infections is through proper travel planning, cooking food thoroughly, consuming clean water, practicing safe sex, and washing hands thoroughly.[18]

Common Parasitic Infections

Enterobiasis (Pinworm infections): common intestinal parasite[12,18]

Giardia: intestinal infection found worldwide especially in areas of poor sanitation and unsafe water; the common causes of waterborne diseases in the United States; found in back-country streams and lakes as well as whirlpools and public swimming pools. Hikers need to take precautions when swimming, camping, and consuming any fresh water without boiling.[12,18]

Malaria (Plasmodium): transmitted by mosquito bites

Pediculosis: head and body lice[12,18]

Pneumocystis pneumonia: lung infections

Toxoplasmosis: transmitted through cats to human; contact with feces and litterboxes[12]

Risk Factors and Transmission of Acquiring Infectious Diseases

In the United States, the leading infectious diseases include viral hepatitis, influenza, and tuberculosis (TB).[19] Anyone can acquire an infectious disease. However, individuals with compromised immune systems are more at risk. For example, individuals are at increased risk when receiving cancer treatments, taking immune suppression medications, have received an organ transplant, have HIV, or suffer from malnutrition. Additionally, infants, with their undeveloped immune systems, and the aging population are at a greater risk for acquiring infectious diseases.[20] Other individuals at-risk include those who are unvaccinated against common infectious diseases, healthcare workers, and those traveling to areas of the world where they may be exposed to mosquitoes that carry infectious diseases, such as malaria, dengue, and Zika viruses.[20]

Infectious diseases do not move without help from humans, animals, and the environment.[20] The four types of infectious disease transmission are direct contact, indirect contact, insect or animal bites, and food or drinking water.

Direct Contact. Direct contact includes person-to-person or skin-to-skin contact with bodily or sexual fluids, such as blood or saliva.[20] It is important to never share personal items, such as toothbrushes, combs, razors, and drinking glasses. Additionally, it is crucial to travel wisely and receive vaccinations as recommended.[20] When an infected individual talks, sneezes, or coughs, the droplets carry the infectious disease germs at least 6 feet, more in some cases. Once the infectious germs land on the susceptible individual, transmission can occur through the eyes, nose, or mouth.[20] At this point, the disease enters the body of the noninfected person, placing them at risk for becoming infected. Infectious diseases that spread through direct contact include COVID-19, TB, polio, pertussis, meningitis, and the rubella measles virus. This mode of transmission is the primary reason why face masks are essential to reduce the transmission of infectious diseases.[20] See **Box 7.1**.

Indirect Contact. Indirect contact is characterized by transmission that occurs when there is no direct human-to-human contact.[20]

For example, an individual's hands become contaminated by touching a surface previously contaminated, such as a doorknob or drinking fountain lever. If individuals fail to use proper hand hygiene, the germs are carried on their hands and transmitted to the next surface. The disease germs remain on the contaminated surface until the next susceptible individual touches the surface. In healthcare settings, it is possible for the infectious disease to be transmitted by medical equipment.[20] For example, when a patient is put on a ventilator for a lung or breathing condition, the ventilator may emit aerosolized germs from the medical device into the room. For this reason, healthcare providers wear PPE—mask, face shield, disposable gown, gloves—when caring for patients on ventilators. If the medical equipment is not properly sanitized after each patient use, the germs may spread from patient to patient.[20]

Other lifesaving medical treatments (e.g., urinary catheters, nasal cannula tubes for oxygen, intravenous [IV] tubes, drainage tubes, and surgery) increase the risk of infection and provide ways for germs to enter the body.[20] For example, a urinary catheter tube is inserted into an individual's bladder through the ureter. The tubing is connected to a plastic bag to collect the urine when the person is unable to excrete urine. The catheter tubing provides a way for germs to travel up the tubing from the skin to the bladder.[20] If the tubing is not cleaned properly, the person has an increased chance of a acquiring a urinary tract infection (UTI), which often leads to a hospital readmission.[20] In addition, infectious disease germs can be transmitted to healthcare workers through unintentional needle sticks or cuts from sharp instruments that were contaminated with a blood-borne infectious disease, such as HIV, hepatitis B, or hepatitis C.[20]

Insect and Animal Bites. Insects and animals bites may transmit infectious diseases to humans. For example, ticks cause diseases such as Lyme disease and Rocky Mountain Spotted fever, while rabies is a life-threatening virus that occurs from the saliva of an infected animal.[20,23] Mosquitoes cause infectious diseases such as malaria, West Nile virus,

Box 7.1 Tuberculosis—Symptoms, Spread, and Treatment

TB is caused by *Mycobacterium tuberculosis*.[21] The bacteria usually attack the lungs. Deaths from TB are concentrated in poor countries in the Global South, with India, China, Nigeria, South Africa, Brazil, and Bangladesh bearing the greatest burdens.[22] Some 40 percent of TB cases are never treated or diagnosed, which means people are passing the disease onto others without realizing it. The death (mortality) rate for TB is 12 percent, but that figure jumps for the millions of patients who do not receive treatment.[22]

However, not everyone infected with TB bacteria becomes sick. However, if symptomatic TB is not treated properly, it can be fatal. The symptoms of TB include a bad cough that lasts 3 weeks or longer, pain in the chest, coughing up blood or sputum, weakness or fatigue, weight loss, poor appetite, fever, chills, and sweating at night.[21] Exposure occurs when an individual with active TB coughs, sneezes, speaks, or sings. TB is not spread through clothing, on drinking glasses, through eating with utensils, via a handshake, through use of toilets, or other surfaces.[21]

If individuals think that they have been in contact with someone with TB disease, they should contact their doctor or local health department and inquire about getting a TB skin test. Only individuals with active TB disease can spread TB bacteria to others.[21] People with TB disease are most likely to spread the bacteria to people they spend time with every day, such as family members, friends, coworkers, or students.

While there is a vaccine for TB called Bacille Calmette-Guérin (BCG), this vaccine is not widely used in the United States, but it is often given to infants and small children in other countries where TB is common. BCG does not always protect people from getting TB. Many people born outside of the United States have been BCG-vaccinated.[21]

Individuals who previously received the BCG vaccine may test positive to a TB skin test.[21] A positive TB skin test or TB blood test reports that an individual has been infected with TB bacteria at some time. Other tests (e.g., a chest x-ray and sputum sample) are required to determine if the individual has active TB. Individuals with a weak immune system (e.g., HIV infection) are at-risk of developing TB.[21]

Treatment requires an antibiotic regimen of multiple drugs taken for a minimum of 6 months.[21] For cases of drug-resistant TB, antibiotics may be recommended for up to 2 years. For highly drug-resistant strains of TB, those treatments can jump to 5 years. It can be challenging for patients to comply with treatment that requires years of medical management. This becomes especially difficult in countries with poor healthcare systems where TB is most prevalent.[21-22]

When people stop antibiotics early, they are at a high risk of developing drug resistance and then passing that resistance on to others. When done correctly, TB treatment is more than 85 percent effective, and since 2000, TB diagnosis and treatment has saved an estimated 54 million lives.[21-22]

yellow fever, and Zika virus. The best protection to prevent infectious disease, especially for international travel, is a vaccine for yellow fever, cholera, hepatitis A and B, and typhoid. Utilizing insect repellant to avoid insect bites and proper insect coverings are additional sources for mitigation.[20]

Food and Drinking Water. Contaminated food and drinking water are prominent sources for acquiring infectious diseases.[20] Food or water may be contaminated with bacterium, viruses, or other microbes. Acquired food-borne diseases such as listeria and salmonella cause mild to severe gastrointestinal symptoms. Additionally, water-borne

diseases such as giardiasis, salmonella, and typhoid fever cause mild to severe gastrointestinal symptoms. The best protection is avoiding contaminated water.[20,24] Do not drink water from rivers, wash all fruit and vegetables thoroughly, peel fresh fruit, and cook food and meat to the proper temperature of 165° F. If bottled water is not readily available, bring water to a full rolling boil for 1 minute (at elevations above 6,500 feet, boil for 3 minutes).[24] See **Figure 7.7**.

When cleaning surfaces, it is important to disinfect dry and wet surfaces.[26] Dry surfaces include countertops, tables, doorknobs, wheelchairs, bed rails, stair rails, elevator buttons, vehicle steering

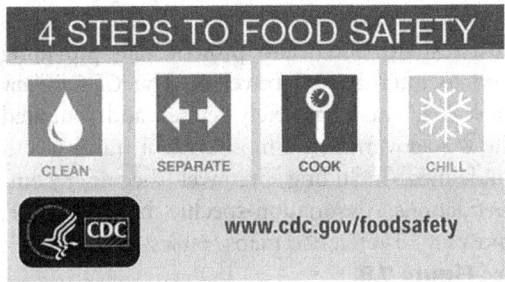

Figure 7.7 Four Steps to Food Safety

Centers for Disease Control and Prevention. Four Steps to Food Safety: Clean, Separate, Cook, Chill. Available at https://www.cdc.gov/foodsafety/keep-food-safe.html. Accessed August 20, 2021. Reference to specific commercial products, manufacturers, companies, or trademarks does not constitute its endorsement or recommendation by the U.S. Government, Department of Health and Human Services, or Centers for Disease Control and Prevention.[25]

wheels and seat covers, medical equipment, fan blades, keyboards, electronic screens, and other hard surfaces. Wet surfaces include faucets, sinks, showers, toilets, drinking fountains, water-proof mattress pads, refrigerator door, shelves, bins, and other wet surfaces. Keep in mind that dust, moisture from leaks, and standing water may harbor bacteria and germs.[26]

Recreational water illnesses are defined as diseases that persons can acquire from the water while swimming and playing in pools, hot tubs, water playgrounds, oceans, lakes, and rivers.[27] The most common symptoms are diarrhea, skin rashes, ear pain, cough or congestion, and eye pain. Swallowing a mouthful of water that contains diarrhea-causing germs can make people sick.[26,27] Individuals can also get sick from contact with other contaminated water sources, such as breathing in the mist from a humidifier.[26,27] See **Box 7.2**.

Box 7.2 **Recreational Water Illnesses**

Infectious Disease Prevention Tips for Swimming or Recreational Water Use:

While swimming, it is important to do our part to keep everyone healthy. Here are a few simple and effective steps to help protect against illness:

- Keep the pee, poop, sweat, and dirt out of the water!
- Stay out of the water if you have diarrhea.
- Shower before you get in the water.
- Do not swallow the water.
- Take children to the restroom breaks every hour.
- During breaks, check diapers, and change them in a bathroom or diaper-changing area—not poolside—to keep germs away from the pool.
- Reapply sunscreen and drink plenty of fluids.

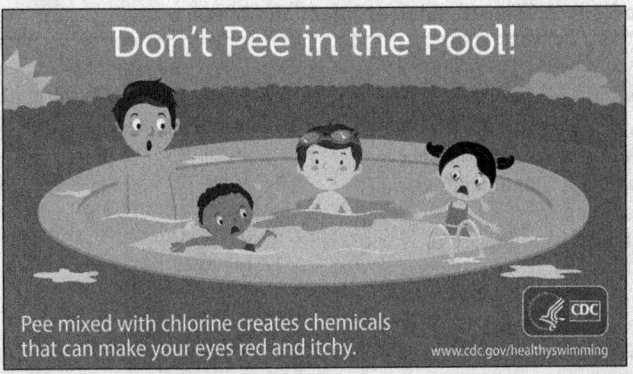

Centers for Disease Control and Prevention. Recreational Water Illness. Available at https://www.cdc.gov/dotw/rwis/index.html. Accessed August 20, 2021. Reference to specific commercial products, manufacturers, companies, or trademarks does not constitute its endorsement or recommendation by the U.S. Government, Department of Health and Human Services, or Centers for Disease Control and Prevention.[27]

Reducing the Transmission of Infectious Diseases

The behavior of humans plays an important role in the spread of infectious diseases. It is essential that people understand how their behavior may increase or decrease the spread of disease.[28] Prevention is the best defense against acquiring or spreading an infectious disease accomplished by reducing the risk of transmission of the disease and is achieved by herd immunity with vaccination rates. See **Box 7.3**.

Herd immunity occurs when a large percentage of the population is immune to a specific disease.[29] If enough individuals are resistant to the cause of the disease, the disease has no way to infect others. Individuals become immune to disease by receiving a vaccine. Some individuals are not able to receive vaccination due to age or health status. Therefore, when enough individuals receive the vaccine, the group has protection, herd immunity is achieved, and those who cannot receive vaccination are protected as well.[29]

When individuals travel outside of the United States, some vaccines are required for reentry to maintain herd immunity. The CDC publishes an online resource guide called the *Yellow Book*.[30]

This book is published every 2 years and serves as a resource for health professionals providing care to international travelers. The *CDC Yellow Book 2020* was completely revised and compiled the U.S. government's most current travel health guidelines, including pretravel vaccine recommendations, destination-specific health advice, and easy-to-reference maps, tables, and charts.[30] See **Figure 7.8**.

Whether staying within the United States or traveling to international destinations, vaccinations are recommended for adults based on age, health status, employment, and other factors. For information about vaccines for children, refer to this website for additional information: https://www.cdc.gov/vaccines/schedules/hcp/imz/child-adolescent.html.[31] For adults, the CDC developed this vaccine assessment tool for adults 19 years or older. Keep in mind that the CDC does not retain any personal information. To take the Adult Vaccine Quiz visit this website: https://www2a.cdc.gov/nip/adultimmsched/Adultquiz_syndicateshell.asp.[32] This quiz will generate a recommended list of the vaccines you may need based on your submitted answers. The list may include vaccines that you have already had. Discuss this list with your primary care doctor or a healthcare professional. See **Figure 7.9**.

Box 7.3 **Steps to Reduce Transmission of Infectious Disease**

To reduce transmission of infectious disease, follow these steps:

1. Wash hands or use hand sanitizer frequently especially after touching a contaminated surface, before and after handling food, and after using the restroom.
2. Wipe surface with disinfectant prior to preparing food and avoid food at room temperature for any extended length of time. Food should be kept cold or hot.
3. Clean kitchen and bathrooms with disinfectant cleaners to remove bacteria and viruses on all surfaces.
4. Do not share items, such as combs, toothbrushes, razor blades, drinking glasses, and utensils.
5. Decrease risk of acquiring sexual transmitted infections (STIs) by obtaining regular medical examinations, using condoms, or abstaining.[3]
6. Take antibiotics when prescribed for bacterial infections and take the full course of treatment. Do not share or save antibiotics for future illness.
7. Obtain vaccinations as recommended.
8. Maintain a strong immune system with an active, healthy lifestyle and eating a nutritious diet.

Data from Felman A. What to know about infections. Available at https://www.medicalnewstoday.com/articles/196271. Accessed September 1, 2021.[3]

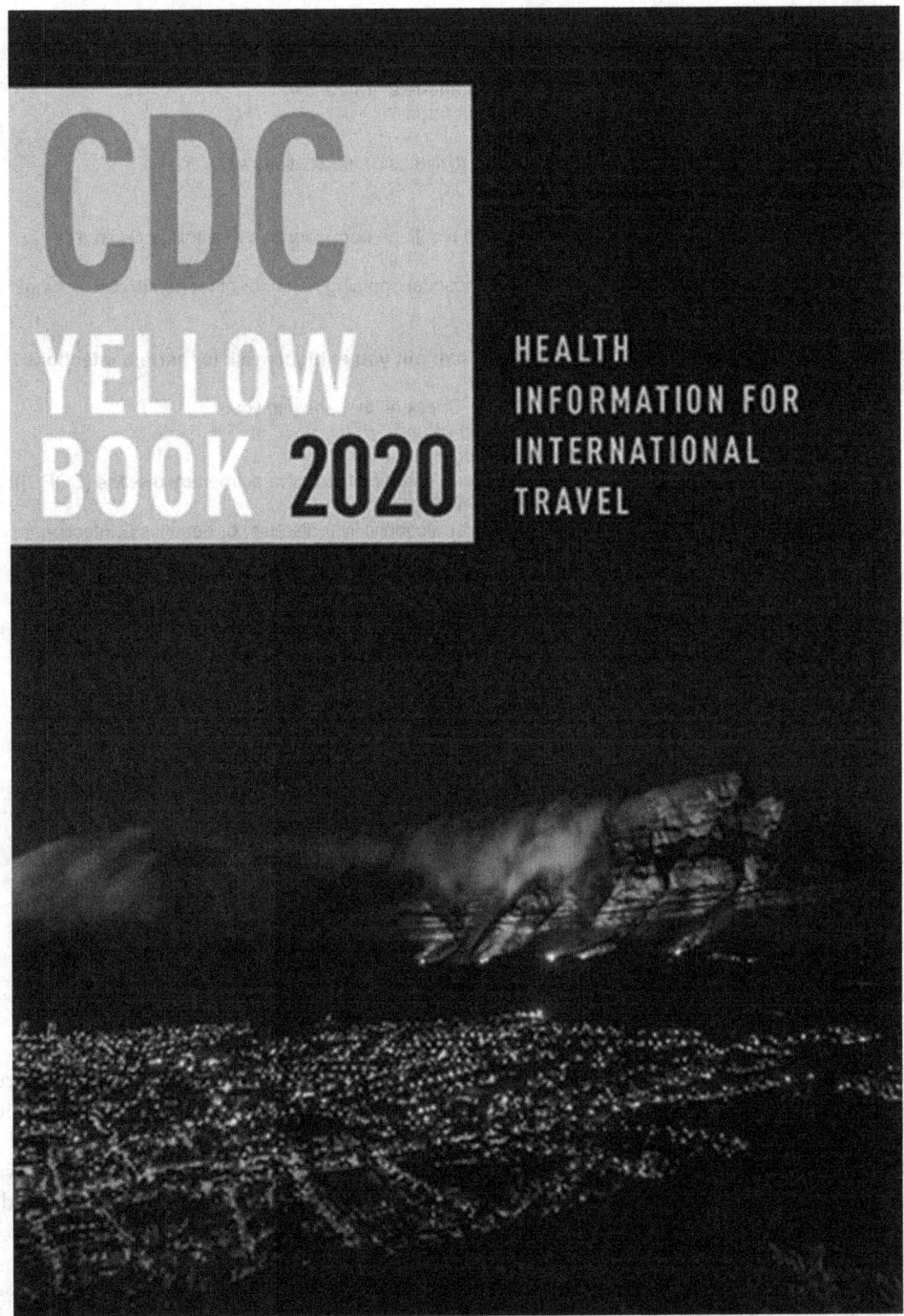

Figure 7.8 The CDC Yellow Book 2020: Health Information for International Travel

Figure from Centers for Disease Control and Prevention. CDC Yellow Book. Available at https://wwwnc.cdc.gov/travel/page/yellowbook-home-2020. Accessed August 22, 2021. Reference to specific commercial products, manufacturers, companies, or trademarks does not constitute its endorsement or recommendation by the U.S. Government, Department of Health and Human Services, or Centers for Disease Control and Prevention.[38]

1. Are you
   ⊙ Male   ⊙ Female
2. What year were you born? (some vaccines are age-related) [2003 ⌄]
3. Will you be traveling outside the U.S. in the near future?
   ⊙ Yes   ⊙ No
4. Do you have a weakened immune system due to illness or medications?
   ⊙ Yes   ⊙ No
5. Do you have HIV infection?   ⊙ Yes ⊙ No
6. Are you a first-year college student who lives in a college dormitory or a new military recruit?
   ⊙ Yes   ⊙ No
7. Do you work with patients in a doctor's office, hospital , nursing home, or other health care setting?
   ⊙ Yes   ⊙ No

Some medical conditions and other situations can put you at higher risk for certain infections.

8. Do you have any of these medical conditions? Check all that apply to you.
   ❑ Heart disease (for example, congestive heart failure)
   ❑ Diabetes mellitus type 1 or 2 (also called "sugar diabetes")
   ❑ Chronic lung disease (for example, asthma and chronic obstructive pulmonary disease [COPD])
   ❑ Kidney failure, end-stage renal disease, or on dialysis
   ❑ Chronic liver disease (for example, cirrhosis or alcoholic liver disease) or hepatitis C infection
   ❑ Spleen has been damaged or removed (for example, due to surgery or sickle cell disease)
   ❑ Cancer or cancer treatment
   ❑ Bone marrow transplant recipient
9. Review the items listed below and check those that apply to you:
   ❑ Alcoholism
   ❑ Smoke cigarettes
   ❑ Man who has sex with men
   ❑ Homeless
   ❑ Factors that can increase your risk for hepatitis A or hepatitis B (such as travel to some countries exposure to blood or bodily fluids, or exposure to contaminated food or drink)
10. Have you had the chickenpox disease or received the chickenpox vaccine?
    ⊙ Yes   ⊙ No   ⊙ Not sure

That's it! Just click "My Results" to find out which vaccines you may need.

Figure 7.9 Adult Vaccine Quiz

Centers for Disease Control and Prevention. The Adult Vaccine Assessment Tool. Available at https://www2a.cdc.gov/nip/adultimmsched/Adultquiz_syndicateshell.asp. Accessed August 22, 2021. Reference to specific commercial products, manufacturers, companies, or trademarks does not constitute its endorsement or recommendation by the U.S. Government, Department of Health and Human Services, or Centers for Disease Control and Prevention.[32]

In some situations, it is not possible to completely control the rapid spread of an infectious disease. For example, during the 2020 COVID-19 pandemic, the world witnessed how rapidly the COVID-19 virus spread globally, despite health education alerts. The population was advised to practice social distancing by maintaining a minimum of 6 feet at gathering, to wear face masks, and to wash hands frequently and practice good hygiene.[33] It was only after the vaccine was developed and distributed that the COVID-19 rate of daily infections began to decrease. As with other similar situations, a portion of the population declined to comply with the health education alerts and chose to rely on alternative protocols or engaged in no safety practices. Since herd immunity was not achieved, the COVID-19 virus mutated with the Delta variant. This variant mutation caused another surge of COVID-19 cases across the globe, but especially in the United States during the summer of 2021. The number of cases surpassed the first surge.

Even without a pandemic, healthcare workers learn the importance of standard safety precautions for all patient care and patient interaction.

These precautions are based on risk assessment, common sense, and use of PPE,.[34] See **Figure 7.10**.

Besides the use of PPE, healthcare facilities provided extra precautions for patients, workers, and families by placing patients in single rooms, limit visiting hours for families, reducing the number of times that patients were moved when possible, and avoiding the use of common equipment for multiple use, such as blood pressure cuffs.[35] Whenever possible, disposable equipment was used or nondisposable equipment was thoroughly cleaned and disinfected before and after each use. All facilities prioritized the cleaning and disinfecting of each room and disinfecting all equipment daily or prior to use by the next patient. Cleaning focused on all frequently touched surfaces and high traffic areas. Also, all racks for paper brochures, magazines, and health information were removed from the exam rooms to eliminate multi-touch paper surfaces.[35] See **Box 7.4**.

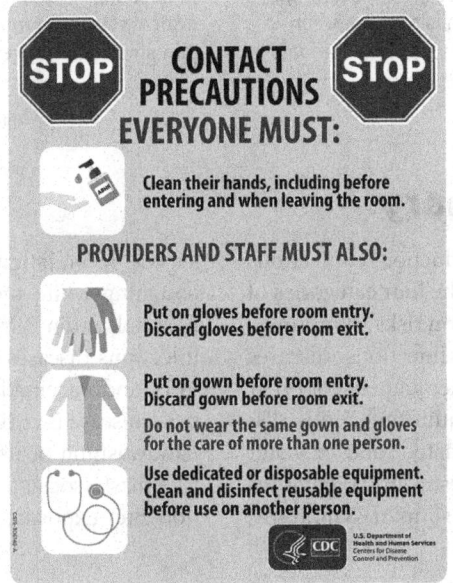

Figure 7.10 Contact Precautions Against Infectious Diseases

Figure from Centers for Disease Control and Prevention. Transmission- Based Precautions. Available at https://www.cdc.gov/infectioncontrol/pdf/contact-precautions-sign-P.pdf. Accessed August 20, 2021. Reference to specific commercial products, manufacturers, companies, or trademarks does not constitute its endorsement or recommendation by the U.S. Government, Department of Health and Human Services, or Centers for Disease Control and Prevention.[34]

Box 7.4 COVID-19 Pandemic and the Vaccines

During the 2020 COVID-19 pandemic, the entire population was urged do their part to stop the spread of the virus including wearing a face mask, washing hands frequently with warm soapy water for at least 20 seconds, using hand sanitizer frequently, maintaining at least 6 feet of distance from others while gathering as a form of social distancing, and staying in isolation if exposed to COVID-19.[36] Even with such efforts to teach and communicate these basic evidence-based public health principles and demonstrate how to decrease the spread of COVID-19, the virus continued to spread rapidly from country to country in a matter of a few months. Many hospitals were overwhelmed with COVID-19 patients for several months.[36]

Across the globe, scientists worked endless hours to build on the foundation of creating an effective vaccine for this newly emerging disease. Individuals volunteered to become study subjects to test the effectiveness of the developing vaccines.[36] By spring 2021, several vaccines were approved for use in the United States and European Union. The race to end the pandemic started as individuals began receiving the vaccine.[36] In the United States, there were many glitches along the way, including the distribution of the vaccine, long waitlists, and uneven supplies within states and across the United States as well as across other countries. As of this writing, more than 3.5 million people have died worldwide from COVID-19, and these numbers are likely conservative comparison to the true global death toll.[36]

Although many individuals were anxious to receive the vaccine, there was a segment of the U.S. adult population that chose not to receive the vaccine. Vaccination opposition is not a new concept. Starting in the early 1800s, some individuals refused to receive the smallpox vaccine.[37] They opposed the idea of injecting the cowpox for protection from smallpox. Other criticism was based on political and religious beliefs. In the 1970s, there was a wave of opposition against the DPT (diphtheria, tetanus, and pertussis) vaccine based on alleged links to neurological disorders that were considered as low risk. As a result, laws have been passed that require vaccinations for circumstances, such as specific travel destinations and school admissions.[28,37] The COVID-19 virus and its global impact showcased how human behavior plays a critical role in promoting infectious disease mitigation strategies to prevent illness or death.[28,37]

Chapter Summary

This chapter presents an introduction to infectious diseases with a discussion of the four categories of infectious diseases, transmission risks, symptoms, and prevention techniques. Infectious diseases are transmitted by insects, other animals, or other humans. It is possible to acquire infectious diseases by consuming contaminated food or water or through exposure to organisms in the environment. Infectious diseases cause mild symptoms, such as fever, fatigue, diarrhea, muscle aches, and coughing while some infectious diseases require hospitalization. Precautions and prevention of infectious diseases include food safety, the use of PPE, and vaccinations.[1] The spread of an infectious disease is reduced by frequent and thorough handwashing or use of hand sanitizer, wearing a face mask, social distancing, and practicing isolation after exposure.

CASE STUDY

Reducing the Spread of Infectious Disease

Belinda is 24 years old and single and lives in Lakeland, Florida, where she was born and raised. Her siblings, parents, and grandparents live within easy driving distance. She lives in a one-bedroom apartment. Belinda became a certified nursing assistant (CNA) during high school and has worked in the assisted living wing of a large retirement community. Belinda enjoyed getting to know the elderly residents and making friends with her coworkers.

About 6 months ago, Belinda completed her CHW training at the Pasco County Community College near her home. She applied for a CHW position and was hired by a community clinic located in the next county. After working in small assisted living facilities as a certified nurse aide, she was thrilled to be working as a CHW. Within 3 months of starting her new position, the COVID-19 pandemic hit the United States. Since the community clinic offered essential services, she was able to work. Belinda's parents and grandparents lived in the same town. However, after Belinda attended a mandatory training on PPE, she realized that her life was limited to working and returning to her apartment with no social contact. Like everyone else, she followed the CDC guidelines to keep herself and others safe. At work, she focused on her new position as much as possible. Belinda is usually an outgoing individual. It did not take long before Belinda started feeling depressed due to the isolation of the pandemic combined with the stress of the new position, living alone, and missing her family and friends. She enjoyed her new job and meeting new colleagues and patients, but she did not feel like herself. Belinda's situation was common during the COVID-19 pandemic. She reviewed her CHW textbooks books and found that new jobs may cause stress and sometimes even depression. The chapter was written before the COVID-19 pandemic, but it did mention ways to adjust to a change in jobs. Belinda tried some of the suggestions after work, such a taking a walk to get some fresh air and exercise or contacting friends and family for a phone conversation or through video capabilities. Belinda began to feel better.

Now that Belinda felt back on track with her personal life, she started to focus on her position as the only CHW at the community clinic. She was limited to the amount of patient contact she would have during the pandemic, so she decided to develop some health education materials. Since she is fluent in English and Spanish, she thought that she could start with developing some health education materials with English on one side and Spanish on the other side. However, she did not know what type of health education information was needed by the healthcare providers or by the patients. Even though the COVID-19 pandemic was raging during the summer of 2020, patients were still coming to the clinic for treatment related to other infectious diseases. Belinda has a few questions for you to answer to help with her job.

Questions

1. If you were recently hired as the first community healthcare worker in a community clinic, what activities would you begin to do?
2. Is it most important for Belinda to focus on the COVID-19 health education materials or to spread her time between COVID-19 patients and those with other infectious diseases?
3. Belinda's clinic is not conducting on-site COVID-19 testing. Where should Belinda look to find the nearest locations to her clinic?
4. Besides following the CDC guidelines, what else can Belinda do, to lower her risk of acquiring COVID-19?

References

1. Infectious diseases. Mayo Clinic Web site. https://www.mayoclinic.org/diseases-conditions/infectious-diseases/symptoms-causes/syc-20351173. Accessed July 29, 2021.
2. Different types of infectious diseases. Nanocellect Biomedical, Inc. Web site. https://nanocellect.com/blog/different-types-of-infectious-diseases/. Accessed August 2, 2021.
3. Felman A. What to know about infections. https://www.medicalnewstoday.com/articles/196271. Accessed September 1, 2021.
4. Food safety for power outages. Centers for Disease Control and Prevention Web site. https://www.cdc.gov/foodsafety/food-safety-during-a-power-outage.html. Accessed September 1, 2021.
5. About antibiotic resistance. Centers for Disease Control and Prevention Web site. https://www.cdc.gov/drugresistance/about.html. Accessed September 1, 2021.
6. 5 things to know. Centers for Disease Control and Prevention Web site. https://www.cdc.gov/drugresistance/about/5-things-to-know.html. Accessed February 1, 2022.
7. How antibiotic resistance happens. Centers for Disease Control and Prevention Web site. https://www.cdc.gov/drugresistance/about/how-resistance-happens.html. Accessed February 1, 2022.
8. How antibiotic resistance happens. Centers for Disease Control and Prevention Web site. https://www.cdc.gov/drugresistance/pdf/threats-report/How-AR-Spreads.pdf. Accessed February 1, 2022.
9. What is sepsis? Centers for Disease Control and Prevention Web site. https://www.cdc.gov/sepsis/what-is-sepsis.html. Accessed February 1, 2022.
10. Germs develop antibiotic resistance. Centers for Disease Control and Prevention Web site. https://www.cdc.gov/drugresistance/pdf/threats-report/Select-Germs-Develop-Resistance-Over-Time.pdf. Accessed February 1, 2022.
11. COVID-19 & antibiotic resistance. Centers for Disease Control and Prevention Web site. https://www.cdc.gov/drugresistance/covid19.html. Accessed February 1, 2022.
12. Seladi-Schulman J. Infections: what you need to know. https://www.healthline.com/health/infections#1. Accessed September 1, 2021.
13. Do I really need antibiotics? Centers for Disease Control and Prevention Web site. https://www.cdc.gov/antibiotic-use/graphics.html. Accessed September 1, 2021.
14. About HIV. Centers for Disease Control and Prevention Web site. https://www.cdc.gov/hiv/basics/whatishiv.html. Accessed February 1, 2022.

15. HIV 101. Centers for Disease Control and Prevention Web site. https://www.cdc.gov/hiv/pdf/library/consumer-info-sheets/cdc-hiv-consumer-info-sheet-hiv-101.pdf. Accessed February 4, 2022.

16. The state of the HIV epidemic in the U.S. Centers for Disease Control and Prevention Web site. https://www.cdc.gov/nchhstp/newsroom/fact-sheets/hiv/state-of-the-hiv-epidemic-factsheet.html. Accessed February 4, 2022.

17. Parasites, health professionals. Centers for Disease Control and Prevention Web site. https://www.cdc.gov/parasites/health_professionals.html. Accessed August 4, 2021.

18. Kinman T. Parasitic infections. Healthline Web site. https://www.healthline.com/health/parasitic-infections. Accessed August 4, 2021.

19. Healthy people 2030: infectious disease. U.S. Department of Health and Human Services, Office of Disease Prevention and Health Promotion Web site. https://health.gov/healthypeople/objectives-and-data/browse-objectives/infectious-disease. Accessed August 6, 2021.

20. Infectious diseases. Cleveland Clinic Web site. https://my.clevelandclinic.org/health/diseases/17724-infectious-diseases. Accessed August 6, 2021.

21. TB risk factors. Centers for Disease Control and Prevention Web site. https://www.cdc.gov/tb/topic/basics/risk.htm. Accessed August 11, 2021.

22. Higgins A. The deadliest infectious disease is becoming drug resistant [online]. https://www.vox.com/policy-and-politics/2018/9/28/17914344/tuberculosis-united-nations-funding-india-china. Accessed September 3, 2021.

23. Rabies. Mayo Clinic Web site. https://www.mayoclinic.org/diseases-conditions/rabies/symptoms-causes/syc-20351821#:~:text=Rabies%20is%20a%20deadly%20virus,%2C%20foxes%2C%20raccoons%20and%20skunks. Accessed August 11, 2021.

24. Boil water advisory. Centers for Disease Control and Prevention Web site. https://www.cdc.gov/healthywater/emergency/drinking/drinking-water-advisories/boil-water-advisory.html#:~:text=Boil%20water%20advisories%20usually%20include%20this%20advice%3A%201,feed%20your%20child%2C%20provide%20ready-to-use%20formula%2C%20if%20possible. Accessed August 19, 2021.

25. Four steps to food safety: clean, separate, cook, chill. Centers for Disease Control and Prevention Web site. https://www.cdc.gov/foodsafety/keep-food-safe.html. Accessed August 20, 2021.

26. How infections spread. Centers for Disease Control and Prevention Web site. https://www.cdc.gov/infectioncontrol/spread/index.html. Accessed August 20, 2021.

27. Recreational water illness. Centers for Disease Control and Prevention Web site. https://www.cdc.gov/dotw/rwis/index.html. Accessed August 20, 2021.

28. Yan QL, Tang SY, Xiao YN. Impact of individual behavior change on the spread of emerging infectious diseases. *Statistics in Medicine*.2018;37(6):948–969.

29. What is herd immunity? WebMD. https://www.webmd.com/lung/what-is-herd-immunity#1. Accessed August 22, 2021.

30. *CDC Yellow Book 2020*. Atlanta, GA: Centers for Disease Control and Prevention; 2020. Available at https://wwwnc.cdc.gov/travel/page/yellowbook-home-2020. Accessed August 22, 2021.

31. Immunization schedules. Centers for Disease Control and Prevention Web site. https://www.cdc.gov/vaccines/schedules/hcp/imz/child-adolescent.html. Accessed August 22, 2021.

32. The adult vaccine assessment tool. Centers for Disease Control and Prevention Web site. https://www2a.cdc.gov/nip/adultimmsched/Adultquiz_syndicateshell.asp. Accessed August 22, 2021.

33. Standard precautions for all patient care. Centers for Disease Control and Prevention Web site. https://www.cdc.gov/infectioncontrol/basics/standard-precautions.html. Accessed August 20, 2021.

34. Transmission-based precautions. Centers for Disease Control and Prevention Web site. https://www.cdc.gov/infectioncontrol/pdf/contact-precautions-sign-P.pdf. Accessed August 20, 2021.

35. Transmission-based precautions. Centers for Disease Control and Prevention Web site. https://www.cdc.gov/infectioncontrol/basics/transmission-based-precautions.html. Accessed August 20, 2021.

36. The true death toll of COVID-19. World Health Organization Web site. https://www.who.int/data/stories/the-true-death-toll-of-covid-19-estimating-global-excess-mortality. Accessed September 5, 2021.

37. Boulanger A. Understanding opposition to vaccines. Healthline Web site. https://www.healthline.com/health/vaccinations/opposition. Accessed September 5, 2021.

Appendix

1. An Overview of Infectious Diseases: https://www.youtube.com/watch?v=9axOFtPqS0c

2. What Is Herd Immunity? https://www.youtube.com/watch?v=8BUCi5Tuzms

Aspects of Aging

Safety for the Aging Population, Elderly, and Community Health Workers

LEARNING OBJECTIVES

1. Explain how addressing community safety is impacted by communication skills, basic need assessments, activities of daily living, falls, and home safety.
2. Describe how the signs and symptoms of elder abuse are linked to the safety and care of the elderly.
3. Describe how to prepare for natural disasters and arrange emergency plans for the elderly.
4. Describe ways that community health workers manage stress, utilize body mechanics to avoid injuries, use personal protective equipment, and resolve conflicts.

KEY TERMS

Maslow's hierarchy of needs
activities of daily living (ADLs)
instrumental activities of daily
    living (IADLs)

fall-related injuries
elder abuse
stress management
body mechanics

personal protective equipment
    (PPE)
conflict resolution

Introduction

This chapter is divided into two sections to discuss various topics of safety related to the elderly population and safety for community health workers (CHW) while on the job. Safety for the elderly begins with becoming acquainted with the elderly clients and practicing adequate communication skills, determining their basic needs, and assessing activities of daily living. Next, adverse circumstances are discussed and include information about fall prevention, home safety, elder abuse, and preparation for natural disasters and emergency planning. The second section discusses safety issues for the community health worker profession and includes stress assessments, stress management tips, proper body mechanics, use of personal protective equipment (PPE), and conflict resolution approaches.

Safety for the Elderly

Before a CHW conducts an initial interview with a new patient at intake, it is important to review the well-known psychological theory known as **Maslow's hierarchy of needs**. The hierarchy of needs is depicted as a pyramid with five levels that build upon each other. In 1943, Maslow stated that an individual's needs must be met in full at one level prior to the individual being able to progress to the next level.[1] However, over time with new research and human observation, this concept was modified to state that satisfying the *majority* of one level in the hierarchy is sufficient prior to moving to the next level. See **Figure 8.1**.

The hierarchy of needs provides a psychological overview of the complexities that surround human needs. Starting at the bottom of the pyramid, one's foundational or physiological needs include the necessities for living such as food, water, rest, and shelter.[1-2] The next level of the pyramid, which builds upon the bottom level showcasing one's basic needs, begins to address the intricacies of human psychological needs. Humans require relationships, interaction, and support structures to build personal self-esteem, experience community, and

achieve emotional security. Continuing upward, after satisfying their physiological and psychological needs, they progress toward self-fulfillment.[1] This self-fulfillment includes feelings or emotions based on sense of accomplishment, desire to achieve, creative output, and other mechanisms that motivate individuals to reach feelings of self-satisfaction. While the hierarchy of needs is a foundational concept in psychology and has wide interpretations across other disciplines, it is important to remember that this pyramid is a simplified visual representation. There are facilitators and barriers to achieving each level due to diverse circumstances and human complexities.[1-2]

For example, homeless individuals need food, water, warmth, and rest. However, they may be able to give up a little food to save money for a safe place to sleep. Individuals without proper housing have difficulty satisfying the foundational physiological needs level, thus they have difficulty promoting to the next level.[1-2] They must have a dependable amount of food, water, shelter, and safety prior to gaining adequate self-determination to seek permanent employment. This example explains why it is difficult for a homeless person to gain sustainable employment or have access to opportunities.

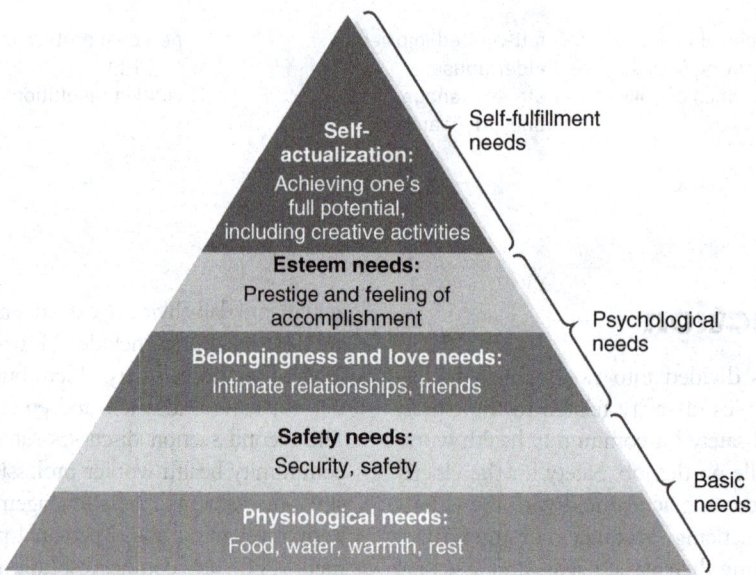

Figure 8.1 Maslow's Hierarchy of Needs

While temporary day-labor positions may offer daily cash as a quick fix, they often subtract some of the wages for transportation, lunch, and use of safety protective gear while on the job (e.g., safety goggles, hard hat, and gloves). The money left may be just enough for food and one night at the local shelter. However, these jobs are not available on a regular schedule and do not offer a sustainable future.

After understanding Maslow's hierarchy of needs, it is time for the CHW to begin reviewing communication skills, basic needs, and **activities of daily living (ADLs)**. Since a CHW is not licensed to conduct a clinical physical exam, they use their communication skills to conduct the initial interview which consists of getting to know the individuals to prepare them for a clinical work-up. This conversation is followed by identifying the individual's basic needs and their ADLs.

Communication Skills

Before meeting with a new client or patient, it is helpful to review some valuable tips for effective interviewing and communication skills.

Establish Rapport. Rapport is established if individuals feel comfortable within the surrounding environment.[3] While walking from the waiting room to the office, greet each individual, and asking if they would like to use the restroom or need to get a drink of water. These few questions allow the CHW to assess the individual's ability to hear and communicate in English. If the CHW shows a calm and professional presence, the person is more likely to be at ease.[3] Once in the office, direct patients to a comfortable chair across from the clinician or CHW. For people with a disability or using a wheelchair, the CHW should safely assist with medical devices or other mobility aids as needed. Now is a good time for the CHW to assess vision and reading by handing the individual a brochure about the services of the clinic.[3] Individuals with low vision will usually place the brochure on the desk. If the CHW noted any hearing issues while walking down the hallway, it will be necessary to speak louder and adjust the seating for closeness. If low vision is noted, more verbal cues are needed rather than brochures and paper forms.

Always sit at the same eye level and directly across from the person. Avoid sitting behind the desk or a computer screen because the distance makes it difficult for people to hear the questions. If a clipboard or tablet is used, have the questions within view, but avoid the need to look down while the patient is speaking. The focus must remain on the patient rather than writing down exact quotes from the conversation. However, casually jotting down a few notes while the person is talking is not distracting.[3] In addition, individuals with memory issues may require special attention to follow a conversation. Always be aware of your professional body language and the body language presented by patients. The goal to establishing a strong rapport is to make individuals feel comfortable, safe to express their thoughts or feelings, and elicit mutual understanding.[3] See **Box 8.1**.

Box 8.1 Communication Needs for Individuals with Memory Deficiency

Ways to enhance communication among those with cognitive difficulty or memory deficiency:

- Approach the individual from the front rather than the back to avoid startling.
- Go slowly to give the individual time to adjust to a new situation.[4]
- Sit at eye-level rather than standing over the individual.
- Give the individual space and watch for reactions or body language cues to determine their needs for space.[4]
- Say the name that the individual prefers, such as Mr. Jones or Robert. Use formal name if a preferred name is not known.[4]
- Make eye contact, display attentiveness and empathy, and listen carefully.[4]
- Be gentle with any touching or moving the patient. As individuals become more familiar with the staff and location, fear of touch or startling diminishes as the individual adjusts. This may take time, so be sure to go at the individual's pace.[4]

Data from National Institute for Occupational Safety and Health. Caring for yourself while caring for others. Cincinnati, OH: U.S. Department of Health and Human Services, Centers for Disease Control and Prevention; 2014. Available at https://www.cdc.gov/niosh/docs/2015-102/pdfs/F14_Handout_5_2015-102.pdf. Accessed September 6, 2021.[4]

Respect the Person's Privacy. Respect for privacy is essential, especially if trust and rapport are not yet established.[3] Near the end of the interview and before asking personal questions, (e.g., financial status, potential substance abuse, family violence, review of health conditions etc.), the CHW may ask if the individual would like a friend or family member to step out of the room. If the person says that the support person may stay, the interview continues.[3] Whenever another person accompanies the patient, the questions are directed to the client. The support person is not there to respond to the answers, unless the patient is unable to communicate or under the age of 18 years old.

Recognize Facial Expressions. Facial expressions often reveal how a person is feeling, particularly if the expression does not match the verbal response.[3,5] The CHW may wish to repeat the question or use different words to further clarify. The individual may not have heard or understood the question or if the individual speaks English as a second language, it may be necessary to rephrase the question or ask the support person to translate. If the person looks away or ignores a specific question, come back to that topic later. Also, discomfort, pain, some medications, and health conditions may impair a person's ability to answer a series of questions. Therefore, facial expressions can help or hinder the interviewing process. If the CHW is distracted, rushed, or looking away, the patient feels a lack of confidence and trust in providing personal information to the CHW. Thus, maintaining a safe environment is important to elicit the best responses and support patients.[5]

Use of Appropriate Body Language. Successful communication involves the use of appropriate body language combined with verbal communication.[3,6] For example, a CHW who is tapping his or her foot or sitting with crossed arms is not maintaining professionalism and is conveying disinterest to what the patient is expressing. This can cause a breach in trust between the patient and clinical staff. However, if the CHW is relaxed,

leaning forward, keeping eye contact, maintaining engagement, and nodding occasionally, the patient feels seen, supported, and cared for.[6]

Ask Open-Ended Questions. If only "yes/no" questions are asked, valuable information is missed.[3] It is more important to ask for comments, thoughts, or opinions:

- Today is the first time that you have visited this clinic. What concerns do you have?
- Tell me why you made an appointment to come to the clinic today.[3]
- What is your most troubling concern today? Any other issues for today's appointment?
- Last week, you talked about moving into another apartment. How is the move going?
- Last week, you described feeling stressed. How are you feeling today?[3]

Focus on One Topic at a Time. Ask questions one topic at a time and wait for an answer before jumping to the next question.[3] Patients may hesitate to think for a few seconds before responding. Questions should be asked in logical order so the patient can follow the conversation. If the patient is feeling ill, they may need additional time to process questions.[3] Ask the most essential questions first and avoid using any medical terminology to prevent confusion. Patients are often embarrassed to say that they did not understand the words that were used, so they will respond incorrectly with a simple yes or no response.[3,6] For example, if a CHW asks a patient if he is interested in receiving any health education materials about his COPD (chronic obstructive pulmonary disease), the patient might respond no. If he has no knowledge about COPD, he might answer no for fear of being asked further questions or might be ashamed to ask.[3]

Listen. Listening is essential to obtain accurate information.[3] Pay attention to each answer before asking the next question. People understand their medical conditions in different ways. For example, one patient may describe his level of daily activity as high because he walks to the end of the driveway to retrieve the mail, while another person describes her activity as high because she bikes six miles. As another example, the patient might use the term "bowel," but the interviewer is using the term "colon," so the patient does not respond correctly or looks puzzled. When in doubt, it is always best to ask for clarification.[3]

Culture, Language, and Geographical Location. Whenever relocating to a new geographical location, it is important take time to learn the local culture, social customs, local holidays, foods, and a few words of the language, such as a simple hello, good-bye, and thank you.

This information allows the CHW to connect with the patients and thus gain their trust.[3] In addition, the agency hiring CHWs should build a culturally competent CHW workforce by hiring workers from within the communities and environments inhabited by the individuals being served by the CHWs. Language is a critical component. Even though an individual's resume states fluent in Spanish, it is beneficial to ask what type of Spanish. For example, Spanish is different across geographical locations, such as Puerto Rico, Nicaragua, Mexico, Texas, New York City, and Spain.

Basic Needs

CHWs meet many individuals and their families within a respective community. It is important to remember that each person has a diverse background with unique needs. For example, when solving a complex problem for one family, the same solution may not resolve a similar problem for the next family due to unique desires or needs. When assessing basic needs or coordinating care, it is necessary to gain in-depth knowledge to provide adequate context to the situation. This section introduces the most common categories that possess important background information to provide context. Information about family, environment, housing, health status (physical, mental, dental, vision, and hearing), legal issues, and social history are important factors to consider addressing basic needs, solve complex problems, and assist patients and their families. These suggested questions are a guide for learning about an individual's

life story. It is essential to listen carefully to individuals' stories and acknowledge any information provided based on their lived experiences.

Before these questions are asked, the CHW needs to review the health history form that was completed prior to the clinic appointment. Individuals never wish to answer the same questions multiple times in a medical setting. These questions are meant to serve as a guide for the conversation. Individuals who mention having a complex medical history, surgical history, or a lengthy list of prescriptions should be told by the CHW that the healthcare provider will review that information them. The CHW does not review medical information because it is outside the CHW's scope of practice.

Conversation Guide
Family

Tell me about your family.

- Are you married?
- Do you have children?
- Are you a caregiver?
- Appropriate other questions.

Environment

Neighborhood

- Do you feel safe in your neighborhood? Are there streetlights and sidewalks?
- Is there public transportation?
- Is the trash collected and placed in dumpsters?

Living Conditions

- Would you like to have someone help you to clean and repairs the outside of your residence (house, rental), such as fix windows, screens, doors, and steps?
- Would you like to have someone help you to make repairs inside of your residence, such as working on plumbing or electrical repair, removing mold or mildew, spraying for insects or address any rodent infestations?
- Would you like to have someone help you keep the inside of your residence, such as clean the kitchen and bathroom or help with laundry?

Housing

- Do you live with anyone? If so, who is that person?
- If you live alone, who would you contact for an emergency or if you need care?
- Do you ever have more monthly bills than you have money to pay each bill? Are you skipping payments (e.g., rent or mortgage or utility bills) or not buying items essential items, such as food, medications, or seeking health care due to financial constraint?
- Do you feel safe at home? *Interviewer Notes: Are there signs of physical, mental, or emotional abuse?*

Legal Issues

- Have you completed your last will and testament? Is the information updated?
- Have you selected a person to be your healthcare advocate to make decisions if you are unable to make the decisions for your care?
- Have you completed your advanced directives and end of life documents?

Interviewer Notes: Check EHR for copy of advanced directives.

- Who is the person that you have chosen to take care of your affairs after you pass?

As these questions are asked, individuals reveal more details about their lives, which is an important aspect of receiving adequate, holistic health care. Additionally, details allow the CHW to better serve as the liaison between the individual, the support person, and the community clinic.

Activities of Daily Living Assessment

There are several definitions for ADLs. Some definitions are more detailed, while other definitions are general.[7] Most organizations use the five basic categories: personal hygiene, dressing, eating, maintaining continence, and transferring/mobility. In other situations, **instrumental activities of daily living (IADLs)** are used and include basic communication skills, transportation, meal preparation, shopping, housework, managing medications, and managing personal finances.[7] As functional IADLs decrease, it is often easier to determine the level of assistance needed.[7] See **Table 8.1**.

Table 8.1 Assessment for ADLs/IADLs

Activities of Instrumental and Daily Living 1= Requires No Assistance; 2= Some Assistance Needed; 3= Complete Assistance Needed		
	Assessment	**Comments**
Bathing		
Climbing stairs		
Communication: talking, expressing feelings, and needs		
Cooking/meal preparation		
Dressing		
Eating and drinking		
Financial management		
Grooming/hygiene		

(continues)

Table 8.1 Assessment for ADLs/IADLs *(continued)*

	Assessment		Comments
Health stability practices: scheduling appointments, stable weight, exercise, vision, and hearing			
Housing stability: cleans, organizes possessions, follows rules of neighborhood			
Laundry			
Legal management			
Oral care			
Medication management			
Phone usage			
Safety: decisions, stove, knives, matches			
Shopping			
Social engagement			
Time management: regular schedule, scheduled activities			
Toileting and hygiene			
Transferring: sitting, standing, using walker, wheelchair, or other mobility aid			
Transportation: driving, bus schedules, taxis			
Walking: inside and outside			
Other			
Totals			

Data from Paying for Senior Care. Activities of daily living checklist & assessments. Available at https://www.payingforseniorcare.com/activities-of-daily-living. Accessed September 8, 2021.[7]

Adverse Circumstances

After getting acquainted with a new patient or client, it is time to discuss some of the common adverse circumstances that impact the aging or elderly population. These circumstances include fall prevention, home safety, signs of elder abuse or mistreatment, preparation for natural disasters, and proper emergency planning.

Fall Prevention

The aging population is vulnerable to **fall-related injuries**. Currently, falls represent the leading cause of injury related deaths among individuals aged 65 years and older.[8] Based on national reports from 2007–2016, fatal falls increased approximately 30 percent each year among older individuals.[8] Every year, one out of four people aged 65 years and older fall.[9] However, these estimates are likely conservative due to underreporting and individuals not disclosing their fall to healthcare providers.[9,13] However, for the aging population, falling once doubles one's chance of losing balance and falling again.[10] Fortunately, many times falls do not cause severe injuries. However, one out of five falls causes a serious injury, defined by broken bones and significant head injuries.[11–12] Head injuries may be serious, especially if the individual is taking blood thinner medications. When a fall involves a head injury, the individual must be evaluated by a physician immediately because falling is the most common cause of traumatic brain injuries (TBIs).[13] Once individuals fall, with or without an injury, they become afraid of falling again. Fear of falling again causes one to become less active, which results in physical weakness, thereby increasing the chance of another fall due to deconditioned muscles, gait issues, and balance-related concerns.[13]

Addressing fall prevention strategies continues to be an important aspect of addressing home and recreational safety concerns and lowering the risk of falling.[10–14] Falls contribute to hospitalizations, increase healthcare costs, cause further injuries, and trigger anxiety related to fears of falling again.[11] Therefore, it is crucial to implement strategies to make communities and homes safer for the aging population to prevent the increase of fall-related deaths and injuries.[13–14] See **Figure 8.2**.

According to the National Institute of Aging, falls can be easily avoided several ways:

Physical Activity. Participate in an exercise program that includes mild weight-bearing activities to strengthen bone density, muscle strength, and balance.[15]

Vision and Hearing. Maintain annual vision and hearing examinations to detect slight changes. Always wear prescribed eyeglasses and hearing aids.[15]

Medication Side Effects. Ask the physician and pharmacist about the side effects of all medications, especially any that cause sleepiness or dizziness.[15]

Adequate Sleep. Quality and quantity of sleep is essential. Adequate sleep is more than time spent in bed. Asking for a sleep apnea assessment is ideal for improving sleep quality.[15]

Limit Amount of Alcohol. Small amounts of alcohol consumption can affect an individual's balance and reaction time. Additionally, be mindful of how alcohol consumption can interfere with medication.[15]

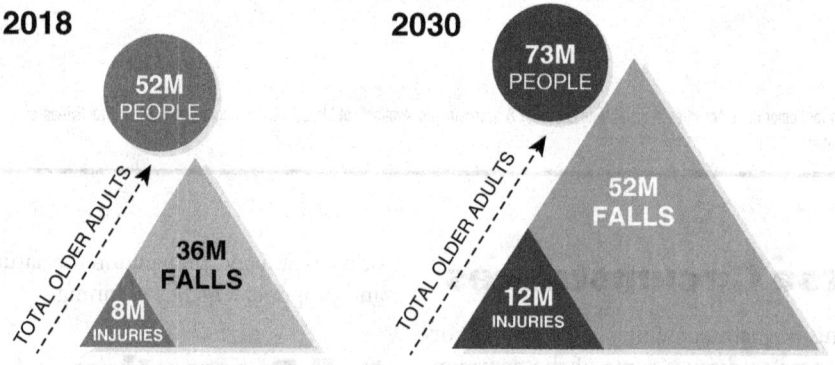

Figure 8.2 Rate of Falls

Figure from Centers for Disease Control and Prevention. Preventing falls: A guide to implementing effective community- based fall prevention programs. Available at https://www.cdc.gov/homeandrecreationalsafety/falls/community_preventfalls.html.Accessed September 8, 2021. Reference to specific commercial products, manufacturers, companies, or trademarks does not constitute its endorsement or recommendation by the U.S. Government, Department of Health and Human Services, or Centers for Disease Control and Prevention.[13]

Stand Up Slowly. When individuals stand up too quickly, their blood pressure drops and can make them feel light-headed, which might cause a fall.[15]

Use of Canes, Walkers or Other Mobility Aids. When individuals are advised by their healthcare provider to use a cane or a walker, a few sessions of proper training with a physical therapist can be useful.[15]

Walking on Wet or Icy Surfaces. Slippery surfaces are a common source of falls. Prepare to spread sand or salt on ice prior to walking on the surface. Avoid dangerous public surfaces while walking alone.[15]

Wearing Appropriate Shoes. Do not walk on floors and stairs while wearing only socks or smooth sole slippers. The best footwear includes nonskid soles, low heels, or laced shoes that support the feet. Adequate footwear is important to prevent falls.[15]

Alert Healthcare Provider After a Fall. Healthcare providers who are notified about a fall may adjust medications, check vision, suggest physical therapy, add walking or other mobility aids, or advise a home health check to prevent future falls.[15]

Home Safety

Numerous objects within the home can be hazardous. At times, common household items are often overlooked but must be considered when determining adequate home safety. For example, adhering to proper oxygen safety is crucial because oxygen containers present numerous household hazards if not correctly stored.

Oxygen Safety. When compressed oxygen is used for medical conditions, it is important that the individual and family realize the dangers and risks of the oxygen causing a fire.[16] Oxygen tanks should be kept 5 feet away from open flames or heaters,

such as candles or hot water heaters. Do not use anything flammable, such as cleaning fluids, gasoline, or aerosol sprays near your oxygen. Do not let anyone smoke in the house or near the oxygen. Do not drink alcohol when using oxygen.[16]

- Keep a fire extinguisher and a phone close by in case of a fire.[16]
- Be sure to notify the fire department that oxygen canisters are within the home when or if they are called. Also, notify the electric company that there is medical equipment in use at the address. The company will add the address to the priority list in the event of a power outage.[16]
- Always keep a backup oxygen tank that does not need electricity in case of a power failure. Call 911 if symptoms occur, such as sudden chest pain, pain when inhaling, tired, confused, inability to think clearly, blue lips and fingernails, or feeling anxious.[16]

Fire Safety. Reminders about fire safety are important for older adults. Here are a few suggestions from the National Fire Protection Association.[17]

- Make sure that smoke alarms are installed in all sleeping areas. If the person is living in a high-rise building, ensure that proper fire alarms and sprinklers are installed and working properly.[17]
- Keep a telephone near sleeping areas in case of an emergency. When calling 911, stay on the phone until emergency personnel arrive.[17]
- If one person in the home is unable to escape due to physical or medical issues, have a plan in place to help them with a designated person and a backup person.[17]
- Make sure that all doors and windows open easily. If windows have security bars, install easy release levers on the inside. If windows are painted or nailed shut, make the necessary repairs to remove the appropriate seals to open windows.[17]

Poison Safety and Control. Approximately 83 percent of older adults take at least one prescription drug, and 50 percent take three or more medications.[18] Of the children treated for medication poisoning, 38 percent accidentally consumed their grandparent's medicine.[19–20] It is important to follow these prevention tips to keep children safe from hazardous items:

- Keep medicines stored away and out of reach of visitors, children, and older adults with dementia.[20]
- Never take medications in a dark room. Always have adequate lighting to read prescriptions labels to prevent taking the wrong medication.[20]
- Use glasses, contact lenses, or a magnifying glass when taking medications to ensure accurate dosing and safety precautions.[20]
- Ask the pharmacist any questions regarding the prescribed medications or use of over-the-counter products to prevent any medication interactions or adverse side effects.[20]
- If an individual has low vision, impaired hearing, or speaks English as a second language, another person should verify understanding the medication (i.e., dose, purpose, side effects, and frequency of use) for extra precaution.[20]
- Store all personal care items (e.g., medications, soap, sunscreen, hair products) separately from household products (e.g., cleaning products, insect repellent, detergents, laundry pods). Also, separate topical

ointments from oral products to avoid misplacement or confusion.[20] See **Figure 8.3**.

Disposal of Sharps and Contaminated Products:. In many homes, individuals use "sharps" which commonly include medical needles, finger stick lancets, or syringes to treat their medical conditions (e.g., insulin administration, glucose testing strips, or injectable prescriptions).[21–22] It is important to teach the individual and caregivers the proper way to dispose of these home-generated medical sharp items. If the CHW is stuck unintentionally with someone else's needle, it is important to act promptly.[21] See **Figure 8.4**.

The Universal Recycling Law allows people to reuse rigid plastic bottles to dispose of their home-generated sharps.[22] To be safe and legal, dispose of home-generated sharps, needles, and syringes in this manner:

- Place sharps in an empty, rigid plastic container, such as a laundry detergent bottle.[22]
- Tape the bottle's cap shut with strong tape. Firmly attach a "Do Not Recycle" label to the bottle. Please see the sample label here: https://dec.vermont.gov/sites/dec/files/wmp /SolidWaste/Documents/Sharps-container -label-example.pdf.[22]
- Dispose of the bottle in the trash.[22] See **Figure 8.5**.

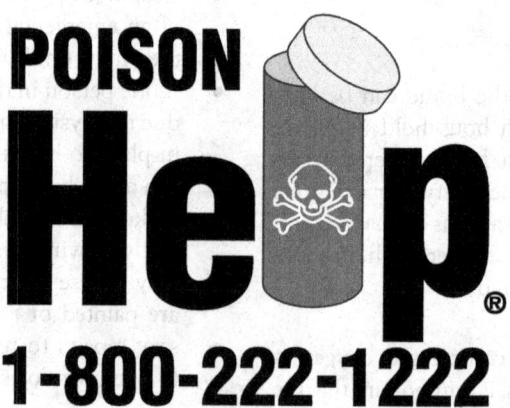

Figure 8.3 Poison Control Information

Centers for Disease Control and Prevention. Tips to Prevent Poisonings. Available at https://www.cdc.gov/homeandrecreationalsafety/poisoning/preventiontips.htm. Accessed September 8, 2021. Reference to specific commercial products, manufacturers, companies, or trademarks does not constitute its endorsement or recommendation by the U.S. Government, Department of Health and Human Services, or Centers for Disease Control and Prevention[18]

What to do if you experience a needlestick injury

If you experienced a needlestick injury or were exposed to the blood or other body fluid of a patient during the course of your work, **immediately follow these steps:**

* Wash needlesticks and cuts with soap and water
* Flush splashes to the nose, mouth, or skin with water
* Irrigate eyes with clean water, saline, or sterile irrigants
* Report the incident to your supervisor
* Immediately seek medical treatment

Figure 8.4 Unintentional Needle Stick with Someone Else's Needle

Centers for Disease Control and Prevention. (2021). Needlestick Injuries are Preventable. Retrieved from https://www.cdc.gov/niosh/newsroom/feature/needlestick_disposal.html. Reference to specific commercial products, manufacturers, companies, or trademarks does not constitute its endorsement or recommendation by the U.S. Government, Department of Health and Human Services, or Centers for Disease Control and Prevention.

WARNING: SYRINGES

DO *NOT* RECYCLE

KEEP OUT OF REACH OF CHILDREN!

LABEL: Apply label to a rigid plastic container with a screw-on lid, such as a laundry detergent bottle. Bottles stamped with ⚠2 on the bottom are best. **DO NOT USE SODA BOTTLES OR ANY OTHER THIN PLASTIC CONTAINER:** Needles can puncture them.

STORE: Carefully put each of your used syringes into the bottle.

SEAL: When bottle is 2/3 full, put heavy tape over the screw-on bottle cap for disposal.

DISPOSE: Dispose of the bottle in your household trash—**NOT in your recycling bin!**

Figure 8.5 Safe Disposal of Sharps

Reproduced from Agency of Natural Resources Department of Environmental Conservation. Warning: Syringes. Available at https://dec.vermont.gov/sites/dec/files/wmp/SolidWaste/Documents/Sharps-container-label-example.pdf. Accessed September 12, 2021.[23]

Signs of Elder Abuse

Abuse of an older person can happen by a loved one, a hired caregiver, or a stranger. Abuse can happen at home, at a relative's home, or in an eldercare facility. There are many types of abuse, including physical, emotional, sexual, abandonment, financial, and neglect.[24] See **Figure 8.6**.

At times, family members do not live close to their elder parents or close relatives. However, they wish to ensure that the elderly relatives are taken care of properly; this concept is labelled as "spotting abuse from afar."[25] In some situations, the afar family member can call the elderly person on a regular basis and take note of any subtle changes, such as mood changes. It is also useful to identify nearby friends or neighbors who can stop by unannounced to serve as the eyes and ears of the distant relative or hire a geriatric care manager to oversee the care.[25] Even though these long-distance solutions attempt to avoid elder abuse, family members need to remain vigilant to ensure quality of care for their older family member.

Elder abuse can occur in any setting and at any socioeconomic level.[24] Abuse may include many forms, including domestic violence, emotional abuse, financial abuse, theft, and neglect.[24–25] The abuser may be a hired caregiver or someone familiar. Keep in mind that for each elder abuse case reported, 23 cases are not reported.[26] The stress of caregiving can take a toll on adult children caring for aging parents or an older person who is caring for an aging spouse or sibling. In some families, abuse may continue due to long-standing family patterns. In other cases, the older

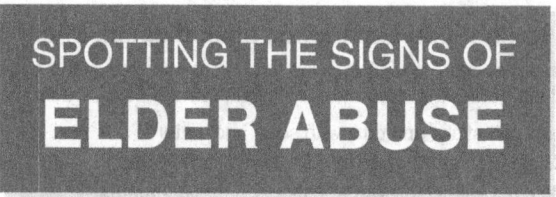

SPOTTING THE SIGNS OF
ELDER ABUSE

Abuse can happen to any older person, by a loved one, a hired caregiver, or a stranger. Abuse can happen at home, at a relative's home, or in an eldercare facility.

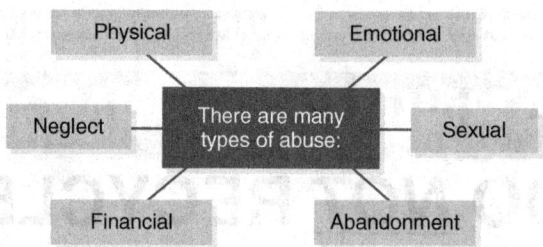

Figure 8.6 Spotting the Signs of Elder Abuse

National Institute of Health, National Institute on Aging. Spotting the Signs of Elder Abuse. Available at https://www.nia.nih.gov/health/infographics/spotting-signs-elder-abuse. Accessed September 12, 2021.[24]

adult's need for constant care can cause a caregiver to lash out verbally or physically.[24–25] Additionally, in the middle to late stages of Alzheimer's disease, the older adult may become difficult to manage and physically aggressive, causing harm to the caregiver. In this situation, the caregiver may respond with anger perhaps out of frustration and exhaustion.[24–25] See **Box 8.2**.

Last, as a CHW, it is your obligation to notify your supervisor immediately if you ever suspect elder abuse. *It is not within your job description to report elder abuse.* The legal side of elder abuse is beyond the scope of this chapter. However, mandated reporting is defined as reporting abuse of older adults and adults with disabilities, and it is generally the legal requirement of a specific profession to report suspected abuse, neglect, and/or exploitation of a person meeting the state's definitions of an adult eligible for special protection under the law.[27] Your employer knows the laws for your state. State laws include and define (1) who is mandated to report, (2) what situations they are required to report on, (3) when they are required to report, and (4) to whom they are required to report.[27] Mandated reporting laws

> **Box 8.2** Watch for These Signs of Elder Abuse
>
> As a CHW, it is important to watch for these signs of elder abuse:
>
> - Seems depressed, confused, or withdrawn[25]
> - Isolated from friends and family
> - Has unexplained bruises, burns, or scars
> - Appears dirty, underfed, dehydrated, overmedicated or undermedicated, or not receiving needed care for medical problems
> - Has bed sores or other preventable conditions
> - Recent changes in banking or spending patterns
>
> Talk with the older adult and then contact the local adult protective services, long-term care ombudsman, or the police.[24]
>
> National Institute of Health, National Institute on Aging. Spotting the Signs of Elder Abuse. Available at https://www.nia.nih.gov/health/infographics/spotting-signs-elder-abuse. Accessed September 12, 2021.[24]

vary greatly across states and there are no federal laws defining abuse of older adults and persons with disabilities.[27]

Preparation for Natural Disaster and Emergency Plans

All types of natural disasters, such as hurricanes, fires, floods, heat waves, and heavy snow fall, place the entire population in the path at risk.[28] Elderly individuals and other vulnerable persons often have trouble preparing for a disaster due to a lack of ability to plan, secure financial resources, isolation, problems with mobility, lack of transportation, and various other circumstances.[28] See **Box 8.3**.

Box 8.3 The Medical Reserve Corps

The Medical Reserve Corps (MRC) is a national network of more than 200,000 volunteers, organized locally to improve the health and safety of their communities. Become a part of the MRC, a national network of volunteer medical professionals, public health experts, and others who help in their communities during disasters and every day. MRC volunteers also promote preparedness in their communities to improve everyday health, reducing potential public health risks and vulnerabilities.

What would I do as a volunteer?
MRC volunteers train to improve their skills, knowledge, and abilities. Sometimes the training is coursework, and other times it is part of a drill or exercise conducted with partner organizations in the community. Continuing education units and credits are even available for some programs.

What do nonclinical individuals do as an MRC volunteer?
Many MRC volunteers assist with activities to improve public health, including increasing health literacy, supporting prevention efforts, and eliminating health disparities.

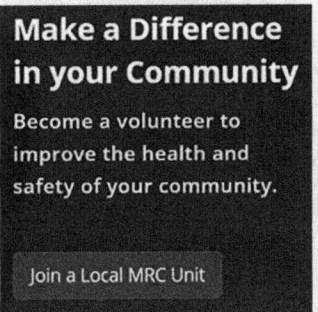

Make a Difference in your Community

Become a volunteer to improve the health and safety of your community.

Join a Local MRC Unit

Assistant Secretary for Preparedness and Response, U.S. Department of Health and Human Services. The Medical Reserve Corps. Available at https://aspr.hhs.gov/MRC/Pages/index.aspx. Accessed February 6, 2022.

Once I become an MRC volunteer, what happens if I am not available all the time?
Volunteer availability is discussed during the MRC volunteer application process. Some volunteers may only be interested in a minimal commitment during times of crisis or for other specific community needs. These preferences are respected. Different people have different amounts of time to give. Local MRC unit coordinators match community needs for emergency medical response and public health initiatives with volunteer capabilities.

I am interested in becoming an MRC volunteer. What do I do first?
The first step in becoming an MRC volunteer is to locate the closest MRC unit to you. Access the list of registered MRC units by visiting: https://geohealth.hhs.gov/arcgis/apps/opsdashboard/index.html#/7570dde7406d4c4abb65ea9be132d5ae to find contact information.[29] Then, contact the local unit coordinator to find out more about volunteer opportunities in your community and the local registration process.

Data from Assistant Secretary for Preparedness and Response, U.S. Department of Health and Human Services. The Medical Reserve Corps. Available at https://aspr.hhs.gov/MRC/Pages/index.aspx. Accessed February 6, 2022.[30]

CHWs are a valuable resource before, during, and after the natural disaster occurs. They are aware of the resources in the local and extended community. Many times, family and friends are willing to assist the elderly, but due to their own situation, they may not be able to actually lend a hand.[28] In such circumstances, the community must depend on the resources available, such as a senior support network. For example, one essential service is transportation for recommended or mandatory evacuation to designated community shelters.

For everyone, but especially for seniors, planning is essential.[28] The time to start planning is months before the disaster is pending. For example, if the geographical location is annually threatened by heavy snowfall, flooding, fires, tornadoes, or hurricanes, emergency planning should become a standard precaution prior to the season.[28] If people wait until the serious weather condition is approaching within a few days, there is limited time to adequately plan, purchase supplies, fill the car with gas, obtain cash, secure important documentation, find shelter, buy groceries and water, and pick-up medications. See **Table 8.2** for questions to consider when planning for potentially dangerous weather condition.[28]

Table 8.2 Questions When Planning for a Potential Natural Disaster

Questions	Yes	No	Not Sure	Comments
Evacuation to Shelters				
Are there likely to be shelters nearby?				
What are the best routes to access shelters?				
Is the elderly individual living in the household able to evacuate without assistance?				
Does someone in the household have a car in good working condition and can drive?				
Can everyone in the household fit in the car, if needed?				
Are there emergency transportation options available?				
Are the individuals able to access cash, such as cashing a check or using an ATM, prior to evacuation?				
Does the individual have family or friends in the same town or across the country in which to stay in touch with daily? Let them know if the plan is to evacuate or shelter in place.				
Has the individual evacuating made a hardcopy list of important contact names (e.g., healthcare providers, pharmacy, family, and friends), phone numbers, and emails in case phone charging becomes unavailable?				

(continues)

Table 8.2 **Questions When Planning for a Potential Natural Disaster** *(continued)*

Questions	Yes	No	Not Sure	Comments
Is there a designated person or community agency that has a list of elderly individuals that would need services when evacuating for a pending disaster?				
Sheltering in Place at Home				
What supplies should be in the house or on hand if it is necessary to leave on short notice?				
Is the home in adequate condition with routine maintenance and capable of withstanding the storm?				
What are the specific risks that individuals might face at home, such as collapsed power lines or power outages, falling trees, closed roads due to flooding, and heavy traffic on evacuation routes?				
What medical needs are required on a regular basis, such as medications, electricity/generator to charge medical equipment (e.g., breathing machines, power wheelchair, refrigeration for medication), daily supplies (e.g., adult diapers, protein drinks, feeding tube supplies, diabetic supplies)?				
Do the individuals living in the household depend on volunteers or government agencies for meal delivery or other services, such as taking an individual to dialysis, cancer treatment appointments, or wound care management appointments?				
Do the individuals living in the household have the capacity to be aware of local weather reports or severity of the pending weather conditions, such as access to television, radio, or internet?				
Does the individual have family or friends in the same town or across the country to stay in touch with daily? Let them know if the plan is to evacuate or shelter in place.				
Has the individual staying at home made a hardcopy list of important contact names (e.g., healthcare provider, pharmacy, family, and friends), phone numbers, and emails in case phone charging becomes unavailable?				

(continues)

Table 8.2 Questions When Planning for a Potential Natural Disaster *(continued)*

Questions	Yes	No	Not Sure	Comments
Is there a designated person or community agency that has a list of elderly individuals that would need services at home for a pending disaster?				
For the elderly living in senior housing, additional questions to should be asked:				
Does the facility have sufficient water, food, and supplies for each resident for at least 2 weeks?				
Does the facility have transportation to evacuate residents, if necessary?				
Have arrangements been made to shelter residents in a safe location, if needed?				
What are the plans for trained staff to stay with residents sheltering in place or evacuating to a shelter?				

Data from Aging.com. Disaster Preparedness: A Complete Guide for Seniors. Available at https://aging.com/disaster-preparedness-for-seniors/. Accessed September 12, 2021.[28]

Building a Disaster Kit

1. Basic Disaster Kit Items

The basic kit includes the minimum supplies for 3 or 4 days:

> Water: one gallon per person per day
> Flashlight with extra batteries
> Food: canned food including can opener and utensils
> Radio with extra batteries
> First-aid kit with up-to-date supplies and equipment

All supplies except for water should be stored in a dedicated container to take for a quick evacuation.[28] See **Figure 8.7**.

Items for Seniors or Individuals with Medical Conditions

In addition to the standard recommendations for a preparedness kit, personal kits should include the following:

- Medications: Ask your healthcare provider or pharmacist for an additional supply of prescription and over-the-counter medications for emergency kit. Be sure to rotate the medications in the kit so that the medications do not expire.[28]
- Medical equipment: Charger for hearing aids or batteries, extra pair of glasses (if available), equipment for monitoring blood sugar or blood pressure.[28]
- Medical documents: Documents stating basic medical information, current treatment plan, such as dialysis and cancer treatment, use of medical equipment, list of prescriptions and dosage, healthcare provider contact information, and copies of your insurance cards, such Medicare, Medicaid, or others.[28]

The basic kit allows survival for a few days, but additional items provide comfort beyond the basics:

- Personal care items, like toothbrushes, soap, shampoo, and other toiletries[28]
- Extra clothing and shoes

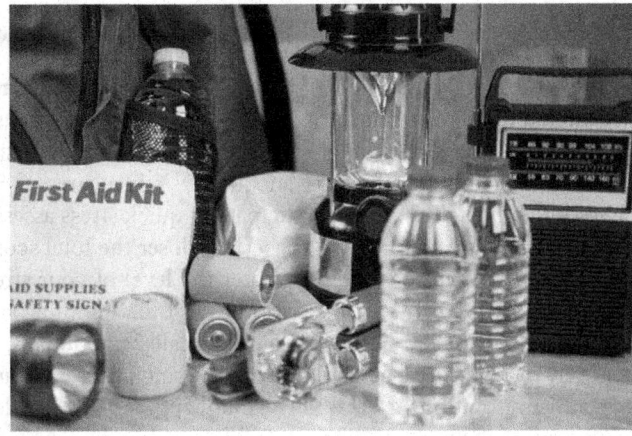

Figure 8.7 Basic Disaster Kit

© Fstop123/iStock/Getty Images Plus/Getty Images.

- Blankets or sleeping bags
- Rain gear
- Light sticks[28]

It is important to note that many of the additional items are likely to be necessary. These items should be packed and placed in the same location as the basic kit. There will not be time to run around the house grabbing items if the evacuation is immediate, such as in the case of a fire.[28]

2. Documents

In addition to the supply kit, it is important to assemble and prepare important documents in advance of a disaster. Make photocopies of personal identification documents (e.g., driver's license and passport) and put all documents into a waterproof bag and place it inside of the basic kit.[28] Other documents, such as legal, insurance, and financial records may be scanned and uploaded to a computer or kept on a smartphone device, placed in a security deposit box, or kept in a safe.[28] In the event of an emergency, these documents should be stored in one location for easy access. Then while preparing, place all files and documents in a resealable waterproof bag before adding to the basic kit. Annually, it is valuable for individuals to take pictures or videos of their belongings, inside rooms, and outside of

their dwelling for insurance companies.[28] These photos should be stored in a safe location (e.g., security deposit box or safe) or mailed to the insurance company. This action takes too long if a storm is pending. In that case, a few quick photos will be useful.[28] Lastly, any individual can save hours of time after a disaster by establishing direct deposits for any or all benefits, such as Social Security, disability benefits, or a pension. This task allows the individual to access money regardless of location.[28]

3. Service Animals and Pets

Documents for service animals needs to be included in the basic kit.[28] For all pets, documents of their immunization records are an essential component to include in the basic kit. This information is also often required for boarding or entry into a shelter location.[28]

Lastly, hurricanes, wildfires, earthquakes, and other natural disaster are alarming. For older adults, these events are dangerous. But with adequate planning, older adults can be prepared for such weather conditions. This preparation takes help from family, friends, and a community support effort to engage in taking care of the elderly during serious weather conditions, so no one is caught off guard and vulnerable community members receive adequate help.[28]

Safety for CHWs

Recognizing the importance of safety for CHW is essential. Safety is not limited to the individual whom the CHW is caring for. Rather ensuring CHWs feel comfortable and safe within their community work role is fundamental to their emotional, spiritual, physical, and mental wellness while on the job. This section introduces how stress management allows CHWs to remain safe and healthy in their lives and on the job along with maintaining proper body mechanics, reviewing PPE, and providing conflict resolution.

Stress Management

When exploring **stress management**, it is useful to identify what causes stress, how stress impacts health, and what strategies are useful to adequately reduce stress.[31] See **Table 8.3** to participate in quick stress assessment.

The closer the total score is to 50 points, the greater the level of your stress.[31] As a CHW, it is important to be mindful of how stress can affect you physically, emotionally, and behaviorally. See **Table 8.4** and see if you can identify with any of the following stress effect identifiers.

Table 8.3 How Stressed Do You Get When

	1 = Not at all	2 = A bit	3 = Some	4 = Quite a bit	5 = Very much	Score
1. Your assignment includes more tasks than you can get done in the amount of time that you have.						
2. You are working despite aches and pains.						
3. You are working too many hours.						
4. You are experiencing tensions and trouble at home.						
5. You work unpaid time to take care of all your client's needs.						
6. The neighborhood feels unsafe to you.						
7. Some aspect of your life has fallen through (your car breaks down or your kids or loved ones get sick) and you cannot get to work on time or at all.						
8. You are worried how things are going with your supervisor.						
9. You are short the money you need to pay bills.						

(continues)

Table 8.3 How Stressed Do You Get When

(continued)

	1 = Not at all	2 = A bit	3 = Some	4 = Quite a bit	5 = Very much	Score
10. You shared your personal problems with a client and now you are nervous.						
					Total score:	

National Institute for Occupational Safety and Health. Caring for yourself while caring for others: Module 6: Tips for Setting Healthy and Safe Boundaries to Reduce Stress. Cincinnati, OH: U.S. Department of Health and Human Services, Centers for Disease Control and Prevention; 2014. Available at https://www.cdc.gov/niosh/docs/2015-102/pdfs/F14_Handout_6_2015-102.pdf. Accessed September 14, 2021.[31]

Table 8.4 The Effects of Stress

How stress affects...		
Body	**Emotions**	**Behavior**
Get headaches more often	Obsessively think about worries and concerns	Not want to do the things that you used to enjoy
Have low energy and feel fatigued	Feel sad and depressed	Have difficulty sleeping
Become sick more often	Feel anger	Eat too much or too little
Have back and chest pain	Feel anxious and tense	Increased use of alcohol, tobacco, or drugs
Have higher risks of heart disease or hypertension	Feel burned out and having difficulty concentrating	Feel angry or tense toward others
Have low immunity against diseases	Feel insecure and uncomfortable around others	Have fewer positive interactions, leading to relationship problems
Have a frequent upset stomach	Feel irritable and restless	Complain about personal problems too often, putting stress on others

National Institute for Occupational Safety and Health. Caring for yourself while caring for others: Module 6: Tips for Setting Healthy and Safe Boundaries to Reduce Stress. Cincinnati, OH: U.S. Department of Health and Human Services, Centers for Disease Control and Prevention; 2014. Available at https://www.cdc.gov/niosh/docs/2015-102/pdfs/F14_Handout_6_2015-102.pdf. Accessed September 14, 2021.[31]

After determining how stress affects health, it is time to explore ways to lower stress in daily activities. See **Table 8.5**.

Body Mechanics

Generally, lifting heavy equipment or assisting individuals while transferring from a wheelchair to a car or chair is not common in the CHW scope of practice. However, such a request may be made occasionally at their place of employment or while working in the community. Therefore, it is important to know proper body mechanics for safety and to avoid injuries while performing daily activities on the job.[33] **Body mechanics** are defined as ways to move oneself or perform daily activities with ease and without sustaining

Table 8.5 Ways to Lower Stress

1. Reprioritize daily actions and focus on accomplishing the most important activities.
2. Express feelings and confide in a trusted person.
3. Organize time to eliminate procrastination. Do things a bit at a time to avoid burnout.
4. Relax and take time to enjoy a book, a movie, or to be alone.
5. Try to maintain adequate sleep, a minimum of 8 hours per day.
6. Stay active and exercise on a regular basis.
7. Learn to say no for relief from unnecessary burdens.
9. Eat healthy and nutritious food. Do not skip meals. Focus on drinking water rather than high calorie drinks.
10. Avoid alcohol, drugs, and caffeine.
11. Stay up to date with receiving recommended vaccines, such as annual flu vaccines.
12. Take time to laugh and find enjoyment in life and relationships.

Data from The Calculator. Stress Management Test. Available at https://www.thecalculator.co/personality/Stress-Management-Test-626.html. Accessed September 14, 2021.[32]

injuries.[33] When moving a heavy object, utilizing proper body mechanics involves three steps. See **Box 8.4**.

Additional suggestions for proper body mechanics include wearing appropriate shoes with low heels, shoes with closed backs, and nonslip soles to prevent falling.[33] Additionally, to maintain proper body alignment, remember to pull a heavy object instead of pushing the object.[33] This will

Box 8.4 Body Mechanics for Moving a Heavy Object and Body Mechanics for Sitting

To protect yourself while moving a heavy object remember the following:

1. The back, neck, pelvis, and feet must align when lifting a heavy object. Never twist or bend at the waist. Always bend at the hips and knees. This alignment maintains balance by dividing the weight evenly between the upper and lower body.
2. Feet should be flat on the floor and about 12 inches or shoulder width apart to maintain side to side balance. One foot should be slightly in front of the other foot.
3. Lift the object using arm and leg muscles. Hold the object close to the body at waist level. Use the same process if there is a need to push or pull a heavy object. Use leg muscles when lifting, and squat rather than bend forward to lift an object to protect the lower back.

When sitting, remember the following body mechanic tips:

1. Sit with a straight back and place extra support behind the lower back.
2. Get up and change positions often when sitting for long periods of time.
3. Ask about exercises to stretch neck and shoulder muscles.
4. Adjust the computer so the top of the monitor is at eye level.
5. Use a paper holder so that documents are at the same level as the computer screen to avoid neck strain due to repetitive movement.
6. Use a headset if talking on the phone frequently or for long periods of time.

Drugs.com. Proper Body Mechanics. Available at https://www.drugs.com/cg/proper-body-mechanics.html. Accessed September 14, 2021.[33]

help reduce the risk of straining the back muscles. Ask for help when moving heavy objects or when transferring patients. When available, use moving devices or equipment to assist and reduce injury.[33]

Personal Protective Equipment

For CHWs, **personal protective equipment (PPE)** is mostly focused on face masks and gloves. First, face masks protect against inhaling various viruses, germs, and bacteria into the respiratory system. After looking at **Figure 8.8**, it is easier to determine why the face mask provides a protective barrier when worn correctly. **Figure 8.9** shows how to properly put on a face mask and remove the face mask safely.

Second, gloves are worn to protect the fingers and hands from becoming contaminated with viruses, germs, and bacteria.[36] However, it is not possible to put on a clean pair of gloves each time a different surface is touched. Therefore, since everyone touches hundreds of surfaces daily, including when using the restroom, it is essential to frequently wash your hands for 20 seconds with soap and warm water and use hand sanitizer frequently.[36] Always avoid touching your face, nose, eyes, and ears prior to hand washing. If gloves are worn, there are proper ways to put on and take off gloves. Review the following steps:

Step 1: Wash (and dry) your hands before touching the gloves.[36] Because bacteria multiply in moist environments underneath gloves, it is important to dry your hands thoroughly before putting on gloves.[36]

Step 2: Put the gloves on slowly to avoid holes or rips.[36]

Step 3: Avoid touching your face while wearing gloves. Remember that the gloves become contaminated during use.[36]

Step 4: Remove your gloves carefully and without touching the outside of the gloves. This action is completed by pinching one from the outside with one gloved hand, then use your clean hand to reach inside the glove to remove the other one.[36]

Step 5: Place the used gloves into a proper receptacle. Never throw the gloves into a hospital or facility laundry bin. Always wash your hands after disposing of the used gloves.[36]

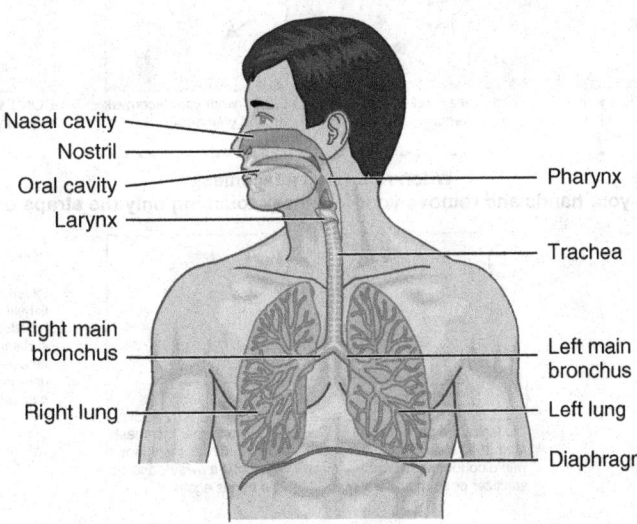

Figure 8.8 Human Respiratory System

Reproduced from Oregon State University. 22.1 Organs and Structures of the Respiratory System. Available at https://open.oregonstate.education/aandp/chapter/22-1-organs-and-structures-of-the-respiratory-system/. Accessed September 14, 2021.[34]

Facemask do's and don'ts
for healthcare personnel

When putting on a facemask
Clean your hands and put on your facemask so it fully covers your mouth and nose.

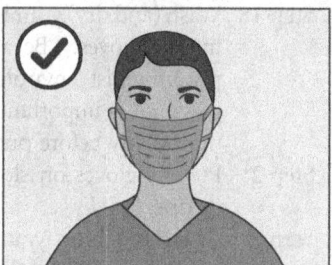

DO secure the elastic bands around your ears.

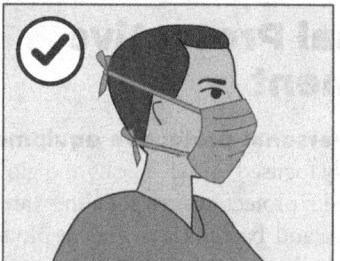

DO secure the ties at the middle of your head and the base of your head.

When wearing a facemask, don't do the following:

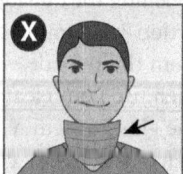

DON'T wear your facemask under your nose or mouth.

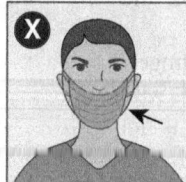

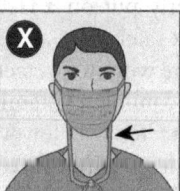

DON'T allow a strap to hang down. DON'T cross the straps.

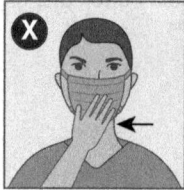

DON'T touch or adjust your facemask without cleaning your hands before and after.

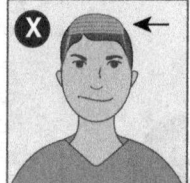

DON'T wear your facemask on your head.

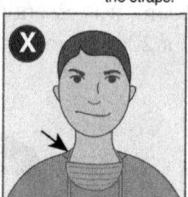

DON'T wear your facemask around your neck.

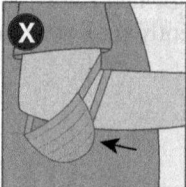

DON'T wear your facemask around your arm.

When removing a facemask
Clean your hands and remove your facemask touching only the straps or ties.

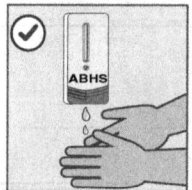

DO leave the patient care area, then clean your hands with alcohol-based hand sanitizer or soap and water.

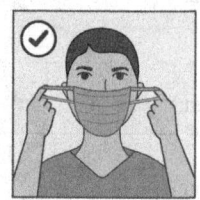

DO remove your facemask touching ONLY the straps or ties, throw it away*, and clean your hands again.

*If implementing limited-reuse: Facemasks should be carefully folded so that the outer surface is held inward and against itself to reduce contact with the outer surface during storage. Folded facemasks can be stored between uses in a clean, sealable paper bag or breathable container.

Figure 8.9 Proper Face Mask Protocol

Figure from Centers for Disease Control and Prevention. Facemask Do's and Don'ts for Healthcare Personnel. Available at https://www.cdc.gov/coronavirus/2019-ncov/downloads/hcp/fs-facemask-dos-donts.pdf. Accessed September 18, 2021. Reference to specific commercial products, manufacturers, companies, or trademarks does not constitute its endorsement or recommendation by the U.S. Government, Department of Health and Human Services, or Centers for Disease Control and Prevention.[35]

Conflict Resolution

CHWs will encounter diverse situations or circumstances where conflict is possible. As a CHW, it is important to understand ways to enhance **conflict resolution** to dissolve tensions and maintain a safe environment for all.[37] Whether the situation occurs at work among employees, between a client and family, in a community setting, or within your own family, it is beneficial to acquire basic skills.[37] One of the main reasons that conflict occurs is due to a lack of communication, which leads to disputes between two or more individuals in a variety of settings. If the situation is between family members involving elder care, it is best to resolve the issue before it escalates within the family. Conflict may be resolved with adequate communication by using the following six step guide. If the individuals involved are unable to reach an agreeable resolution, they may utilize a mediator to guide further conversations.[37]

1. Be Calm and Stop Arguing

Even if only two individuals are involved in the disagreement, it is likely that other members of the family or organization will become involved or be affected by the disagreement. Finding a way for all individuals to stay calm is an excellent place to begin to resolve the conflict.[37] Continuous arguing intensifies the conflict and thus causes anger, resentment, helplessness, and further breakdown of communication.[37] Select a time and location that is agreeable for involved individuals to gather. Individuals attending the meeting are asked to abide by the rules, such as talking to one person at a time, being willing to listen without interrupting, staying calm, and talking without imposing blame or retribution. In some cases, the family may select or hire an individual who is not involved in the situation to mediate the meeting.[37]

2. Identify the Issues in Their Own Words

Everyone describes the specific problem in their own words without blaming anyone without interruption. One family member is selected to write each specific problem as stated on a white board or a single piece of poster paper.[37] All problems are listed as separate issues until the discussion begins. No one may change or alter how another person stated the problem in their own words. For example, the individual writes the identified issues at the top of the column and includes the person's name, such as "lack of family finances for home health services for Mom and Dad" (Joe, son), "time management: balancing work and caregiving" (Kathy, daughter).[37]

3. Discuss Information Peacefully

The discussion of the information is conducted in a calm and orderly manner.[37] As individuals express their concerns, the other participants remain quiet and focus on listening to the speaker rather than mentally preparing a rebuttal before the speaker is finished. Honest speaking and listening are critical for communication.[37] The new comments are added under the appropriate column on the white board or poster paper, such as on Kathy's poster board: family could designate the role of each sibling in caring for parents (Joe's comment).[37]

4. Express Realistic Assessment Statements

When it is each person's turn to speak, the participants speak in a factual and nonemotional way. Each comment is written on the board and expresses a realistic assessment statement or goals for a resolution to reduce future conflicts.[37] The use of anger, resentment, self-pity, being "right," or assigning blame serves no purpose and only derails what could be a calm conclusive discussion.[37]

5. Compromise Is Not the Same as Giving Up

It is important to discuss that compromise is not the same as giving up.[37] When participants view compromise as a form of giving up, giving in, or getting out, the conclusion is not a healthy way to resolve any conflict. If compromise is not viewed as winning or losing, this attitude results in a complete failure to end the conflict in any satisfactory way. Participants should not hide the way they feel about the results of the conflict.[37] The participants are allowed to respectfully speak about their dissatisfaction with said result. If one participant sees that others are willing to reach a solution, that individual may consider the possibility of reexamining and letting go of underlying issues, such as negative feelings or emotions that have nothing to do with the current conflict, such as a past unpaid debt or obligation.[37] The family concludes that when the next conflict arises, the participants will consider the tools of conflict resolution prior to allowing the issue to escalate out of control.[37]

6. Continuing the Conversation Is a Priority to Maintain Positive Relationships

Interactions with family members, friends, neighbors, and coworkers are a part of daily life. Resolving conflict is a priority to maintain positive relationships.[37] It is useful to learn to see the best in others, avoid all assumptions, and accept the natural faults and limits in others and in yourself. Use the tools of conflict resolution to allow everyone to step back and think through the situation without anger and resistance.[37] Heightened emotions may be unavoidable, and feelings are natural; however, continued anger fuels conflict. Resolving all problems requires a tailored, collaborative effort from all parties involved. If professional assistance or guidance is required, there is no shame or fear in seeking help. Most communities have support networks available for such services.[37]

Chapter Summary

This chapter discusses multiple topics regarding safety for individuals and safety for CHWs. The first section explores safety for individuals by including tips for adequate communication skills, identifying basic needs, and assessing ADLs. Next, adverse circumstances are examined, including information about fall prevention, home safety, elder abuse, preparation for natural disasters, and emergency planning. The second section discusses work-related safety issues for CHWs, including stress management techniques, body mechanics, use of PPE, and conflict resolution strategies.

CASE STUDY

Meeting a New Client Patient

Janis brought her mother, Mrs. Mary Williams, to the clinic today to establish a healthcare provider for her mother. Mrs. Williams is 79 years old, has been a widow for 12 years, takes medications for hypertension and high cholesterol, and recently moved to Hillview. Currently, she is living with Janis, her recently divorced daughter. Janis has two adolescent sons who live with her part-time and part-time with their father. Mrs. Williams sold her condo of 22 years when she decided to move across the state to be closer to Janis. Mrs. Williams also has a son, Jackson. He is single, 39 years old, travels for work, and does not have time to stay closely connected to his mother or his sister. Mrs. Williams has not lived in the same town with either of her two children since they were in high school. They are not a close family, and Mrs. Williams often lacks social support. Mrs. Williams is not interested in buying another condo and would prefer to rent. She retired from the school district after teaching middle school for many years. Her financial situation is secure, since she has her state teacher's pension, Social Security benefits, deceased husband's life insurance benefits, and the profit from selling her condo. Mrs. Williams' health insurance includes Medicare, a supplemental plan, and a long-term care policy if needed in the future.

When Cindy, the clinic's CHW, called Mrs. Williams from the waiting room, Janis said that she would like to listen to the visit. Mrs. Williams politely told Janis, her daughter, to stay in the waiting room because she was able to handle her healthcare interview and examination. Mrs. Williams completed the health history questionnaire prior to the appointment. Cindy talked to Mrs. Williams about the clinic and gave her a packet of new patient information and services. Cindy went over the social questions on the health history form, asked about Mrs. Williams current living situation as well as asked if she had any other questions for Cindy. Mrs. Williams hesitated and said that she was a bit concerned about her memory loss. Cindy said that she would put a note in Mrs. Williams' electronic health record (EHR) for the physician.

Mrs. Williams was glad that she was finally going talk with a physician about her memory loss concern. She was nervous as she waited in the exam room. When Dr. Charlotte Hoffman came in the room, Mrs. Williams relaxed and felt like she had met a new friend. Dr. Hoffman completed a thorough physical exam and reviewed her medication list. Lastly, she gently asked Mrs. Williams to describe her concern about her memory loss. She started crying and said that for the past several years, she frequently got lost driving in the city where she had lived for 25 years. She limits the time spent with family because she was afraid and embarrassed of anyone noticing her memory loss. Her biggest fear is being placed in a memory care center. Dr. Hoffman explained that Mrs. Williams needed to be evaluated by Dr. Missam Patel, the neurologist at the clinic. Mrs. Williams made it clear that Dr. Hoffman did not have permission to tell her daughter or son any information related to her health or need of further testing. She stated that her close friend, Nancy Mitchell, serves as Mrs. Williams' health advocate and is legally in charge of her medical and legal affairs. Dr. Hoffman typed Nancy's contact information into Mrs. Williams's EHR while explaining that her health records would not be shared or discussed with anyone else.

At the end of Mrs. Williams appointment, Dr. Hoffman walked her back to Cindy's office. Cindy offered Mrs. Williams some chilled water, while Cindy reviewed Dr. Hoffman's EHR notes. Cindy asked Mrs. Williams if she had any immediate questions before Cindy scheduled her next appointments. Mrs. Williams asked Cindy if she was aware of any rental senior retirement communities that offered independent living at a reasonable monthly rate. Cindy gave her brochures for three retirement communities in the area. They chatted for about 15 minutes after Cindy scheduled an appointment with Dr. Patel and Dr. Hoffman on the same day in 2 weeks. Mrs. Williams had a few more questions but decided that those could wait until her next appointment. Cindy assured Mrs. Williams that they would meet each time that Mrs. Williams had a clinic appointment. Lastly, Cindy gave Mrs. Williams her business card and told her that she could email or call and leave a message during the clinic hours of operation. As Cindy walked Mrs. Williams back to the waiting room, Janis was waiting. She was eager to talk to Cindy.

1. How should Cindy handle Janis, Mrs. Williams's daughter, after this first appointment?
2. What other brochures and information should Cindy have available for Mrs. Williams' next appointment?

References

1. Maslow A. H. A theory of human motivation. *Psychological Review.* 1943;50(4):370–396.
2. McLeod S. Maslow's hierarchy of needs. https://www.simplypsychology.org/maslow.html#gsc.tab=0. Accessed September 6, 2021.
3. Putts M. 10 tips for a better patient interview. https://www.hmpgloballearningnetwork.com/site/emsworld/article/10319762/10-tips-better-patient-interview. Accessed September 6, 2021.
4. National Institute for Occupational Safety and Health. Caring for yourself while caring for others. Cincinnati, OH: U.S. Department of Health and Human Services, Centers for Disease Control and Prevention; 2014. https://www.cdc.gov/niosh/docs/2015-102/pdfs/F14_Handout_5_2015-102.pdf. Accessed September 6, 2021.
5. Sharpley CF, Jeffrey AM, McMah T. Counsellor facial expression and client-perceived rapport. *Counselling Psychology Quarterly.* 2006;19(4):343–356.

6. Griffith CH, Wilson JF, Langer S, Haist SA. House staff nonverbal communication skills and standardized patient satisfaction. *J Gen Intern Med.*2003;*18*(3):170–174.

7. Activities of daily living checklist & assessments. Paying for Senior Care Web site. https://www.payingforseniorcare.com/activities-of-daily-living. Accessed September 8, 2021.

8. Burns E, Kakara R. Deaths from falls among persons aged ≥ 65 years—United States, 2007–2016. *MMWR.*2018;67(18):509–514.

9. Bergen G, Stevens MR, Burns ER. Falls and fall injuries among adults aged ≥ 65 years—United States, 2014. *MMWR.*2016;*65*(37):993–998.

10. O'Loughlin JL, Robitaille Y, Boivin JF, Suissa S. Incidence of and risk factors for falls and injurious falls among the community-dwelling elderly. *American Journal of Epidemiology.*1993;137(3):342–354.

11. Alexander BH, Rivara FP, Wolf ME. The cost and frequency of hospitalization for fall–related injuries in older adults. *American Journal of Public Health.* 1992;82(7):1020–1023.

12. Sterling DA, O'Connor JA, Bonadies J. Geriatric falls: injury severity is high and disproportionate to mechanism. *Journal of Trauma and Acute Care Surgery.* 2001;50(1):116–119.

13. Important facts about falls. Centers for Disease Control and Prevention Web site. https://www.cdc.gov/homeand-recreationalsafety/falls/adultfalls.html. Accessed September 8, 2021.

14. Preventing falls: A guide to implementing effective community-based fall prevention programs. Centers for Disease Control and Prevention Web site. https://www.cdc.gov/homeandrecreationalsafety/falls/community_preventfalls.html.Accessed September 8, 2021.

15. Prevent falls and fractures. National Institute of Health, National Institute on Aging Web site. https://www.nia.nih.gov/health/prevent-falls-and-fractures. Accessed September 8, 2021.

16. Using oxygen at home. Drugs.com. https://www.drugs.com/cg/using-oxygen-at-home.html. Accessed September 8, 2021.

17. Older adults. National Fire Protection Association Web site. https://www.nfpa.org/Public-Education/Fire-causes-and-risks/Specific-groups-at-risk/Older-adults. Accessed September 8, 2021.

18. Tips to prevent poisonings. Centers for Disease Control and Prevention Web site. https://www.cdc.gov/homeandrecreationalsafety/poisoning/preventiontips.htm. Accessed September 8, 2021.

19. Poison prevention, seniors. Poison Control Web site. Available at https://www.poison.org/poison-prevention-tips-by-age/seniors. Accessed September 12, 2021.

20. Poison prevention tips: a guide for older adults. Children's Hospital of Philadelphia Web site. https://www.chop.edu/health-resources/poison-prevention-tips-guide-older-adults. Accessed September 12, 2021.

21. Vermont Needle Disposal Initiative. What to do with a found needle. Vermont Department of Health Web site. https://www.healthvermont.gov/sites/default/files/documents/pdf/HS_VermontNeedleDisposalInitiative_Factsheet.pdf. Accessed September 12, 2021.

22. Safe disposal of sharps. Agency of Natural Resources Department of Environmental Conservation Web site. https://dec.vermont.gov/content/safe-disposal-sharps#:~:text=Safe%20Disposal%20of%20Sharps%20Home-Generated%20Sharps%2C%20Syringes%2C%20and,plastic%20container%2C%20such%20as%20a%20laundry%20detergent%20bottle. Accessed September 12, 2021.

23. Warning: syringes. Agency of Natural Resources Department of Environmental Conservation Web site. https://dec.vermont.gov/sites/dec/files/wmp/SolidWaste/Documents/Sharps-container-label-example.pdf. Accessed September 12, 2021.

24. National Institute on Aging. Spotting the signs of elder abuse. National Institute of Health Web site. https://www.nia.nih.gov/health/infographics/spotting-signs-elder-abuse. Accessed September 12, 2021.

25. National Institute on Aging. How to spot elder abuse from afar: signs and solutions for long-distance caregivers. National Institute of Health Web site. https://www.nia.nih.gov/health/how-spot-elder-abuse-afar-signs-and-solutions-long-distance-caregivers. Accessed September 12, 2021.

26. Moran Elder Law. *What Is Elder Abuse—How and Why It's Occurring.* https://www.youtube.com/watch?v=QAsk6g9OHvQ. Accessed September 12, 2021.

27. National Adult Protective Services Association. Mandated reporting of abuse of older adults and adults with disabilities. National Center on Elder Abuse Web site. https://ncea.acl.gov/NCEA/media/Publication/NCEA_NAPSA_MandatedReportBrief.pdf?time=164223953337#:~:text=Mandated%20reporting%20of%20abuse%20of%20older%20adults%20and,of%20a%20specific%20profession%20to%20report%20suspected%20abuse%2C. Accessed February 8, 2022.

28. Disaster preparedness: a complete guide for seniors. Aging.com. https://aging.com/disaster-preparedness-for-seniors/. Accessed September 12, 2021.

29. Medical Reserve Corps (MRC) unit locations. Geo Health Web site. https://geohealth.hhs.gov/arcgis/apps/opsdashboard/index.html#/7570dde7406d4c4abb65ea9be132d5ae. Accessed February 6, 2022.

30. The Medical Reserve Corps. Assistant Secretary for Preparedness and Response, U.S. Department of Health and Human Services Web site. https://aspr.hhs.gov/MRC/Pages/index.aspx. Accessed February 6, 2022.

31. National Institute for Occupational Safety and Health. *Caring for Yourself While Caring for Others: Module 6: Tips for Setting Healthy and Safe Boundaries to Reduce Stress.* Cincinnati, OH: U.S. Department of Health and Human Services, Centers for Disease Control and Prevention; 2014. https://www.cdc.gov/niosh/docs/2015-102/pdfs/TrainersGuide_6_2015-102.pdf. Accessed September 14, 2021.

32. Stress management test. The Calculator Web site. https://www.thecalculator.co/personality/Stress-Management-Test-626.html. Accessed September 14, 2021.

33. Proper body mechanics. Drugs.com. https://www.drugs.com/cg/proper-body-mechanics.html. Accessed September14, 2021.

34. 22.1 organs and structures of the respiratory system. Oregon State University Web site. https://open.oregonstate.education/aandp/chapter/22-1-organs-and-structures-of-the-respiratory-system/. Accessed September 14, 2021.

35. Facemask do's and don'ts for healthcare personnel. Centers for Disease Control and Prevention Web site. https://www.cdc.gov/coronavirus/2019-ncov/downloads/hcp/fs-facemask-dos-donts.pdf. Accessed September 18, 2021.

36. Lee YJ. A doctor shares the right way to take off gloves amid coronavirus. Business Insider Web site. https://www.businessinsider.com/how-to-put-on-wear-and-take-off-gloves-2020-4#:~:text=1%20Wash%20%28and%20dry%29%20your%20hands%20before%20touching,this%20article%20it%27s%20this%3A%20Wash.%20Your.%20Hands.%20. Accessed September 19, 2021.

37. A six step guide to family conflict resolution. United Families International Web site. https://www.united families.org/family/a-six-step-guide-to-family-conflict-resolution/. Accessed September 24, 2021.

Appendix

1. Maslow's Hierarchy of Needs: https://www.youtube.com/watch?v=O-4ithG_07Q
2. Elder Abuse: https://www.youtube.com/watch?v=QAsk6g9OHvQ
3. Conflict Resolution: https://www.youtube.com/watch?v=QyXFirOUeUk

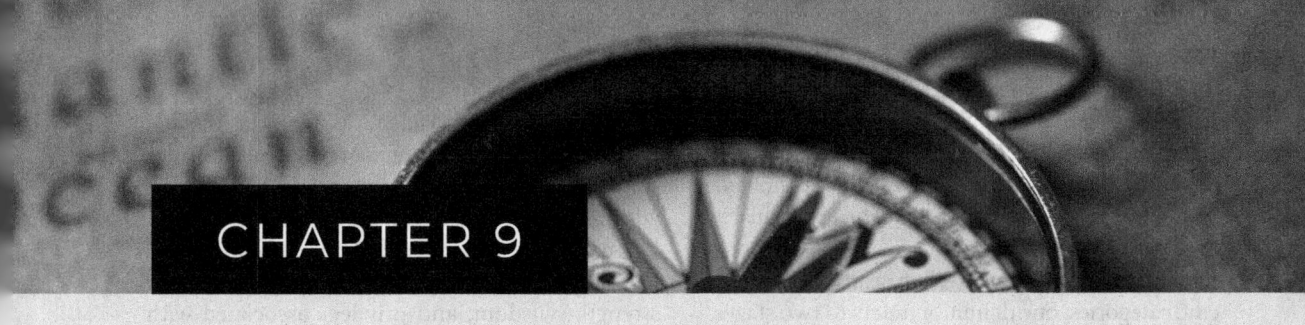

CHAPTER 9

Aspects of Aging

LEARNING OBJECTIVES

1. Define "elderly" and describe the cultural views of the elderly across countries.
2. Explain three reasons why elderly adults need to receive an annual physical examination.
3. Describe four physical body systems, including how each body system changes with aging.
4. Define the symptoms and care management of Alzheimer's disease.
5. List two positive and two adverse behaviors that are affected by aging.
6. List the common economic difficulties that affect the financial aspects of aging.

KEY WORDS

elderly	hysterectomy	prostatectomy
longevity	mastectomy	annual mental status examination

Introduction

This chapter covers information about the aspects of aging. The chapter begins with the definitions of elderly and factors impacting longevity. The next section provides an overview of changes in body systems across the aging process, starting with a typical physical examination by a healthcare provider that includes a history interview, review of medications, and a physical examination. The next section provides a detailed description of the various changes that occur among the elderly, particularly the aspects of aging related to physical, mental, behavioral, financial, and functional activities.

Who Are Considered the Elderly?

When looking for a definition of the word "elderly," many synonyms or common phrases were provided, such as senior, older, ancient, as old as the hills, geriatric, golden oldie, retiree, gray-haired, wrinkly, senile, old fashioned, later in life, pensioner, not as young as one used to be, decrepit, doddering, past one's prime, and the list continues.[1] One source showed respect by defining an elderly person as one who is older or higher in rank than oneself, an aged person, and an influential member of a tribe or community, often a chief or ruler or someone superior.[2]

Conversely, another source provided a simple, two-part definition as (1) rather old especially being past middle age and (2) old fashioned.[3] A medical definition of an **elderly** individual is defined as someone over 65 years old who has functional impairments.[4] When searching for specific categories, one definition refers to two stages: those individuals between the ages of 65 to 74 years old are called the early elderly, and those that are over the age of 75 years old are defined as the late elderly, while another system of age classification noted 75–90 years of age is considered old age and over 90 is advanced old age.[5-6]

From a social perspective, it is important to recognize how labels and the language used to define older persons can produce stigma, stereotypes, foster ageism as a form of discrimination, and present disrespectful attitudes toward the aging population. For example, additional searches revealed how the English language suggests the elderly as frail and often lacks positive terminology that recognizes the strength, wisdom, and privilege associated with chronological age. Many cultures revere their elders and look to them for wisdom, guidance, and identify older individuals as respected pillars within their respective cultural community. Cultures that value youth and physical appearance have a different perspective and struggle with inevitable aging. See **Table 9.1** to better understand how different countries and cultures view older individuals.

Table 9.1 Views of the Elderly Across Countries

Country	View of Elderly
Australia	"The process of maintaining a positive attitude, feeling good about yourself, keeping fit and healthy, and engaging fully in life as you age."[8]
China	"The criteria are sufficiently inclusive, encompassing physical health, mental health, social engagement, and nutritional status, which in principle are in conformity with both the WHO definition and the Rowe and Kahn model."[9]
Eastern Europe	"Active aging is concerned with facilitating the rights of older people to remain healthy (reducing the costs of health and social care), remain in employment longer (reducing pension costs), while also participating in community and political life."[10]
Japan	"Old age is understood as a socially valuable part of life, even a time of 'spring' or 'rebirth' after a busy period of working and raising children."[11]
New Zealand	"Positive aging reflects the attitudes and experiences older people have about themselves and how younger generations view the process of aging. It considers the health, financial security, independence, self-fulfillment, personal safety and living environment of older New Zealanders."[12]
United Kingdom	"A way of living rather than a state of being."[12]
United States	"Successful aging is multidimensional, encompassing the avoidance of disease and disability, the maintenance of high physical and cognitive function, and sustained engagement in social and productive activities."[12]
World Health Organization (WHO)	"The process of developing and maintaining the functional ability that enables wellbeing in older age."[13]

The Demographics and Global Views of the Elderly

The elderly population is approximately 15 percent of the U.S. population. The number of people who are age 65 and older in the United States has grown rapidly over most of the 20th century. The aging population grew from 3.1 million in 1900 to 35 million in the year 2000. In 2018, 52 million people were 65 years and older.[14-16] Baby boomers are the generation of Americans born during the post–World War II period, between 1946 and 1964.[15] Due to a demographic shift, the elderly population is likely to double from approximately 52 million in 2018 to 95 million by 2060.[14-17]

Important Aspects of Longevity

This section focuses on aspects affecting **longevity**, the geriatric assessment instrument, and how to conduct a nutritional assessment. First, nine factors may impact longevity.

1. Gender: According to the Institute and Faculty of Actuaries (IFA), women live longer than men, on average. The current overall life expectancy for U.S. men is 76.4 years and for U.S. women is 81.2 years.[18]
2. Genetics: Genetics are known contributors to nine of the top 10 causes of death, according to the Centers for Disease Control and Prevention (CDC).[19]
3. Prenatal and childhood conditions: Poor conditions in utero, at birth, and in very early childhood are associated with higher mortality even at advanced ages, according to the IFA.[18]
4. Education: For individuals with a bachelor's degree or higher, life expectancy at age 25 increased by 1.9 years for men and 2.8 years for women, according to the CDC.[20]
5. Socioeconomic status: Socioeconomic status can affect a person's ability to access adequate medical care and participate in healthier lifestyle behaviors, such as exercise, not smoking or smoking cessation, and maintaining a healthy weight.[21]
6. Marital status: Married people have lower mortality rates than those who were never married, are divorced, or are widowed, according to the IFA.[18]
7. Ethnicity/immigrant status: According to the CDC, life expectancy ranged from 71.7 years for non-Hispanic Black males and 83.7 years for Hispanic females. Additionally, ethnicity or immigrant status may also be associated with socioeconomic changes influencing life expectancy.[22]
8. Lifestyle: Historically, lifestyle factors that affect mortality include an unhealthy diet, inadequate exercise, tobacco use, excessive use of alcohol, risky behaviors, food safety, workplace environment, and motor vehicle safety. Currently, the largest lifestyle factor that affects mortality is obesity.[23]
9. Medical technology: Development of antibiotics, immunizations, improvements in imaging, surgery, cardiac care, and organ transplants have increased the average life expectancy higher.[23] Along with the nine factors, the Geriatric Assessment Instrument is utilized as a comprehensive assessment instrument to examine the holistic aspects of age. This assessment is important for community health workers (CHWs) to have available as a reference guide to thoroughly assess how age can affect the total person.[24] See **Table 9.2**.

Many individuals have the desire to stay healthy and live to be 100 years old even though only 1 person in every 6,000 (0.0173 percent) reach their 100th birthday.[25] However, 50 years ago, only 1 person in every 67,000 reached the century mark.[25] Following are three resources that show how age can vary based on where one lives.

1. The living to 100 Life Expectancy Calculator: Please see the figure available at https://livingto100.com/calculator.2620. With this link, it is possible to learn about health-related behaviors that individuals may control.

Table 9.2 A Geriatric Assessment Instrument

Domain	Item
Daily function ability	Degree of difficulty eating, dressing, bathing, transferring between bed and chair, using the toilet, and controlling bladder and bowel. Degree of difficulty shopping.
Assistive devices	Use of personal devices (e.g., cane, walker, wheelchair, oxygen); use of environmental devices (e.g., grab bars, shower bench, hospital bed)
Caregivers	Use of paid or unpaid caregivers (e.g., nurses, aides)
Drugs	Name of prescription drugs and nonprescription drugs used
Nutrition	Height, weight stability over past 6 months
Preventive measures	Regularity of blood pressure measurements; sigmoidoscopy or colonoscopy, immunizations (influenza, pneumococcal, tetanus, shingles, pertussis, COVID-19), thyroid-stimulating hormone assessment, and dental care; intake of calcium and vitamin D; regular exercise; use of smoke detectors
Cognition	Ability to remember three objects after 1 minute and draw a clock face (Mini-Cog©)
Affect	Feelings of sadness, depression, or hopelessness; lack of interest or pleasure in doing things
Advance directives	Possession of a living will; establishment of durable power of attorney for health care
Substance abuse/ misuse	Moderate use of alcohol; avoid use of all tobacco and vaping products; avoid overuse of prescribed or unprescribed drugs
Gait and balance	Number of falls in the past 6 months; time required to rise from a chair, walk 10 feet, turn around, return, and sit down; extent of maximal forward reach while standing
Sensory ability	Ability to report three numbers whispered 2 feet behind the head; ability to read eye exam chart at 20/40 or better with corrective lenses, if needed
Upper extremities	Ability to clasp hands behind the head and back

Data from Besdine RW. Evaluation of the older adult. Available at https://www.merckmanuals.com/professional/geriatrics/approach-to-the-geriatric-patient/evaluation -of-the-older-adult. Accessed September 20, 2021.[24]

2. The Life Expectancy by ZIP Code link: https:// www.rwjf.org/en/library/interactives/where youliveaffectshowlongyoulive.html illustrates the location of neighborhoods affects life expectancy.[27] See **Figure 9.1**.

It is easy to see that multiple factors impact the aging process and aspects of longevity.[28] According to the Danish Twin Study, approximately 20 percent of an individual's life-span is defined by genes, while the remaining 80 percent is determined by lifestyle choices and healthy behaviors.[29] Evidence-based research has shown that food consumption, the surrounding environment, social influences, access to safe places, and practicing healthy behavior plays a critical role in life expectancy.[29]

This section provides information about dietary guidelines and nutrition assessments for individuals at each stage of life. The 2020–2025 Dietary Guidelines for Americans encourages healthy eating patterns at each stage of life and recognizes that individuals will need to make

Enter your street address or zip code (Example: "1234 Main Street, Anytown, NY 12345")

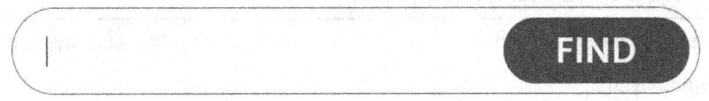

FIND

NOTE: YOUR INFORMATION WILL NOT BE STORED RWJF PRIVACY POLICY

Your Census Tract life expectancy is not available. The results below are based on your ZIP code only.

EXAMPLE RESULT

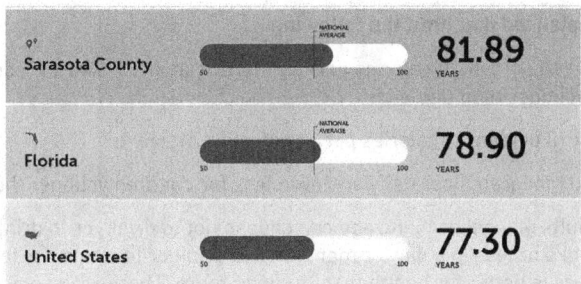

Figure 9.1 Life Expectancy by ZIP Code

Visit: https://www.rwjf.org/en/library/interactives/whereyouliveaffectshowlongyoulive.html[77]
Reproduced from Robert Wood Johnson Foundation. Life Expectancy: Could where you live influence how long you live? Available at https://www.rwjf.org/en/library/interactives/whereyouliveaffectshowlongyoulive.html. Accessed October 22, 2021.[77]

shifts in their food and beverage choices to achieve a healthy pattern.[30] The guidelines also explicitly emphasize that a healthy dietary pattern is not a rigid prescription. Rather, the guidelines are a customizable framework of core elements within which individuals make tailored and affordable choices that meet their personal, cultural, and traditional preferences.[30]

A healthy dietary pattern can benefit all individuals regardless of age, race, or ethnicity, or current health status. The Dietary Guidelines provides a framework intended to be customized to individual needs and preferences as well as the food from the diverse cultures in the United States.[30] Focus on meeting food group needs with nutrient-dense foods and beverages and stay within calorie limits. See **Table 9.3**.

Important Dietary Guidelines for Consideration in Adults Ages 60 and Older

Hydration. Many older adults do not drink enough fluids to stay hydrated. One reason for this is that the sensation of thirst tends to decline with age.[30] Concerns about bladder control or issues with mobility also may hinder intake of fluids among older adults. It is important that older adults drink plenty of water to prevent dehydration and aid in the digestion of food and absorption of nutrients. In addition to water, choosing unsweetened beverages can support fluid intake to

Table 9.3 The Core Elements for a Healthy Diet

Vegetables of all types—dark green; red and orange; beans, peas, and lentils; starchy; and other vegetables

Fruits, especially whole fruit

Grains, at least half of which are whole grain

Dairy, including fat-free or low-fat milk, yogurt, and cheese, and/or lactose-free versions and fortified soy beverages and yogurt as alternatives

Protein foods, including lean meats, poultry, and eggs; seafood; beans, peas, and lentils; and nuts, seeds, and soy products

Oils, including vegetable oils and oils in food, such as seafood and nuts

To maintain a healthy, balanced diet limit the following:

Added sugars—Less than 10 percent of calories per day starting at age 2. Avoid foods and beverages with added sugars for those younger than age 2.

Saturated fat—Less than 10 percent of calories per day starting at age 2.

Sodium—Less than 2,300 milligrams per day—and even less for children younger than age 14.

Alcoholic beverages—Adults of legal drinking age can choose not to drink, or to drink in moderation by limiting intake to two drinks or less in a day for men and one drink or less in a day for women, when alcohol is consumed. Drinking less is better for health than drinking more. There are some adults who should not drink alcohol, such as women who are pregnant.

United States Department of Agriculture. Dietary Guidelines for Americans 2020–2025. Available at https://www.dietaryguidelines.gov/sites/default/files/2021-03/Dietary_Guidelines_for_Americans-2020-2025.pdf. Accessed January 14, 2022.[30]

prevent dehydration. The water that is contained in foods such as fruits, vegetables, and soups contributes to hydration status and is a contributor to total fluid intake.[30]

Alcoholic Beverages. To help older adults move toward a healthy dietary pattern and minimize risks associated with drinking, older adults can choose not to drink or drink alcohol in moderation with a limit of two drinks or less in a day for men and one drink or less in a day for women.[30] Drinking alcohol puts older adults at higher risk of falls, car crashes, and other injuries. In addition, older adults tend to have a greater number of comorbid health conditions, and alcohol use or misuse may adversely affect

the condition or interfere with management of the disease.[30] Certain older adults should avoid drinking alcohol completely, including those who do the following:

- Plan to drive or operate machinery, or participate in activities that require skill, coordination, and alertness[30]
- Take certain over-the-counter (OTC) or prescription medications[30]
- Have certain medical conditions
- Are recovering from alcohol use disorder or are unable to control the amount they drink[30]

Additional factors should also be considered when supporting healthy eating for older adults:

Table 9.4 **Government Resources for Older Adults**

Congregate Nutrition Services: The Older Americans Act authorizes meals and related services in congregate settings for any person aged 60 and older and their spouse of any age. Program sites offer older individuals' healthy meals and opportunities to socialize. Congregate meals are typically provided in senior centers, schools, churches, or other community settings.

Supplemental Nutrition Assistance Program (SNAP): Older adults with limited income may qualify for SNAP, a federal program that provides temporary benefits to help individuals purchase foods and beverages to support a healthy dietary pattern when resources are constrained.

Commodity Supplemental Food Program (CSFP): The CSFP supplements the diets of low-income older adults by providing nutritious USDA packaged food to support a healthy dietary pattern. The CSFP is federally funded, and private and nonprofit institutions facilitate the distribution of monthly CSFP packages to eligible older adults.

Home-Delivered Nutrition Services: The Older Americans Act authorizes meals and related services in a person's home for individuals ages 60 and older and their spouse of any age. Older adults who have trouble leaving the home due to frailty, health concerns, or certain medical conditions may benefit from home-delivered meals offered under the Older Americans Act.

Child and Adult Care Food Program (CACFP): The CACFP is a federal program that provides reimbursements for nutritious meals and snacks to older adults enrolled in daycare facilities. Older adults receiving care at nonresidential care centers may receive meals and snacks that meet CACFP nutrition standards.

United States Department of Agriculture. Dietary Guidelines for Americans 2020–2025. Available at https://www.dietaryguidelines.gov/sites/default/files/2021-03/Dietary_Guidelines_for_Americans-2020-2025.pdf. Accessed January 14, 2022.[30]

- Enjoyment of food by sharing meals with friends and family
- Ability to chew or swallow foods, including good dental health
- Food safety: Older adults are prone to a decline in immune system function, increasing the risk of foodborne illness[30]

Additional resources to support older adults exist at the community level. See **Table 9.4**. For example, the Senior Farmers Market Nutrition Program (SFMNP) provides many low-income seniors with access to fruits and vegetables grown in their local communities.[30] SNAP Education (SNAP-Ed) programming may also be offered and teach older adults cooking and shopping skills.[30] See **Figure 9.2**.

To take the MyPlate Quiz, visit: https://www.myplate.gov/my/quizzes/2360621/863077a6a60380144f7e7653f73d1827.[31]

Changes in Body Systems amid the Aging Process

This section has two main parts. First, an overview of the annual physical examination for an elderly person by a healthcare provider, which includes a history interview, review of medications, and a physical examination.[24] Second, a description of the various changes that occur among the elderly regarding the aspects of aging related to physical, mental, behavioral, financial, and functional activities.[24] The physical changes of aging occur inside the body long before those changes become noticeable to the individual or to others. Such changes are the reasons why it is important for all aging individuals to have an annual physical exam with a primary care physician.

Are you making every bite count?

Take the MyPlate Quiz to find out!

New! Levels have been added to the MyPlate Quiz. Take the quiz today to find out your level and get personalized resources to *Start Simple with MyPlate*.

(A)

Start Quiz   Empieza la prueba

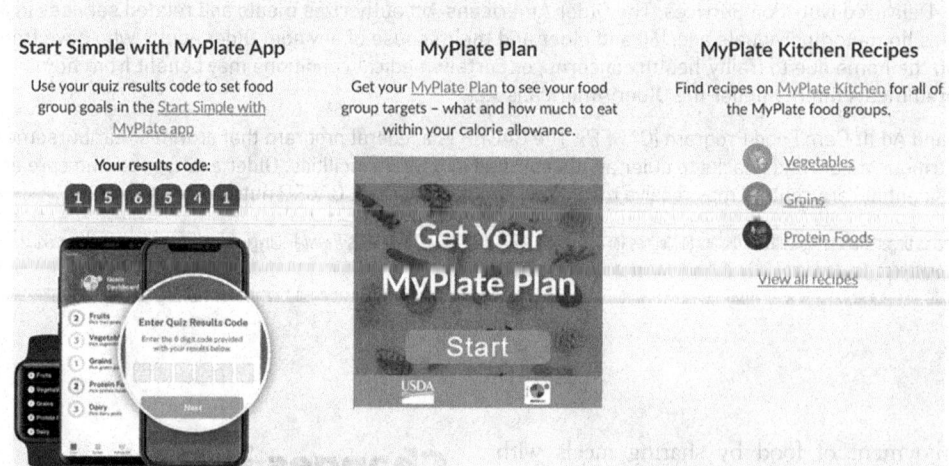

Free resources and tools for you

Start Simple with MyPlate App

Use your quiz results code to set food group goals in the Start Simple with MyPlate app.

Your results code:

1 5 6 5 4 1

MyPlate Plan

Get your MyPlate Plan to see your food group targets – what and how much to eat within your calorie allowance.

MyPlate Kitchen Recipes

Find recipes on MyPlate Kitchen for all of the MyPlate food groups.

Vegetables

Grains

Protein Foods

View all recipes

(B)

Figure 9.2 Nutritional Assessment—My Plate Quiz

Figures from United States Department of Agriculture. Your MyPlate Quiz Results. Available at https://www.myplate.gov/my/quizzes/2360621/863077a6a603801447e7653f73d1827. Accessed March 1, 2022.[31]

Patient History Interview. The healthcare provider's knowledge must be updated regarding the patient's current everyday concerns, whether it is the first visit or an established patient's return visit. This interview includes immediate questions, social circumstances, mental function, emotional state, and overall sense of well-being (e.g., sleep patterns, weight loss or gain, depression, fall history, recent surgery, medical interventions).[24] The interview establishes rapport with the patient and the family member at the visit. This interview allows the clinician to assess the patient's mental status, reliability of providing accurate responses, and how the patient describes his or her current health.[24] In addition, the verbal and nonverbal clues (e.g., tempo of speech, tone of voice, eye contact, body movements) provide additional information for the healthcare provider.[24]

Review of Medications. At every clinic visit, it is useful for patients to bring all bottles of their prescriptions, OTC medications, herbs, and dietary supplements.[24] The drug name, dose, dose schedule, name of prescriber, reason for prescribing the drug, and any specific drug allergies are essential. The drug history is recorded with a is given to patients and/or the caregiver.[24] Following this discussion, patients are asked to read the labels, open the containers, and recognize the drugs to verify their skill level in taking medication. Healthcare providers investigate drug interactions and the use of drug to ensure appropriate utilization for each individual. In addition, providers should ask about vaccines (e.g., flu, pertussis, shingles, and COVID-19) received and make a note of any vaccines that are due.[24]

Physical Examination. Older patients may have diagnosable disorders, but the disorders may not be known or recognized without further investigation by the physician via scans, lab tests, preventative interventions (e.g., colonoscopy) or specialty referrals. Early diagnosis frequently depends on the healthcare provider's familiarity with the patient's behavior and history, including mental status.[24] Commonly, the first signs of a physical disorder are behavioral, mental, emotional, or functional decline. For example, if the clinician asks about joint symptoms, the patient may deny pain.[24] However, when asked about a change in activities, the patient may report that she no longer takes a morning walk or volunteers at the hospital. Changes in activities warrant further investigation and opportunities to restore function, such as physical therapy, may be recommended to build strength, address other issues, and assist in maintaining one's independence.[24] If clinicians are unaware of this possibility and attribute these signs to dementia, diagnosis and treatment can be delayed. This example showcases how important it is to gather a patient's social history.[24]

A disorder in one organ system often weakens another system, which leads to disability, discomfort, or a lack of independence.[24] For example, heart disease may involve the kidneys, lungs, and contribute to other symptoms related to the primary disease. Multiple disorders complicate diagnosis, treatment, and the effects of the disease process.[24] As the comorbidities (numerous diagnoses) increase, all other aspects of the patient's life change, such as activities of daily life, isolation, nutritional status changes, financial stability, physical weakness, and increased risk of falling. For example, an elderly patient who is bedridden can lose 1 to 3 percent of muscle mass and strength each day. The more days that a person spends in bed leads to a greater risk of reduced mobility.[24]

1. Physical Aspects

Heart. The heart is an essential organ that pumps day and night without the individual's awareness. As people age, the blood vessels throughout the body begin to lose elasticity and fatty deposits build up against artery walls. These conditions make the heart work harder to circulate the blood throughout the body.[32] These conditions lead to high blood pressure (hypertension) and atherosclerosis (hardening of the arteries). Individuals of all ages need to be aware of taking care of their heart, which can be accomplished through regular exercise, eating heart-healthy foods, refraining from smoking or tobacco use, or stopping the use of tobacco use.[32] See **Case Study 9.1**.

Case Study 9.1 CHW and Heart Failure (HF)

Clare, a CHW, works in the community health clinic. This morning Ann, an ARNP (nurse practitioner), told Clare that Mr. Sam Williams was recently in the hospital with heart failure (HF) diagnosis. His first appointment after being discharged from the hospital is today. Ann tells Clare that Mr. Williams has agreed to meet with Clare after his appointment to learn more about the community resources available for his HF diagnosis. Clare enjoys conversing with Mr. Williams and his wife, Sara. They have met previously to review his hypertension (high blood pressure). Clare remembers that their literacy skills are proficient. Mr. Williams owned a plumbing business, and Sara was the administrator. They both have associate degrees from the local community college. Before the scheduled appointment with Mr. and Mrs. Williams, Clare gathers written information about HF.

At the CHW appointment, Clare provides a simple overview by saying that HF happens when the heart muscle is no longer working properly to meet the needs of the body. She gives Mr. and Mrs. Williams a brochure about the common signs and symptoms of heart failure. See **Box 9.1**.

Box 9.1 Heart Failure Signs and Symptoms

Heart Failure includes the following signs and symptoms:

- Shortness of breath: the heart is unable to pump enough to keep up with the body's current blood supply. Therefore, due to poor circulation, the excess fluid backs up into the lungs causing pressure.
- Swelling in the legs, feet, and ankles: The fluid gathers in the legs, feet, and ankles due to gravity, and the heart is unable to pump enough to handle the excess fluid.
- Dry and hacking cough that does not go away: The cough is the body's response to the excess fluid collecting in the lungs. The heart is unable to pump hard enough to keep up with the excess fluid.
- Trouble sleeping when lying flat: The excess fluid builds up in the lungs, causing pressure related to the excess fluid.
- Rapid weight gain (3 or more pounds in a day): Since the heart cannot keep up with the excess fluid, the body stores the excess in the tissues.
- Feeling tired: Since the heart is not pumping adequately, any activity causes more stress on the heart and causes fatigue. Also, if the individual is not sleeping well, then he or she feels tired most of the time.

Data from Keep It Pumping. About Heart Failure: What Is Heart Failure? Available at https://www.us.keepitpumping.com/what-is-heart-failure?utm_source=bing&utm_medium=cpc&utm_campaign=sitelink&utm_term=Sitelink_What_is_Heart_Failure?gclid=8b663f6aaf7910bc079060e2f6340213&&msclkid=8b663f6aaf7910bc079060e2f6340213&gclid=CMCtvq_ktuwCFUrBHwodn_QEtw&gclsrc=ds. Accessed October 19, 2021.[34]

Clare reminds Mr. and Mrs. Williams to contact the healthcare provider immediately if new or worsening symptoms appear. During the meeting, Mr. and Mrs. Williams asked Clare a few questions. Clare states that she is not licensed to answer their specific questions, but she will ask Ann to answer that question before they leave. However, she does suggest that they begin a notebook to track Mr. Williams's food and fluid intake and weight each day. Clare said that they have a follow-up appointment in 2 weeks, so they could bring the notebook. The food and fluid log will provide the physician valuable information about whether Mr. Williams's medication dosage needs adjusted. As Ann walks by, Clare asks her to step into her office for a few minutes, so she can answer their questions. Clare gives Mr. and Mrs. Williams a folder of community resources for HF support groups at the local YMCA plus a few brochures about appropriate diet and exercise for HF.

Questions

1. What causes a person with HF to have a dry and hacking cough?
2. Why would Ann, ARNP, suggest that Mr. Williams weigh himself each day before breakfast?

Answers

1. The cough is the body's response to the excess fluid collecting in the lungs. The heart is unable to pump hard enough to keep up with the excess fluid.
2. Since the heart cannot keep up with the excess fluid, the body stores the excess in the tissues, and the patient may experience a rapid weight of up to 3 pounds in one day.

Bones, Muscles, and Joints. As people age, the density of their bones decreases, making the bones brittle, fragile, and prone to fractures. A bone density scan is performed every 1–2 years to determine the degree of bone loss.[34] In addition, muscles and tendons lose strength and flexibility. Low impact forms of exercise, such as walking, are excellent ways to slow or prevent the problems with bones, muscles, and joints while maintain strength and flexibility. In addition, a healthy, calcium-rich diet maintains bone strength.[34] See **Table 9.5**.

Table 9.5 Foods Rich in Calcium

Vegetables		
Collard	Broccoli	Spinach
Okra	Kale	Bok Choy
Legumes		
White Beans	Chickpeas	Red Beans
Green Beans	Lentils	Kidney Beans
Fruits		
Orange	Raisins	Dried Figs
Currant	Apricot	Kiwi
Dairy Products		
Cheese	Almond Milk	Yogurt
Milkshake	Whole Milk	Ice Cream
Seeds and Nuts		
Sunflower	Sesame	Chia
Almonds	Hazelnuts	Walnuts
Others		
Eggs	Tofu	Cereal (fortified)
Sardines	Shrimp	Salmon

Data from Bone Health & Osteoporosis Foundation. A Guide to Calcium-Rich Foods. Available at https://www.nof.org/patients/treatment/calciumvitamin-d/a-guide-to-calcium-rich-foods/. September 20, 2021[35]

Digestive System. The reflexive process of chewing, swallowing, and digesting begins to slow as a part of the body's natural aging process. Chewing is the first step in the digestion process. However, if the individual does not have healthy teeth and gums, chewing becomes a problem, usually due to tooth decay and gum disease. Swallowing may become more difficult as the esophagus contracts less forcefully.[32] For individuals at risk of aspiration due to swallowing difficulties (dysphagia), thickening additives may be put in thin liquids to increase the viscosity (thickness) of the fluid. Thin liquids include soda, coffee, tea, juice, and soup broth. Products are available to thicken foods to improve swallowing issues.[36] The flow of secretions that help digest food in the stomach, liver, pancreas, and small intestine decreases over time. The reduced flow results in digestive issues ranging from constipation to intermittent diarrhea.[32] For some conditions, individuals are more comfortable wearing adult diapers to avoid unexpected mishaps.

Kidneys and Urinary Tract. With age, the kidneys may become less efficient in removing waste from the bloodstream due to a decrease in size.[32] Chronic diseases such as diabetes or high blood pressure (hypertension) many also cause kidney damage. In addition, urinary incontinence may occur due to a variety of health conditions, including changes in hormone levels in women and having an enlarged prostate in men. Both conditions are examples of contributing factors related to urinary incontinence.[32]

Brain and Nervous System. With age, the number of brain cells decreases, causing changes to the brain's composition and memory loss or the ability to access long-term memory. The brain attempts to compensate for the loss of cells by increasing the number of connections between the cells to preserve brain function. These new connections may cause slower reflexes, mental distraction, and difficulties with body and mind coordination.[32]

Parkinson's Disease. One of the most common diseases related to the nervous system is Parkinson's disease, which is a progressive nervous system disorder that affects movement. The symptoms start gradually with tremors (shakiness), stiffness, or slowing of movement. Speech may also be affected.[37] Symptoms worsen as the condition progresses over time. Parkinson's disease is not curable, but medications may significantly improve the symptoms, quality of life, and cognitive function.[37] Parkinson's disease causes certain nerve cells (neurons) in the brain to gradually break down or die.[37] The symptoms are the result of losing neurons that produce a chemical messenger in your brain called dopamine. When dopamine levels decrease, it causes abnormal brain activity, leading to impaired movement and other symptoms related to Parkinson's disease.[37] The cause of Parkinson's disease is unknown, but several factors appear to play a role, including genes, exposure to certain toxins or environmental factors, and identified clumps of specific substances within the brain cells called Lewy bodies. Though research is ongoing, the risk factors of Parkinson's disease currently include age (usually over 60 years), heredity/genetics (small risk), male gender, and the possible exposure to toxins, such as herbicides and pesticides.[37]

Alzheimer's Disease. Alzheimer's disease is the most common type of dementia. Alzheimer's disease is one of the top 10 leading causes of death in the United States.[38] It is a progressive disease beginning with mild memory loss and involves parts of the brain that control thought, memory, and language. Over time, it seriously affects a person's ability to carry out daily activities.[38] Researchers do not yet fully understand what causes Alzheimer's disease. There likely is not a single cause but rather several factors that can affect each person differently.[38] See **Figure 9.3**.

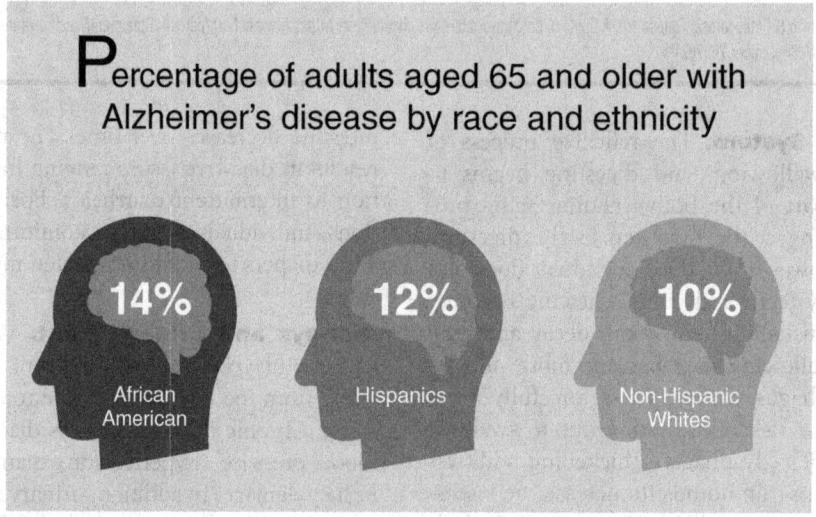

Figure 9.3 Who Has Alzheimer's Disease?

Figure from Centers for Disease Control and Prevention. Alzheimer's Disease and Related Dementias. Available at https://www.cdc.gov/aging/aginginfo/alzheimers.htm#AlzheimersDisease?. Accessed October 29, 2021. Reference to specific commercial products, manufacturers, companies, or trademarks does not constitute its endorsement or recommendation by the U.S. Government, Department of Health and Human Services, or Centers for Disease Control and Prevention.[38]

Despite the common misconception, Alzheimer's disease is not a normal part of aging. Memory problems are typically one of the first warning signs of Alzheimer's disease and related dementias.[38] The number of people living with the disease doubles every 5 years beyond age 65, and this number is projected to nearly triple to 14 million people by 2060.[38] Symptoms of the disease can first appear after age 60, and the risk increases with age. In addition to memory problems, someone with symptoms of Alzheimer's disease may experience one or more of the following:

- Memory loss that disrupts daily life, such as getting lost in a familiar place or repeating questions
- Trouble handling money and paying bills
- Difficulty completing familiar tasks at home, at work, or during leisure
- Decreased or poor judgment
- Misplacing things and being unable to retrace steps to find them
- Changes in mood, personality, or behavior

Even if an individual has several or even most of these signs, it does not mean that the individual has Alzheimer's disease.[38] Alzheimer's disease is diagnosed by a team of physicians after the person undergoes a series of brain scans and tests. Medical management can improve quality of life for individuals living with Alzheimer's disease and for their caregivers. There is currently no known cure for Alzheimer's disease.[38] Treatment addresses includes helping people maintain brain health, managing behavioral symptoms, and slowing or delaying symptoms of the disease.[38] Currently, many people living with Alzheimer's disease are cared for at home by family members. Although most people willingly provide care to their loved ones and friends, caring for a person with Alzheimer's disease at home can be a difficult task and may become overwhelming at times.[38] As the disease gets worse, people living with Alzheimer's disease often need intensive full-time care, such as a memory care facility. Death rates for Alzheimer's disease are increasing, while other diseases such as heart disease and cancer-related deaths decline.[38]

Sexual Health. There are many potential barriers concerning sexuality in older age, such as the lack of a healthy sexual partner, depression, the monotony of a repetitive sexual relationship, a spouse's physical changes, hormone variability, and illness.[39] However, it is usually assumed that older adults do not have sexual desires, and elderly people often find it difficult to discuss this topic with their doctor. Many older adults wish to be close to others as they grow older. Aging may mean adapting sexual activity to accommodate physical, health, and other changes.[39]

Normal aging brings physical changes in both men and women. These changes sometimes affect the ability to have and enjoy sex.[39] For women, if vaginal dryness is an issue, water-based lubricating jelly or lubricated condoms may increase comfort. For men, impotence (also called erectile dysfunction, or ED) becomes more common.[39] ED is the loss of ability to have and keep an erection. In both situations, communication with partner may improve enjoyment. Also, a physician may have suggestions to improve intimacy. In addition, some illnesses, disabilities, medicines, and surgeries can affect the ability to have and enjoy sex. For example, these conditions may decrease sexual enjoyment: arthritis (joint pain), chronic pain, dementia, diabetes, heart disease, incontinence, stroke, depression, and surgery.[39]

Types of surgeries that may affect sexual intimacy may include the following:

Hysterectomy is surgery to remove a woman's uterus, and perhaps the ovaries, because of pain, bleeding, fibroids, or other reasons. The surgeon will discuss any concerns about sexual intimacy after the surgery.[39]

Mastectomy is surgery to remove all or part of a woman's or man's breast because of breast cancer. This surgery may cause some women to lose their sexual interest due to feeling less desirable or attractive to their partner. Programs like the American Cancer Society's "Reach to Recovery" can be helpful. Also, some women choose to have breast reconstruction.[40] To learn more about Reach to Recovery, visit: https://www.cancer.org

/treatment/support-programs-and-services/reach -to-recovery.html.[40]

Prostatectomy is surgery that removes all or part of a man's prostate because of cancer or an enlarged prostate.[41] This surgery may cause urinary incontinence or ED.[42] Communicate with the physician and partner before surgery about any concerns.

Additionally, some medications can cause sexual problems or influence sexual desires. These include some blood pressure medicines, antihistamines, antidepressants, tranquilizers, medications for Parkinson's disease, cancer medications, appetite suppressants, drugs for mental problems, and ulcer drugs.[43–44] Discuss any concerns with the physician to determine if there is an alternative drug without this side effect. Additionally, excessive alcohol consumption may can cause erection problems in men and delay orgasm in women.

Age does not protect individuals from sexually transmitted infections.[45] Older people who are sexually active may be at risk for diseases such as syphilis, gonorrhea, HIV/AIDS, chlamydial infection, genital herpes, hepatitis B, genital warts, and trichomoniasis. Individuals who are engaging in non-monogamous sexual activity, should have regular checkups and testing. People are never too old to be at risk for sexually transmitted infections.[45]

Eyes. As people age, changes in vision are common.[32] Eyeglasses are usually needed for reading. Older individuals find it difficult to see in low-light conditions, such as when driving at night. Additionally, due to less tear production in older individuals, they are likely to experience chronic dry eyes, and the eye's lenses located behind the iris become cloudier.[32] See **Figure 9.4**.

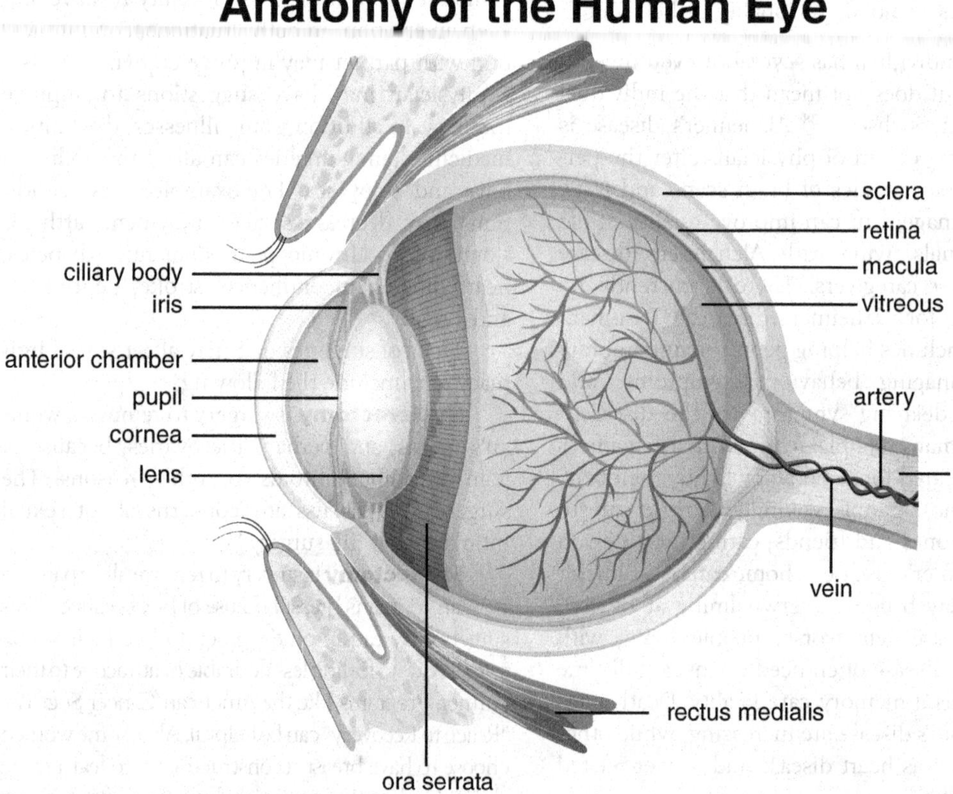

Anatomy of the Human Eye

Figure 9.4 Anatomy of a Normal Human Eye

Figure from American Macular Degeneration Foundation. What is macular degeneration? Available at https://www.macular.org/what-macular-degeneration. Accessed September 20, 2021.[46]

The most common eye problems associated with age include the following:

Cataracts: A cataract causes clouding (e.g., looking through fog or frosted glass) of the normal clear lens of the eye.[47] Cataracts develop slowly over time and make it difficult to read or to drive at night. Fortunately, cataract surgery is generally a safe and effective procedure.[47]

Glaucoma: Glaucoma is an eye condition that damages the optic nerve caused by abnormally high pressure in the eye. Glaucoma is one of the leading causes of blindness for people over the age of 60.[48] Many forms of glaucoma have no warning signs. The effect is so gradual that the individual may not notice a change in vision until the condition is at an advanced stage.[48] Because vision loss due to glaucoma is not reversible, it is important to have regular eye exams that include measurements of the eye pressure. If glaucoma is recognized early, vision loss can be slowed or prevented. Once an individual is diagnosed, treatment is required for the rest of the person's life.[48]

Diabetic retinopathy: Diabetes retinopathy is caused by diabetes and is the leading cause of blindness for adults with diabetes. Since diabetes retinopathy may not have early symptoms, it is recommended that all adults schedule an annual comprehensive eye exam including dilation to look for early signs of diabetes retinopathy. When an individual has diabetes, unregulated or high blood sugar levels may cause damage throughout the body including the retina of the eyes. The symptoms of diabetic retinopathy are blurred vision, difficulty seeing colors and eye floaters in field of vision. Without treatment, diabetic retinopathy causes blindness. Prevention is most important by managing blood glucose levels and scheduling annual eye examinations.

Macular degeneration: Macular degeneration is caused by the deterioration of the central portion of the retina, the inside back layer of the eye that records the images and sends them via the optic nerve from the eye to the brain for recognition.[46] The central portion of the retina is known as the macula and is responsible for focusing central vision in the eye, controlling the ability to read, drive a car, recognize faces or colors, and see objects in fine detail.[46] Macular degeneration is the leading cause of vision loss more than cataracts and glaucoma combined. At present, macular degeneration is considered an incurable eye disease. Individuals with advanced macular degeneration are considered legally blind. However, they retain some peripheral vision since the sides of the retina still work.[46]

For all older patients, an eye examination by an ophthalmologist is recommended every year to detect and prevent common eye disorders (e.g., glaucoma, cataracts, retinal disorders).

Ears. Excessive noise throughout the lifetime may cause hearing loss later in life.[32] Older adults have difficulty hearing high pitched voices and sounds, experience trouble hearing in busy places, and often have an overproduction of earwax.[32] When hearing loss occurs, it can have a negative effect on one's self-esteem, impact the ability to communication, enjoy relationships, interact socially, and may hurt emotional well-being.[49] Properly fitted hearing aids can help in many listening situations.[50] There are two basic types of hearing aids: analog and digital.[50] Analog hearing aids are programmed during the fitting process, and some have multiple listening profiles that the patient can select with a button on the hearing aid component. Digital hearing aids are also programmable during the fitting process, have multiple listening profiles, and allow for a more advanced signal processing to aid in noise reduction, filtering, and acoustic feedback (ringing) control.[50] Digital hearing aids are more popular because of the increased performance and flexibility over the analog versions.[50]

Skin Concerns. The common skin changes in the aging process include dry skin, bruises, wrinkles, age spots, and skin cancer.[32,51] Some skin changes are caused by not drinking enough liquids, spending too much time in the sun, smoking, medical conditions, and medications.

Skin cancer is a very common type of cancer in the United States.[51] Skin cancer may be cured if it is found before it spreads to other parts of the body.[51] Skin cancer can happen anywhere on the body but is usually found on parts of the skin most exposed to sun, such as head, face, neck, hands, and arms. It is recommended that everyone check their skin once a month for changes, such as a new growth, a sore that does not heal, or a bleeding mole.[51] Good skin care includes not being in the sun for long periods of time, wearing protective clothing, using sunscreen, and staying hydrated. In addition, individuals should schedule an annual skin examination by a licensed dermatologist (skin physician).[51] See **Box 9.2**. Whenever a CHW is asked about skin concerns, he or she should refer the individual to a healthcare provider for examination and treatment.

Foot Problems. The diagnosis and treatment of foot problems help elderly people maintain their independence and increase quality of life.[52-53] Common age-related foot problems include bunions, calluses and corns, hammer toe, ingrown toenails, dry or cracked heels, and foot deformities from rheumatoid arthritis, diabetes, or neurologic disorders.

Box 9.2 Check Moles, Birthmarks, or Other Parts of the Skin for the "ABCDEs"

A = Asymmetry (one half of the growth looks different from the other half)
B = Borders that are irregular
C = Color changes or more than one color
D = Diameter greater than the size of a pencil eraser
E = Evolving; this means the growth changes in size, shape, symptoms (itching, tenderness), surface (especially bleeding), or shades of color

See your doctor right away if you have any of these signs to make sure it is not skin cancer.

U.S. Department of Health and Human Services, National Institute of Health. Skin Care and Aging. Available at https://www.nia.nih.gov/health/skin-care-and-aging. Accessed October 29, 2021.[51]

Additionally, foot ulcers can result from diabetes or other illnesses.[52-53] Patients with foot problems should be referred to a podiatrist (foot specialist) for regular evaluation for prevention, treatment, or interventions.[52-53]

2. Mental Health

Although mental health has many aspects, this section explores the need for an annual mental health status examination and describes the effects of depression and lack of sleep on an individual's overall mental health status as aging occurs.

Mental Health Status Examination. With aging, information processing and memory retrieval slows. However, with extra time and encouragement, patients do perform tasks satisfactorily unless there is a neurological abnormality present.[34] An **annual mental status examination** is important for people over 70 years old. Patients who are anxious about this test should be reassured that it is routine. The examiner must ensure that patients can hear.[54] Hearing deficits that prevent patients from hearing and understanding questions may be mistaken for cognitive dysfunction.[54] It useful to record the baseline results and repeat the examination annually for comparison or when a change in mental status is suspected. Most tests take about 30 minutes to administer and cover the following assessments: orientation, short-term memory, long-term memory, basic math or computational skills, word finding, attention and concentration, naming objects, following commands, writing, spatial orientation, abstract reasoning, and judgment.[54]

Depression and Aging. Mental health problems are not easily detected in aging patients. Because of this, it is important to closely monitor for any behavioral change or a change in a person's desire to participate in a previously enjoyed activity.[24,54] Depression may be exhibited by sadness, hopelessness, crying, or anxiety; irritability may be the primary affective symptom of depression.

These symptoms may also represent cognitive dysfunction.[24,54] Many circumstances, such chronic medical illness, chronic minor daily stress, chronic pain syndrome, family history of depression, low income or job loss, low self-esteem, low social support, prior depression, single/divorced/widowed, or traumatic brain injury, may contribute to depression.[24,54] Remember, answers to questions can be subjective and circumstantial. Therefore, asking follow-up questions is recommended to increase accuracy and ensure correct diagnostics. See **Table 9.6**.

Sleep. Along with nutrition and exercise, maintaining a consistent sleep schedule is critical for physical, mental, and emotional health. Poor sleep is often responsible for mood changes and decreases the ability to recall details and process new information.[56] In addition, chronic lack of sleep causes more negative emotional reactions and fewer positive ones. Insomnia increases the chance of developing a mood disorder such as depression, anxiety, or panic symptoms.[56] Physical affects from inadequate sleep include increased blood pressure, stroke, and heart disease.[56] Poor sleep is linked to increased weight gain, obesity, calorie intake and type 2 diabetes. However, adequate sleep and rest improves many aspects of daily physical performance, concentration, and endurance. Additionally, sleep improves the immune system function and decreases inflammation.[56]

3. The Impact of Positive and Adverse Health Related Behaviors

This section examines the activities that have positive and adverse impacts on aging. The positive behaviors include consistent exercise, dietary habits, and water consumption, while adverse behaviors cover tobacco use, alcohol consumption, and recreational drug use.

Exercise and Physical Activity. Everyone can experience the health benefits of physical activity regardless of age, ability, ethnicity, shape, or size.[57] Individuals over the age of 65 should aim for a total of 150 minutes per week of moderate intensity aerobic activity (e.g., brisk walking) and 2 days of muscle strengthening activities.[57-58] All physical activity can be creatively tailored to meet the needs of the individual. For example, low impact exercises such as seated leg raises without weight or engaging in light walking may be more appropriate for

Table 9.6 Geriatric Depression Scale (Short Form)

Question	Response	
	Yes	No
1. Are you basically satisfied with your life?		
2. Do you often get bored?		
3. Do you often feel helpless?		
4. Do you prefer to stay at home rather than going out and doing new things?		
5. Do you feel worthless the way you are now?		
Scoring: A "no" response to question 1, or a "yes" response to questions 2 through 5 counts as one point. A score of two or more points is considered a positive screen.		

Hoyl MT, Alessi CA, Harker JO, et al. Development and testing of a five-item version of the Geriatric Depression Scale. *J Am Geriatr Soc.* 1999;47(7):873–878.[55]

an individual who is recovering from a fall or is experiencing weakness due to an illness, or injury.[57–58] Regular physical activity is one of the most important things that individuals can do to maintain their health. A few of the most important benefits of exercise include improving brain health, supporting healthy weight management, reducing or slowing the disease process, strengthening bones and muscles, and improving the ability to perform everyday basic activities.[57] Although exercise benefits all ages, the specific benefits of exercise among seniors includes a lowered risk of heart disease, stroke, hypertension, and type 2 diabetes, improved bone health, a lowered risk of dementia or cognitive decline, improved quality of life, and lowered risk of depression.[58–59] **Figure 9.5** showcases the benefits of incorporating exercise into one's lifestyle and indicates the long-term benefits of exercise as an individual ages.

Maintaining physical activity stabilizes flexibility and stimulates the metabolism to prevent gaining weight as people age.[32] However, many elderly people exercise less, become more sedentary, and continue to eat the same type of diet. Since the body is unable to burn off the caloric intake, the extra calories are stored as fat. Too often, people do not choose to reduce their exercise routine, but their health conditions, injuries, and medications interfere with daily activities. A routine of walking is an important starting point to maintain strength or regain former activities.[32,58]

It is important to recognize that some individuals may require one or more mobility aids to support their body weight, prevent loss of balance, and reduce falling.[60] Falling is a serious safety hazard, and wheelchairs, motorized scooters, walkers, canes, or crutches play a vital role in the promotion of senior safety. Individuals who utilize mobility aids can effectively participate in tailored exercises.[60] Even if a person uses a wheelchair, there are sitting exercise routines that improve strength and posture. See **Figure 9.6**.

Even if the activity is limited to walking inside with a walker or cane, it is more beneficial than

reclining. However, it is common for people to decide that they need a cane for increased balance, so they purchase a cane at a drug store without consulting a healthcare provider. As a result, they may use the cane improperly. See **Box 9.3** to learn how to properly measure a cane to be effectively used.

Dietary Habits and Water Consumption.

Healthcare providers should ask their elderly patients about their daily dietary habits, including type, quantity, and frequency of food consumption, and patients should be assessed based on nutritional status. Typically, individuals who eat less than two meals a day may be at risk of malnutrition depending on the quality and quantity consumed at each meal.[24] Here are a few questions related to food and water consumption:

1. Is the person on any special diet (e.g., low salt, low carbohydrate, low fat, low calorie) that was prescribed by a provider?[24]
2. Is the person on any self-prescribed fad diets, such as keto, juice cleanses, grapefruit, military diet, intermittent fasting?
3. Does the person consume enough high fiber foods? Is the patient using any prescription medication or OTC medication for constipation?
4. Has the person unintentionally lost weight or gained weight over the last few months? Do the person's clothes fit?[24]
5. Approximately how much money does the person spend per week on food? Does the person have access or participate in SNAP, Meals on Wheels, or a local food bank?[62]
6. Does the person have access to grocery stores with a variety of fresh fruits and vegetables? Does the person have suitable kitchen facilities for preparing food?[24]

Finally, the healthcare provider evaluates the patient's ability to eat, including chewing and swallowing.[24,32] Dental problems, such as tooth decay, missing or poor fitting dentures, and gum disease among the elderly are not uncommon. Too often dental care is neglected due to lack of money. Without annual dental examination, a small dental issue, such as a cavity, turns into a necessary tooth extraction and

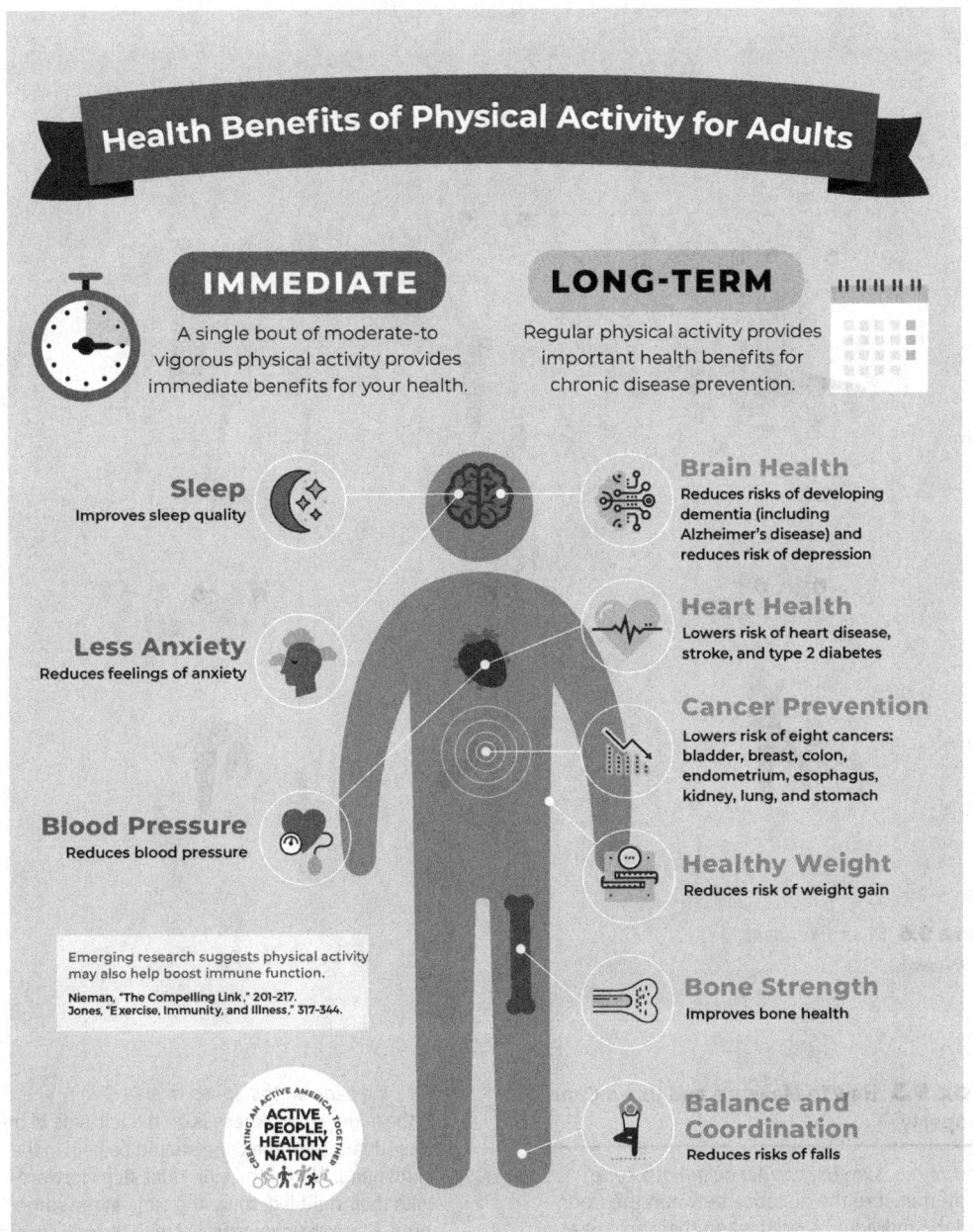

Figure 9.5 Health Benefits for Physical Activity for Adults

Figure from Centers for Disease Control and Prevention. Health Benefits of Physical Activity for Adults. Available at https://www.cdc.gov/physicalactivity/basics/adults/health-benefits-of-physical-activity-for-adults.html. Accessed October 29, 2021. Reference to specific commercial products, manufacturers, companies, or trademarks does not constitute its endorsement or recommendation by the U.S. Government, Department of Health and Human Services, or Centers for Disease Control and Prevention.[99]

gum disease.[24] Patients with decreased vision, arthritis, immobility, or tremors have difficulty preparing meals. Patients with urinary incontinence may reduce their fluid intake, especially if the individual has difficulty getting to the restroom. In addition, patients living alone experience little pleasure in eating with no social contact.[24]

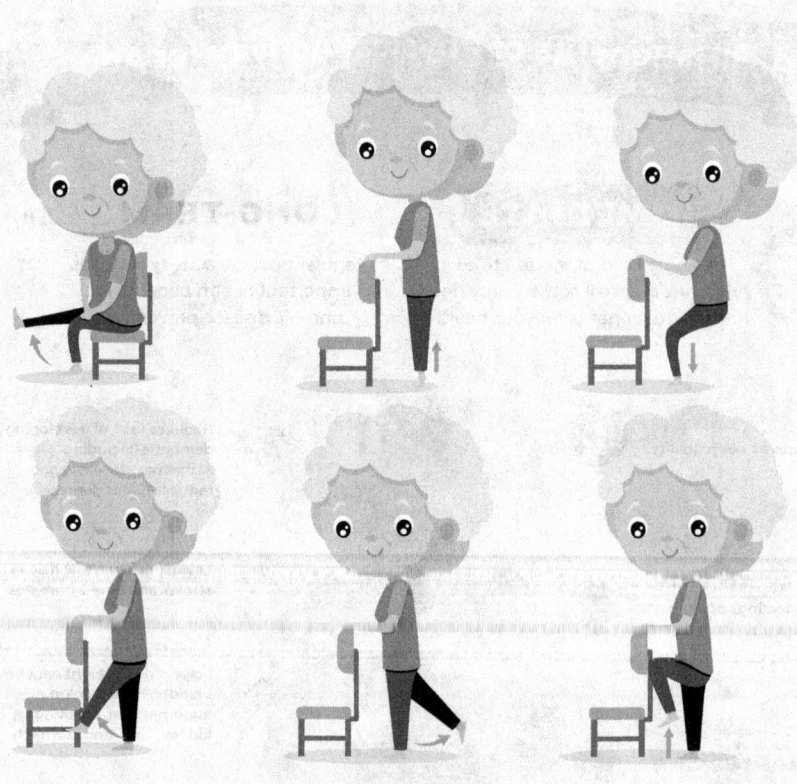

Figure 9.6 Chair Exercises

© Thetor.P/Shutterstock

Box 9.3 How to Measure and Use a Cane Properly

How to measure the correct height of a cane:
First, measure the distance between the floor and the individual's wrist when their arm is at their side. Second, measure the distance from the floor to the individual's hand when their arm is bent at a 15-degree angle. The two measurements should be approximately the same plus/minus an inch. Most canes are adjustable and allows the individual to shorten or lengthen the cane within the appropriate range of height measurement.

Use the cane on the opposite side of injury:
If the injury or weakness is on the left-side of the individual's body, the cane should be held in the right hand. Also, if the individual steps forward with their right leg, move the cane at the same time. Place the cane parallel with the individual's opposite foot, not in front or behind the foot.

Walking up and down stairs when using a cane:
When walking up stairs with a cane, plant the weak leg and cane on the ground, use the strong leg to take a step-up. The cane and weak leg will assist with balance. Take each step one at a time, always starting with the strong leg first.

Tobacco, Alcohol, and Recreational Drug Use. The use of tobacco, alcohol, and recreational drugs should be discussed with the primary care provider when taking the patient's medical or social history.[24] Some substances interfere with prescribed medications or limit medication effectiveness, causing numerous issues with patient health outcomes. Older individuals who participate in such activities should be strongly encouraged to discuss this information with their trusted primary care provider in a safe space.[24] For patients who smoke, the healthcare provider should encourage smoking cessation products or classes to stop for a variety of health reasons. Patients who refuse to stop smoking should be counseled to avoid smoking inside and completely refrain from smoking in bed because older adults are more likely to fall asleep while smoking.

As for alcohol consumption, patients should be checked for signs of alcohol use disorders, including confusion, anger, hostility, alcohol odor on the breath, impaired balance and gait, tremors, peripheral neuropathy, and nutritional deficiencies. See **Table 9.7** for questions that can be asked to start a conversation about alcohol use and abuse.

The topic of recreational drug use, especially marijuana, has changed considerable over the past few years. As of 2017, marijuana for medical use is legal in 26 states and the District of Columbia.[64] Where and how an individual can purchase and use marijuana varies widely, even among the states that have legalized marijuana. However, marijuana remains illegal on federal lands, including national parks.[56] The use of recreational and medical marijuana has grown exponentially in the general population. Among the older adults, it is used for pain relief in the form of topical creams, oils, and edibles. Healthcare providers need to ask about the use of marijuana as well as other recreational drugs during the medical appointment. In some states, the patients are asking their healthcare providers for a prescription to receive a medical marijuana license to purchase the products.[64-65]

Table 9.7 Alcohol Screening Test for Seniors

Questions	Response	
	Yes	No
After drinking, do you tend to skip eating?		
After drinking, do your tremors go away?		
Do you tell people you drink less than you actually do?		
After drinking, do you sometimes forget things that happened during the day?		
Do you drink to forget problems or heartaches?		
Do you convince yourself that tomorrow you won't drink before or after a certain time of day?		
After drinking, do your feelings of loneliness go away?		
Do you prefer to drink when you are home rather than attending social events?		
Do you drink to help you sleep?		

Data from Short Michigan Alcoholism Screening Test--Geriatric Version (SMAST-G). University of Michigan Alcohol Research Center, 1991.

Financial Aspects of Aging

Aging adults may encounter economic difficulties due to lay-off, job loss, retirement, inability to work due to a physical or mental condition, a fixed income, or the death of a spouse or partner.[66] Financial or health problems may result in the loss of a home, social engagement, recreational activities, or independence.[66] Most younger individuals have more financial freedom compared to elderly individuals because their incomes are not necessarily fixed. Many elderly adults have one source of income per month, such as a pension, retirement plan, and sometimes only a monthly Social Security check. Due to health issues, lack of transportation, or simply an inability to adequately perform certain job functions, many elderly people cannot find a part-time job to supplement their incomes.[66–67] When prices increase or the elderly individual incurs unexpected expenses, their fixed budget must stretch further. Each month they must make difficult decisions regarding what is essential and what is optional, such as food, utilities, rent, healthcare, transportation, or medications. Unfortunately, food, healthcare, and medication are too often dropped from the essential list due to lack of money.[67]

Methods of saving and planning for retirement used by previous generations no longer work for many older persons today due to economic changes, increased costs, and inflated prices.[67] For example, the workers of today are not likely to stay at the same company for their entire career. The companies experience mergers, downsizing, buy-outs, closures, and bankruptcy. Employees are forced to seek employment elsewhere.[67] This situation may include moving to other cities or states. During the process, there may be a gap in income, so it necessary to cash out their savings while seeking new employment, which creates a myriad of financial problems. If such circumstances happen several times between the ages of 30 to 60 years, these working adults are left with limited funds and no pensions for retirement.

If the working adults are married, both parties must find new employment or sustain a long-distance relationship.[67] If children are involved, the financial burden, stress, and emotional impact increase quickly.[67] See **Figure 9.7** for money-saving tips.

As of January 2022, approximately 70 million Americans received a 5.9 percent increase in their Social Security benefits and Supplemental Security Income (SSI) payments.[70–71] This increase means that the average Social Security check benefit for retired workers increased from $1,522.70 to $1,612.54 per month or $18,264 to $19,341.57 annually.[66,69–70] The 2022 benefits change is the largest increase since 1982.[70] The average retirement income in the United States is $42,264.[66,69–72] This amount is calculated by adding the average retirement saving and/or pension of $24,000 per year plus the average Social Security payment of $18,264 per year.[70–72] See **Critical Thinking 9.1**.

Another financial burden for the elderly is healthcare costs. Due to advances in medical care, better nutrition, and generally higher standards of living, more people are living longer. Living longer is not always financially beneficial because it creates a unique challenge for the elderly populations living on a fixed income. As healthcare costs increase with age, costs of housing, food, and other necessities may also increase, further contributing to the financial burden. In addition, aging individuals with physical and mental decline may become impoverished through financial abuse by relatives or caregivers, such as stealing cash and jewelry, relatives offering to manage bank accounts for their personal gain and illegally using credits cards, increasing debt burden.[69–73]

It is important to explore the actual costs of healthcare for the elderly. Many individuals and families assume that Medicare pays for all healthcare costs. This assumption is false.[66–67] Medicare pays for a large portion of medical care but leaves other costs unpaid. It is essential to contact Medicare to determine exactly what health services, benefits, or products are fully covered, partially covered, covered for a specific

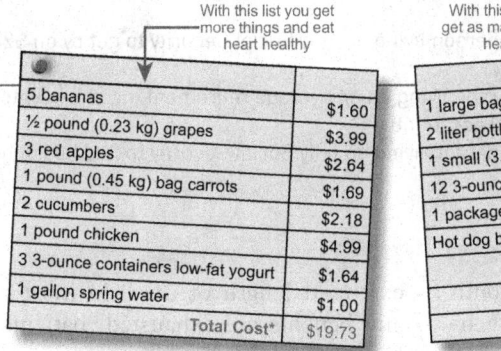

Money-Saving Tips

You and your family can cook healthy meals, even on a tight budget.
Here are some tips that can help.

— Plan Ahead —

- Think about what foods you already have in the house.
- Make a list of meals that you can make with those items.
- Make a list of other foods you still need to buy.
- Make your cooking plan for the week.
- Find coupons. Check food sale ads.
- Figure out where you will shop. This may vary depending on weekly specials.

— Be a Smart Shopper —

- Buy what is on your list. You are more likely to buy too much or buy things that you do not need when you do not use a list.
- Buy only the amount of food your family can use, even if a larger size costs less.
- Buy fruit and vegetables that are in season.
- Shop alone when possible. Family members or friends may try to get you to buy items you do not need.
- Do not shop when you are hungry. You may buy things you do not need.
- Watch for errors at the cash register. Sometimes sale items do not ring up on sale.
- Look for cheaper store brands. They usually are just as nutritious as more expensive name brands.

What Can $20 Buy?

Healthy foods do not have to be expensive! Compare these two shopping lists. The list on the left is the smart choice. It has healthier foods and better buys.

With this list you get more things and eat heart healthy

5 bananas	$1.60
½ pound (0.23 kg) grapes	$3.99
3 red apples	$2.64
1 pound (0.45 kg) bag carrots	$1.69
2 cucumbers	$2.18
1 pound chicken	$4.99
3 3-ounce containers low-fat yogurt	$1.64
1 gallon spring water	$1.00
Total Cost*	$19.73

With this list you do not get as many things or eat heart healthy

1 large bag (10 oz.) potato chips	$2.89
2 liter bottle cola	$1.79
1 small (3.25 oz.) bag beef jerky	$6.49
12 3-ounce packages noodle soup	$1.98
1 package hot dogs	$4.79
Hot dog buns	$2.40
Total Cost*	$20.34

* Costs based on prices in the metropolitan Washington, DC area.

Figure 9.7 Money Saving Tips

Figure from National Institutes of Health, National Heart, Lung, and Blood Institute. Money Saving Tips. Available at https://www.nhlbi.nih.gov/health/educational/healthdisp/pdf/tipsheets/Money-Saving-Tips.pdf. Accessed October 29, 2021.[68]

number of days, or not covered at all.[67,69–73] For example, Medicare does not pay for the cost of assisted living or custodial care. Assisted living facilities are available for the elderly who do not require 24-hour skilled nursing care but are not independent enough to remain living alone safely.

The monthly costs for assisted living facilities for a one-bedroom averages $3,300 per month. If the individual chooses home health, the cost is about $21 per hour depending on geographical location. The cost of a 24-hour skilled nursing facility (SNF) with a semi-private room in a

Critical Thinking 9.1 Monthly Comparison Budget for an Elderly Person

Category	Average Monthly Retirement Income $35,22 per month	Social Security $1,612 per month	Difference
Housing and Utilities	$1,094	$650	–$444
Transportation	$571	$100	–$471
Healthcare and Prescriptions	$480	$275	–$205
Food	$459	$272	–$187
Entertainment	$205	$30	–$175
Personal Life Insurance	$228	$50	–$178
Mandatory Costs: Alimony, Debt, Cell Phone, etc.	$191	$140	–$51
Other: Clothing, Shoes, Haircuts, Toiletries, etc.	$294	$95	–$199

Data from Stoffell B. Here's What the Average Retired American's Budget Looks Like. Available at https://www.fool.com/retirement/general/2016/01/25/heres-what-the-average-retired-americans-budget-lo.aspx. Accessed October 11, 2021.[72]

Questions

1. As a CHW, how would you advise an elderly person living on only Social Security to get by on $272 per month for food, which is about $9.00 per day?
2. As a CHW, what would you tell an elderly person living on an average retirement income how to afford his two new prescriptions, which total over $500 per month?
3. As a CHW, how would you advise an elderly person living on only Social Security to find housing and utilities for $650 per month?

nursing home averages about $6,000 per month or higher. To qualify for the Medicare SNF benefit, the elderly individual must be enrolled in Medicare, have been an inpatient in a hospital for at least 3 days, and enter the SNF within 30 days. The Medicare benefit covers up to 100 days per year in a SNF.[69–73]

Other limited options can cover a portion of the cost of assisted living facilities, such as long-term care insurance, employment-related insurance, and Veteran's benefits.[66–67] However, it is important to review such policy documents carefully before committing to a monthly payment fee. Even with the best policies, there are likely some limitations regarding paying the total cost of assisted living facilities for an extended length of time. In most cases, after any benefits are exhausted, patients and their families pay the costs from their own resources or by liquidating their assets, such as selling property. For the surviving spouse or family members, the cost of assisted living greatly affects their long-term finances.[70–73]

Functional and Social Activities of Aging

Elderly individuals may or may not feel lonely at times. Here are a few examples. Sally may live alone and function independently, but experiences bouts of loneliness because her spouse died last year. Mark has a home health aide that helps him with activities of daily living (ADLs) each morning and evening. Mark has been single for decades and attends activities at the local senior center. He does not feel lonely because he has a large circle of community friends. Lastly, Mary lives in the assisted living facility in her retirement community. She moved into the retirement community after her husband died about 15 years ago. She adjusted easily to the assisted living portion of the retirement community without loneliness because she is acquainted with most residents. Aging is a subjective experience and can be a unique or difficult transition for some older persons. Many elderly adults live independently, but they have limited social interaction.[24,76] For example, Janice lives in an inner-city home that needs repair, including leaking plumbing, deteriorating electrical wiring, and a front porch that is detaching from the main housing structure. She has no money for repairs, is embarrassed to ask for help, and no longer invites friends to visit because of her home conditions. She stopped going to church because even though she has a driver's license, the car is not reliable and needs tires. Last, she dropped and broke her dentures, so eating has become an issue.

If the CHW does not have the opportunity to visit the patient's home, it is important to have patients describe a typical day from the time they wake up to the time they go to sleep. A typical day should include activities unique to them, such as reading, television viewing, computer work, household chores, exercise, hobbies, and interactions with other people.[24,73] This conversation provides valuable information and provides a social assessment, which also indicates factors that may influence one's overall health.[24,73] It is useful to observe patients walking across the waiting room, rising from a chair, and taking off their shoes to get weighed to better understand how they function daily. Observing their personal hygiene adds additional information about their living situation (e.g., condition of clothing, cleanliness, odor, use of adult diapers, urinary catheter, use of walker or cane). This assessment is performed without asking a single question but by merely observing.[24]

As individuals grow older, they may search for activities that promote a deeper sense of connection, wholeness, meaning, and purpose.[73] Additionally, connection promotes better health outcomes, fosters emotional processing, allows for better coping practices, and contributes to positive self-esteem and determination.[73] For those individuals linked to a specific religion, they may find activities such as praying, chanting, fasting, taking part in rituals, celebrating special milestones, and holidays promote new perceptions, renew outlooks, and provide inner strength. However, it is not essential to follow a specific religious practice to feel enlightened. Any activity that an individual enjoys doing makes them feel enriched and energized, including the following activities: volunteering, spending time outside, walking, meditating, participating in a prayer group, attending a support group, sharing stories, listening to music, playing an instrument, dancing, yoga, reading or writing, learning to do crafts, or joining a book club.[24,73] See **Table 9.8**.

Table 9.8 Financial Assistance Organizations for Senior Citizens

Organization	Description
Volunteers of America	Provides senior benefits and programs
Senior Living	Senior living database from independent living to hospice care
Feeding America	Nationwide network of food banks to meal distribution
Retirement Jobs	Helps seniors searching for employment

(continues)

Table 9.8 Financial Assistance Organizations for Senior Citizens   *(continued)*

Organization	Description
Dental Lifeline Network	Nonprofit network dedicated to access to dental care
iCanConnect	Nationwide organization provides vision and hearing equipment
USDA Housing Repair Grants	Provides government grants and loans for housing repairs
Housing and Urban Development (HUD) Programs	Programs for low-income seniors who have paid off mortgage and qualify for the HUD reverse mortgage program
Low Income Home Energy Assistance Program	Government funds for low-income seniors needing assistance with home energy bills
Medicaid	Government funding for low-income seniors in need of health care
Medicare	Benefits for seniors eligible for prescription cost assistance up to $5000 per year
Senior Farmers' Market Nutrition Program	Provides low-income individuals with locally grown produce
Commodity Supplemental Food Program	Eligible seniors receive food packages
Social Security	Benefits for eligible senior over 62 that worked the required amount time to pay into the system
Benefits Checkup	Nationwide directory of government programs benefitting seniors
IRS Elderly Tax Credit	If meeting the eligibility criteria, program may reduce tax owed
Meals on Wheels	Nationwide programs providing nutritious meals to seniors over 60
AmeriCorps Seniors	Volunteer opportunities for seniors in a variety of programs
National PACE Association	Offers at-home health and personal services to those in need

Data from GoFundMe. 25 Resources That Provide Financial Help for Seniors. Available at https://www.gofundme.com/c/blog/financial-help-for-seniors. Accessed March 22, 2022.[75]

Chapter Summary

This chapters examines multiple aspects of the aging process. The chapter begins with the definitions of elderly and discusses factors impacting longevity. Next, an overview is provided to discuss changes in body systems during aging, beginning with a typical physical examination by a healthcare provider that includes a personal medical history interview, review of medications, and a physical examination. The next section provides a detailed description of the various changes that occur within the elderly regarding the aspects of aging related to physical, mental, behavioral, financial, and functional activities. Last, the chapter outlines a variety of resources that every CHW should be familiar with to better serve the community's aging population.

CASE STUDY

CHW Role in the Aspects of Aging

George Myers, age 64, and Joan Myers, age 63, live in St. Louis, Missouri. They have been happily married for 40 years. George is an industrial engineer at a small consulting company, and Joan is a paralegal for a large law firm. They have four children: three girls and one son. Their children have graduated from college. Two of their daughters are married with children and moved out of state for employment opportunities. Their one son and youngest daughter are in graduate school. Their home mortgage is paid off, and they have saved some money for retirement after supporting their children in college and are hoping that it will be sufficient.

George and Joan have many friends since they have lived in St. Louis for more than 35 years. Frequently, they get together with friends for dinner, tailgates parties, and picnics. George and Joan are overweight, but they are not concerned. They state that "they enjoy their midwestern food and beer." Midwestern food includes beer, plenty of grilled meat, and high caloric sides, such as loaded baked potatoes, fries, mac and cheese, and luscious homemade desserts. Their friends are mostly overweight with sedentary desk jobs. No one in their group smokes cigarettes, but occasionally the gentlemen smoke cigars by the firepit.

As for exercise, George does not exercise except for yard work in the summer. He pays to have the snow shoveled off their driveway and sidewalks because his father died of a heart attack while shoveling snow. Joan belongs to the local YMCA. She tries to go at least once or twice a week after work, but she allows work to get in the way of exercise many times each month.

The Myers family has been involved in their faith-based communities for many years. George and Joan saw the value of raising their children in a defined religious community to provide them with basic values. The youth group provided a firm foundation for their children. As their children left for college, George and Joan began to drop out of the religious community. They admit that they participated only for their children and their close friends are not connected to the religious community.

Since George and Joan are planning to retire within 2 years, they are starting to plan for retirement. They want to downsize and move to a smaller home, but with enough space for the grandchildren to visit. They have discussed the need to lose weight, exercise more, and consume less alcohol. They decided that a good first step would be to schedule a physical exam with their primary care physician. Since they stay busy at work, their annual physical exams have been neglected for several years. However, they admit to each other that they are afraid of what may be found during the physical exam. Mark scheduled his appointment for Monday, and Joan schedule her appointment for Tuesday. Since their former primary care physician retired, they decided to go to a new internal medicine physician group close to their home. Before the appointment, they completed the online medical history form. Neither George nor Joan has had any major medical problems in the past. George had knee surgery in college, and Joan had a cesarean section for the last two children's births. Joan has not had a pap test or mammogram for over 5 years, and neither of them has ever had a colonoscopy. Both sets of parents died in their mid-70s. Prior to their appointments, the CHW reviewed their medical history, so he would be prepared to meet them. George and Joan took off Monday and Tuesday, so they would be available to accompany each other at the appointments.

Questions

1. What questions should the CHW ask each of them during the first visit prior to meeting the physician?
2. What packet of information should the CHW compile for George's appointment and for Joan's appointment?
3. What referrals will the physician likely recommend? Since the CHW schedules the referral appointments, how should he/she proceed?

References

1. Elders. Thesaurus.com. https://www.thesaurus.com/browse/elders. Accessed September 12, 2021.
2. Elder. Dictionary.com. https://www.dictionary.com/browse/elder. Accessed September 12, 2021.
3. Elderly. Merriam Webster Web site. https://www.merriam-webster.com/dictionary/elderly. Accessed September 12, 2021.
4. Elderly. The Free Dictionary Web site. https://medical-dictionary.thefreedictionary.com/elderly. Accessed September 12, 2021.
5. What age is legally considered elderly? Informed Senior Living Web site. https://informedseniorliving.com/what-age-is-legally-considered-elderly/. Accessed September 12, 2021.

6. Advanced age. The Free Dictionary Web site. https://encyclopedia2.thefreedictionary.com/Advanced+age. Accessed September 12, 2021.

7. Taylor A. Older adult, older person, senior, elderly, or elder: a few thoughts on the language we use to reference aging. British Columbia Law Institute Web site. https://www.bcli.org/older-adult-older-person. Accessed September 12, 2021.

8. Positive aging. Positive Psychology Institute Web site. https://www.positivepsychologyinstitute.com.au/positive-ageing. Accessed September 12, 2021.

9. Zhou B, Liu X, Yu P. Toward successful aging. *The Chinese Health Criteria for the Elderly. Aging Medicine.* 2018; 1(2):154–157.

10. Foster L, Walker A. Active and successful aging: A European policy perspective. *The Gerontologist.* 2015;55(1):83–90.

11. Karasawa M, Curhan KB, Markus HR, Kitayama SS, Love GD, Radler BT, Ryff CD. Cultural perspectives on aging and well-being: A comparison of Japan and the U.S. *Int J Aging Hum Dev.* 2011;73(1):73–98.

12. Miller KD. What is positive aging? 10 tips to promote the positive aspects of aging. Positive Psychology Web site. https://positivepsychology.com/positive-aging/. Accessed September 13, 2021.

13. Ageing: healthy ageing and functional ability. World Health Organization Web site. https://www.who.int/westernpacific/news/q-a-detail/ageing-healthy-ageing-and-functional-ability. Accessed September 13, 2021.

14. 2020 Census will help policymakers prepare for the incoming wave of aging boomers. United States Census Bureau Web site. https://www.census.gov/library/stories/2019/12/by-2030-all-baby-boomers-will-be-age-65-or-older.html. Accessed September 20, 2021.

15. Baby boomers. History.com. https://www.history.com/topics/1960s/baby-boomers-1. Accessed September 20, 2021.

16. Promoting health for older adults. Centers for Disease Control and Prevention Web site. https://www.cdc.gov/chronicdisease/resources/publications/factsheets/promoting-health-for-older-adults.htm?CDC_AA_refVal=https%3A%2F%2Fwww.cdc.gov%2Fchronicdisease%2Fresources%2Fpublications%2Faag%2Falzheimers.htm. Accessed September 20, 2021.

17. Mather M, Scommegna P, Kilduff L. Fact sheet: aging in the United States. PRB Web site. https://www.prb.org/resources/fact-sheet-aging-in-the-united-states/. Accessed September 20, 2021.

18. The actuarial profession, longevity bulletin. The Institute and Faculty of Actuaries Web site. https://www.actuaries.org.uk/system/files/documents/pdf/longevitybulletin03201205.pdf. Accessed January 12, 2022.

19. Khoury MJ. Geography, genetics, and leading causes of death. Centers for Disease Control and Prevention Web site. https://blogs.cdc.gov/genomics/2014/05/15/geography/#:~:text=Genetic%20factors%20are%20known%20to%20play%20a%20role,chronic%20diseases%20such%20as%20cancer%20and%20heart%20disease. Accessed January 12, 2022.

20. Life expectancy. Vedantu Web site. https://www.vedantu.com/biology/life-expectancy. Accessed January 13, 2022.

21. Beckman K. Nine factors that affect longevity. ThinkAdvisor Web site. https://www.economiapersonal.com.ar/nine-factors-that-affect-longevity/#:~:text=Socio-economic%20status%20As%20socio-economic%20status%20decreases%2C%20so%20does,more%2C%20smoking%20less%20and%20maintaining%20a%20healthy%20weight. Accessed January 13, 2022.

22. Arias E. Changes in life expectancy by race and Hispanic origin in the United States, 2013–2014. Centers for Disease Control and Prevention Web site. https://www.cdc.gov/nchs/products/databriefs/db244.htm. Accessed January 13, 2022.

23. Beckman K. 9 factors that affect longevity. ThinkAdvisor Web site. https://www.thinkadvisor.com/2016/05/27/9-factors-that-affect-longevity/?slreturn=20220021100733. Accessed January 13, 2022.

24. Besdine RW. Evaluation of the older adult. Merck Manual Web site. https://www.merckmanuals.com/professional/geriatrics/approach-to-the-geriatric-patient/evaluation-of-the-older-adult. Accessed September 20, 2021.

25. How many people live to 100? GiT Magazine Web site. http://www.genealogyintime.com/GenealogyResources/Articles/how_many_people_live_to_100_page1.html. Accessed October 20, 2021.

26. Perls T. The living to 100 life expectancy calculator [online]. https://www.livingto100.com/calculator. Accessed October 21, 2021.

27. Life Expectancy: Could where you live influence how long you live? Robert Wood Johnson Foundation Web site. https://www.rwjf.org/en/library/interactives/whereyouliveaffectshowlongyoulive.html. Accessed October 22, 2021.

28. History of blue zones. Blue Zones, LLC Web site. https://www.bluezones.com/about/history/. Accessed October 30, 2021.

29. Buether D, Skemp S. Blue zones. *American Journal of Lifestyle Medicine.* 2016;10(5):318–321.

30. Dietary guidelines for Americans 2020–2025. U.S. Department of Agriculture Web site. https://www.dietaryguidelines.gov/sites/default/files/2021-03/Dietary_Guidelines_for_Americans-2020-2025.pdf. Accessed January 14, 2022.

31. Your MyPlate quiz results. U.S. Department of Agriculture Web site. https://www.myplate.gov/my/quizzes/2360621/863077a6a60380144f7e7653f73d1827. Accessed March 1, 2022.

32. 9 physical changes that come with aging. Johnson Memorial Health Web site. http://blog.johnsonmemorial.org/9-physical-changes-that-come-with-aging#:~:text=%209%20Physical%20Changes%20That%20Come%20With%20Aging,slow%20down%20as%20we%20age.%20Swallowing...%20More%20. Accessed September 20, 2021.

33. About heart failure: what is heart failure? Keep It Pumping Web site. https://www.us.keepitpumping.com/what-is-heart-failure?utm_source=bing&utm_medium=cpc&utm_campaign=sitelink&utm_term=Sitelink_What_is_Heart_Failure?gclid=8b663f6aaf7910bc07

9060e2f6340213&&msclkid=8b663f6aaf7910bc079 060e2f6340213&gclid=CMCtvq_ktuwCFUrBHwodn _QEtw&gclsrc=ds. Accessed October 19, 2021.

34. Bone density exam/testing. Bone Health & Osteoporosis Foundation Web site. https://www.nof.org/patients /diagnosis-information/bone-density-examtesting/. Accessed September 20, 2021.

35. A guide to calcium-rich foods. Bone Health & Osteoporosis Foundation Web site. https://www.nof.org /patients/treatment/calciumvitamin-d/a-guide-to-calcium -rich-foods/. Accessed September 20, 2021.

36. Hayes K. How to thicken liquids for a medical diet. https://www.verywellhealth.com/what-are-thickened -liquids-1192165. Accessed September 20, 2021.

37. Parkinson's disease. Mayo Clinic Web site. https://www .mayoclinic.org/diseases-conditions/parkinsons-disease /symptoms-causes/syc-20376055. Accessed September 20, 2021.

38. Alzheimer's disease and related dementias. Centers for Disease Control and Prevention Web site. https://www.cdc .gov/aging/aginginfo/alzheimers.htm#Alzheimers Disease?. Accessed October 29, 2021.

39. Inelman EM, Sergi G, Girardi A, Coin A, Toffanello ED, Cardin F, Manzato E. The importance of sexual health in the elderly: Breaking down barriers and taboos. *Aging Clin Exp Res.* 2012;24(3):31–34.

40. How does the Reach to Recovery program support people facing breast cancer. American Cancer Society Web site. https://www.cancer.org/treatment/support-programs-and- services/reach-to-recovery.html. Accessed March 1, 2022.

41. Prostate problems. . National Institute on Aging Web site. https://www.nia.nih.gov/health/prostate-problems. Accessed March 1, 2022.

42. Urinary incontinence in older adults. National Institute on Aging Web site. https://www.nia.nih.gov/health/urinary -incontinence-older-adults. Accessed March 1, 2022.

43. High blood pressure and older adults. National Institute on Aging Web site. https://www.nia.nih.gov/health/high -blood-pressure-and-older-adults. Accessed March 7, 2022.

44. Parkinson's disease. National Institute on Aging Web site. https://www.nia.nih.gov/health/parkinsons-disease. Accessed March 7, 2022.

45. Sexuality later in life. National Institute on Aging Web site. https://www.nia.nih.gov/health/sexuality-later-life. Accessed March 7, 2022.

46. What is macular degeneration? American Macular Degeneration Foundation Web site. https://www.macular. org/what-macular-degeneration. Accessed September 20, 2021.

47. Cataracts. Mayo Clinic Web site. https://www.mayoclinic. org/diseases-conditions/cataracts/symptoms-causes/syc -20353790. Accessed September 20, 2021.

48. Glaucoma. Mayo Clinic Web site. https://www.mayoclinic .org/diseases-conditions/glaucoma/symptoms-causes/syc -20372839. Accessed September 20, 2021.

49. Hearing aids. U.S. Food and Drug Administration Web site. https://www.fda.gov/medical-devices/consumer-products /hearing-aids. Accessed September 23, 2021.

50. DiCristina J. *Introduction to Hearing Aids and Important Design Considerations.* https://pdfserv.maximintegrated .com/en/an/AN4691.pdf. Accessed September 23, 2021.

51. Skin care and aging. U.S. Department of Health and Human Services, National Institute of Health Web site. https://www.nia.nih.gov/health/skin-care-and-aging. Accessed October 29, 2021.

52. Amarantos GT. Common foot problems in elderly people. https://footcreamreviews.com/common-foot-problems -elderly-people/#:~:text=Common%20Foot%20 Problems%20in%20Elderly%20People%201% 20Bunions.,related%20to%20deformities.%20...%20 7%20Heel%20pain.%20. Accessed September 23, 2021.

53. Elderly foot care. Advanced Foot and Ankle Care Centers Web site. https://www.afacc.net/foot-problems/treatment /geriatric-foot-care/. Accessed September 23, 2021.

54. Newman G. How to assess mental status. Merck Manuals Web site. https://www.merckmanuals.com/professional /neurologic-disorders/neurologic-examination/how-to -assess-mental-status#v1030587. Accessed October 11, 2021.

55. Hoyl MT, Alessi CA, Harker JO, et al. Development and testing of a five-item version of the Geriatric Depression Scale. *J Am Geriatr Soc.*1999;47(7):873–878.

56. Ellis RR. Surprising reasons to get more sleep. WebMD. https://www.webmd.com/sleep-disorders/benefits-sleep -more. Accessed October 29, 2021.

57. Benefits of physical activity. Centers for Disease Control and Prevention Web site. https://www.cdc.gov /physicalactivity/basics/pa-health/index.htm. Accessed September 25, 2021.

58. U.S. Department of Health and Human Services. *Physical Activity Guidelines for Americans.* 2nd ed. https://health .gov/sites/default/files/2019-09/Physical_Activity _Guidelines_2nd_edition.pdf. Accessed September 30, 2021.

59. Health benefits of physical activity for adults. Centers for Disease Control and Prevention Web site. https://www.cdc .gov/physicalactivity/basics/adults/health-benefits-of-physical -activity-for-adults.html. Accessed October 29, 2021.

60. Leonard J. What types of mobility aids are available? Medical News Today Web site. https://www.medicalnewstoday .com/articles/318463. Accessed September 30, 2021.

61. Kuslikis T. Senior strength: 5 minute chair workout to tone your muscles. https://www.feelgoodlife.com/chair -workout-for-seniors/. Accessed October 28, 2021.

62. Supplemental Nutrition Assistance Program (SNAP). Food and Nutrition Service, U.S. Department of Agriculture Web site. https://www.fns.usda.gov/snap/supplemental -nutrition-assistance-program. Accessed October 4, 2021.

63. Short Michigan Alcoholism Screening Test—Geriatric Version (SMAST-G). University of Michigan Alcohol

Research Center Web site. https://www.westongroupinc
.com/westime/ops_docs/PQRS/12-Short%20
Michigan%20Alcoholism%20Screening%20Test%20
Geriatric%20Version.pdf. Accessed September 25, 2021.

64. Mahvan TD, Hilaire ML, Mann A, Brown A, Linn B, Gardner T, Lai B. Marijuana use in the elderly: Implications and considerations. *The Consultant pharmacist: The Journal of the American Society of Consultant Pharmacists.* 2017;32(6):341–351.

65. Harrar S. Older adults fuel recreational pot use. AARP Web site. https://www.aarp.org/health/drugs-supplements/info-2019/recreational-marijuana.html. Accessed October 3, 2021.

66. Neely CK. Financial problems that are associated with the elderly. https://www.sapling.com/7343940/financial-problems-associated-elderly. Accessed October 9, 2021.

67. Monthly Statistical Snapshot November 2011. Social Security Administration Web site. https://www.ssa.gov/policy/docs/quickfacts/stat_snapshot/2020-11.pdf. Accessed October 9, 2021.

68. Money saving tips. National Institutes of Health, National Heart, Lung, and Blood Institute Web site. https://www.nhlbi.nih.gov/health/educational/healthdisp/pdf/tipsheets/Money-Saving-Tips.pdf. Accessed October 29, 2021.

69. Bogle D. Social Security benefits increase in 2022. https://blog.ssa.gov/social-security-benefits-increase-in-2022/. Accessed October 30, 2021.

70. Probasco J. 6 Social Security Changes for 2022. Investopedia.comhttps://www.investopedia.com/retirement/social-security-changes/. Accessed October 30, 2021.

71. Grant N. What is the average monthly retirement income? https://goodlifehomeloans.com/resources/what-is-the-average-monthly-retirement-income/#:~:text=KEY%20TAKEAWAYS%201%20Median%20retirement%20income%20for%20seniors,of%20your%20pre-retirement%20monthly%20income.%20More%20items...%20. Accessed October 9, 2021.

72. Stoffell B. Here's what the average retired American's budget looks like. The Motley Fool. https://www.fool.com/retirement/general/2016/01/25/heres-what-the-average-retired-americans-budget-lo.aspx. Accessed October 11, 2021.

73. Find local elder law assistance. Elder Law Answers Web site. https://www.elderlawanswers.com/#:~:text=Medicare%20Part%20A%20covers%20institutional%20care%20in%20hospitals,is%20eligible%20for%20Medicare%20Part%20A%20without%20charge. Accessed October 11, 2021.

74. Shah K. Social connectedness: A key to healthy aging. https://www.healthinaging.org/blog/social-connectedness-a-key-to-healthy-aging/. Accessed October 29, 2021.

75. 25 resources that provide financial help for seniors. GoFundMe. https://www.gofundme.com/c/blog/financial-help-for-seniors. Accessed March 22, 2022.

CHAPTER 10

Quality of Life, Advance Directives, and End-of-Life Planning

LEARNING OBJECTIVES

1. Compare and contrast the landmark cases of Karen Quinlan, Nancy Cruzan, and Terry Schiavo.
2. Describe the differences and similarities between palliative care and hospice care.
3. Examine the aspects of end-of-life planning including cultural and religious beliefs, pain management, language barriers, and communication.
4. Describe three burial options that are available in most U.S. states.
5. Define the difference between grief and bereavement.

KEY WORDS

advanced directive	proxy	quality of life
executor	palliative care	end-of-life planning
healthcare power of attorney	hospice care	bereavement
living will	quantity of life	grief

Introduction

This chapter begins with an explanation of the U.S. landmark cases involving three younger, white women under the age of 30 and regarding end-of-life decisions after tragic circumstances. The next discussion defines legal terms used in end-of-life planning including the differences between palliative care and hospice care. After exploring the differences between quality of life and quantity of life, the focus changes to the aspects of end-of-life planning, including diverse cultural and religious beliefs, alternative pain management, language barriers, communication and accommodation, and the conversation regarding these topics. The next focus describes burial options, including embalming, cemetery burial, cremation, green burial, and other available burial options. Last, there is a discussion about differences between grief and bereavement.

History

According to the Center for Disease Control and Prevention, approximately 70 percent of Americans are without an advanced directive and do not have an active end-of-life care plan.[1] Additionally, most individuals do not consider end-of-life care decisions or wishes while they are in their 20s. However, the following three landmark cases may encourage individuals to rethink the benefits of having early discussions to openly communicate one's wishes regarding end-of-life decisions and preparing necessary documentation.[1] Note from author: It is noted that the following three examples of young white women lack diversity. While not specifically leaving anyone out, these landmark cases changed federal law regarding end-of-life decisions and received significant media attention.

Karen Ann Quinlan

At the early age of 21, Karen Ann Quinlan fell unconscious after swallowing alcohol and the common sedative, Valium, on April 14, 1975, near her home in New Jersey. She was rushed to a hospital where doctors saved her life, but she suffered brain damage and lapsed into a "persistent vegetative state."[2] She was kept alive on a ventilator for several months without improvement. Her parents asked the hospital staff to discontinue active care and allow her to die. Karen was quoted as saying she never wanted to be kept alive by extraordinary means. The hospital refused, and subsequent legal battles made the headlines.[3] Her family waged a prominent, publicized legal battle for the right to remove her from life-support machinery. Through perseverance, the family finally won the right to discontinue use of ventilator after a 7–0 decision by the New Jersey Supreme Court on March 31, 1976.[2] Eventually the court allowed removal of Karen's breathing tube, establishing a groundbreaking legal precedent. However, Quinlan kept breathing after the respirator was removed. She was moved to a New Jersey nursing home, where she remained in a coma for the next 9 years until her 1985 death. Karen Ann Quinlan was the first modern icon considering the right-to-die debate.[2]

Karen's case is also credited with the development of formal ethics committees in hospitals, nursing homes, palliative care protocols, hospice, and the development of advance health directives.[3]

Nancy Cruzan

In 1983, Nancy Cruzan was a 25-year-old Missouri woman who was ejected from her car when it flipped over.[4] Three years after sustaining major injuries, Nancy remained in a rehabilitation hospital operated by the State of Missouri. Her physicians and family members concluded she would never return to full consciousness, and her family began a long legal battle to have her feeding tube removed so she could die.

After 8 years, the family won the case. Nancy's tube was removed, and she died 12 days later December 26, 1990.[4] The Court's ruling affirmed that all adults with decision-making capacity have the right to (1) choose or refuse any medical or surgical intervention, including artificial nutrition and hydration, (2) make advance directives, and (3) name a surrogate to make decisions on their behalf.[4]

The Court said that surrogates can decide on a certain course (e.g., treatment or not) even when all concerned are aware that such measures would hasten death. The Cruzan case was the first so-called "right to die" case to be reviewed by the U.S. Supreme Court.[4]

Terri Schiavo

On February 25, 1990, 26-year-old Terri Schiavo, a resident of St. Petersburg, Florida, collapsed in the hallway of the apartment she shared with her husband, Michael Schiavo. It is unclear what caused her to lose consciousness, but she did have abnormally low potassium levels.[5] While she was unconscious, she was without sufficient oxygen necessary for optimal brain function. Though doctors revived her, the only thing she could do was breathe on her own. The doctors said she had no thoughts or emotions. Her body was alive, but everything else was gone.[5]

In 1998, Michael said the feeding tube should be removed because that is what she would have wanted. Her parents, Robert and Mary Schindler, instead said she would have chosen to remain on the feeding tube because they thought she might wake up from her persistent vegetative state.[5]

The court ruled in Michael's favor, agreeing that Terri was in a persistent vegetative state and would not wish to continue life-prolonging measures. On April 24, 2001, Terri's feeding tube was removed—only to be reinserted several days later.[5] The parents and the husband battled over Terri's life for the next 7 years. The courts sided with Michael, but the parents appealed, prolonging Terri's life. In 2005, in the last appeal, five doctors testified, two chosen by Michael, two by the Mr. and Mrs. Schindler (Terri's parents), and one by the court. The doctors chosen by the parents said there was a chance she could wake up. The other three said that there was no chance. The feeding tube was removed on March 18, 2005, and Terri died within 13 days on March 31, 2005. After she died, an autopsy showed that the brain damage had been irreversible, and she would never have woken up.[5-6]

In summary, a 1988 medical publication posed the question of who should rightly decide quality of life versus quantity of life questions as related to health care. Currently, more than 30 years later, the same unresolved questions are asked by healthcare professionals, academics, clergy, bioethics committees, and families. Healthcare professionals regard themselves as the legal decision-makers. In addition to the three landmark cases, there are many more cases where patients' lives have been maintained by extraordinary means without their direct informed consent and against their will.[7]

Definitions

When learning about end-of-life planning, it is essential to become familiar with the terminology and how it pertains to the individual in the state of residence.

Advanced Directives. Individuals plan their future health care by designating a trusted individual to speak for them when they are no longer able to speak for themselves. A clear and well-written **advanced directive** document eases stress and the emotional burden for families during an end-of-life event.[8] Advance directives must be in writing and each state within the United States has different forms, requirements, and legal criteria for creating these legally binding documents. Some states require the document to be signed and witnessed, while other states require notarization. It is important for individuals to review the advance directives with their doctor and their healthcare advocate. After the documents are reviewed and approved, it is necessary to keep the original documents in a safe place that is easily accessible. Additionally, a copy should be provided to one's healthcare provider and health advocate. It is important to discuss healthcare wishes with family members and to carry a wallet-size card that indicates where a copy of the advanced directives is located.

Advance directives may be changed at any time. When changes are made, it is important to repeat the process of distribution (e.g., updating physician, healthcare facilities, health advocate, and family) and destroy outdated copies. The advance directives should be reviewed in the following situations: a new diagnosis, change of marital status, and updated approximately every 10 years because to options regarding end-of-life care changes over time.[9]

Executor (Legal Guardian). An **executor** is defined as the person named to carry out the directions of a will. This person has the legal authority and the corresponding duty to care for the interests of another person. Such interests may include personal or property depending on the jurisdiction and state. In some states, the proxy (healthcare decision-maker) and executor (property decision-maker) may be the same person. In other states, it must be two separate individuals.[8]

Healthcare Power of Attorney. A **healthcare power of attorney (POA)** is a close family member or other trusted person appointed as person's healthcare agent. The POA may make healthcare decisions for the named person when he or she can no longer speak for him or herself or no longer has decisional capacity. End-of-life professionals agree that talking with loved ones and naming a durable power of attorney for healthcare decisions provides the greatest assurance that an individual's wishes will be known and honored.[8]

Living Will. Living wills are documents that provide instructions about life-sustaining treatment and other end-of-life care that individuals desire to be followed when they can no longer speak for themselves.[8-9] A living will is a written legal document indicating specific medical treatments one would and would not desire to be used to be kept alive. The document also contains the following preferences related to other medical decisions, such as providing cardiopulmonary resuscitation, mechanical ventilation for breathing, tube feeding, dialysis, pain management, or organ donation.[9] For example, a living will typically include phrases, such as, "If I am terminally ill, there shall be no heroic measures."[8] It is important to remember that living will documents do not give an individual the right to choose and refuse treatment, since that right is stated in the U.S. Constitution and was affirmed in the Nancy Cruzan case. The main purpose of a living will document is primarily to provide protection to health care professionals from criminal or civil prosecution when following directives.[8]

Proxy. A person who is designated and legally permitted to make healthcare decisions for a specific individual is called a **proxy**. Other terms used include agent, surrogate, healthcare representative and can be designated in a durable power of attorney for health care.[10]

Palliative Care and Hospice Care

The terms palliative care and hospice care are often confused and even used interchangeably. To eliminate the confusion, it is useful to define both terms for clarification.

Palliative Care. Palliative care is specialized medical care that focuses on providing patients relief from pain and other symptoms related to a serious illness or condition, regardless of the diagnosis or stage of disease.[11] Palliative care teams consist of physicians, nurses, social workers, chaplains, and case managers. The palliative team aims to improve the quality of life for both patients and their families. Palliative care can be provided along with curative treatment and may begin at the time of diagnosis.

Palliative care may be offered to patients of any age who are experiencing a serious or life-threatening illness, such as cancer, heart disease, cystic fibrosis, Alzheimer's or other forms of dementia, end-stage liver disease, kidney failure, Parkinson's disease, chronic obstructive pulmonary disease (COPD), stroke, and Amyotrophic Lateral Sclerosis (ALS).[11] The palliative care team manages symptoms, including pain, nausea or vomiting, anxiety or nervousness, depression or sadness, constipation, difficulty breathing, anorexia, fatigue, and trouble sleeping.

Palliative care teams focus on quality of life.[11] See **Figure 10.1** and **Figure 10.2**.

Palliative care is provided in hospitals, nursing homes, outpatient palliative care clinics and certain other specialized clinics, or even at home. Medicare, Medicaid, and private health insurance policies may cover palliative care. Veterans may be eligible for palliative care through the Department of Veterans Affairs.[12] A community health worker (CHW) may find the following list useful when working with patients with a serious illness and their families. See **Table 10.1**.

Palliative Care and Mental Health

When exploring the literature regarding palliative care and mental health, there are several overlaps among individuals with pre-existing mental health problems, individuals with diagnosed dementia, and individuals without a pre-existing mental health issue but struggling with a terminal diagnosis. The investigation revealed gaps in the research for individuals with a pre-existing

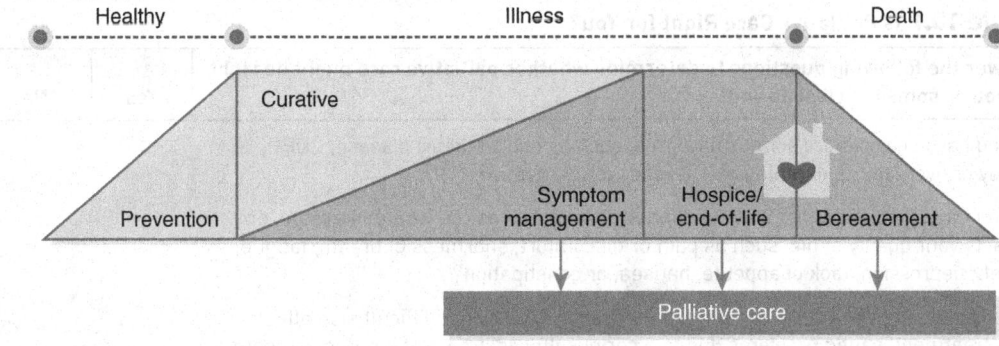

Figure 10.1 The Palliative Care Timeline

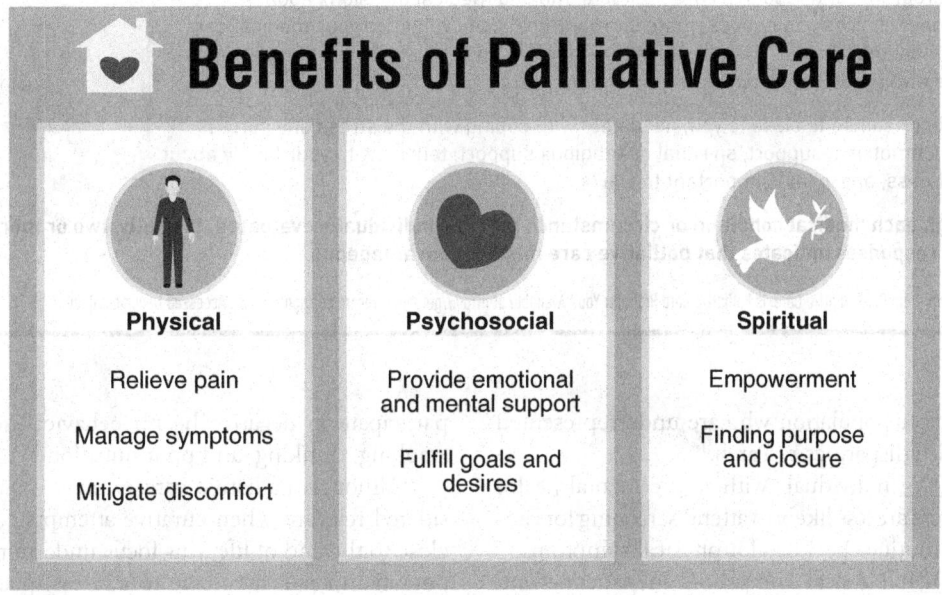

Figure 10.2 The Benefits of Palliative Care

mental health disorders, such as schizophrenia, bipolar disorder and severe clinical depression.[15] The following list reveals the limited available research:

2019: There are misperceptions that individuals with serious mental disorders do not have the capacity to provide consent or participate in decision-making related to treatment such as chemotherapy or surgery or that treatment could potentially disrupt the individuals' mental state.[15]

More research is needed to explore the possible relationship between mental health conditions and palliative care.

Patients with schizophrenia are less likely to receive chemotherapy, surgery, or blood transfusions, to be admitted to acute care units, and to die in intensive-care units or emergency departments than were patients without a diagnosis of mental illness.[16] People with serious mental illnesses and life-limiting physical health comorbidities are a

Table 10.1 Is Palliative Care Right for You?

Answer the following questions to determine whether palliative care might be right for you or someone close to you:	Yes	No
Do you have one or more serious illnesses, such as cancer, heart disease, COPD, kidney or liver failure, neurological diseases, or dementia?		
Do you have symptoms that make it difficult to be active as you would like to be, or impacts your quality of life, such as pain or discomfort, shortness of breath, fatigue, anxiety, depression, lack of appetite, nausea, or constipation?		
Have you, or someone close to your experienced the following: difficult side effects from treatment, eating problems due to a serious illness, frequent emergency room visits, or three or more admissions to the hospital within 12 months and with the same symptoms?		
Do you, or someone close to you, need help with knowing what to expect, knowing what programs and resources are available, making medical decisions about treatment choices and options, matching your goals and values to your medical care, understanding the pros and cons (benefits, burden, and risks) of medical treatments (e.g., dialysis, additional cancer treatment, surgery)?		
Do you, or someone close to you, need help with coping with the stress of a serious illness, emotional support, spiritual or religious support, talking with your family about your illness, and what is important to you?		

Though each medical condition or circumstance must be individually evaluated, typically, two or more "Yes" responses indicates that palliative care might be advantageous.

Reproduced from Get Palliative Care. Is Palliative Care Right for You? Available at https://getpalliativecare.org/rightforyou/. Accessed November 8, 2021.[14]

vulnerable population who are underrepresented in health disparities research.[16]

2006: Individuals with severe mental health disorders are less likely to attend screening for cancer or routine checkups for physical symptoms.[15]

2004: Physical complaints in patients with known psychiatric disorder can be ascribed to their underlying mental illness and not given sufficient attention.[15] However, it is important that the physical complaint be taken seriously by all healthcare professionals.

1999: There is a high rate of substance misuse in this population. One explanation for this is that people with mental health problems attempt to self-medicate symptoms of illness and the uncomfortable adverse side effects of psychiatric medications.[15]

1979: Individuals with severe and long-term mental health disorders typically lead to less healthy lifestyles, have limited exercise, and participate in negative health behaviors such as smoking, drinking, and poor nutrition.[15]

Although palliative care is most often considered relevant when curative attempts cease or close to the end of life, this focus undermines the potential of palliative care to address quality-of-life issues in a wide spectrum of chronic health conditions and earlier in illness trajectories. More recently, palliative care is viewed with a focus on improving the quality of life and psychological needs of patients and families rather than on symptom management at the end of life.[17] In addition, psychologists and psychiatrists are needed to meet the complex mental health needs of palliative care patients and reduce demands on treatment teams by focusing on integrated care teams, changing attitudes about mental health, and increasing interest and training opportunities for psychologists and psychiatrists to be involved in palliative care teams.[17] At the system level, the divisions between physical and psychiatric medicine result in confusion and fragmentation in management of individuals with complex health needs. This barrier of care integration is associated with a serious risk of poor health outcomes.[16]

Hospice Care. Hospice care is introduced when a serious illness, diagnosis, or condition is incurable, or the patient decides to discontinue or refuses treatment.[12] When beginning hospice care, individuals understand that their illness is not responding to medical attempts to cure or slow disease progress. Thus, hospice does not focus on curing the diagnosis or condition. Often people choose hospice care at end of life because hospice care focuses on the care, comfort, and the quality of life related to a total person with a serious illness. Hospice care is popularly understood as a death sentence.[12,18] However, hospice seeks to enhance one's quality of life so that the individual is emotionally, mentally, physically, and spiritually comfortable and has more time to enjoy the company of family and friends.[18] Often patients live longer because they are more comfortable. Like palliative care, hospice provides comprehensive care and comfort measures directly to the patient and resources for the family. Hospice is provided when a physician determines that a person likely has 6 months or less based on the current diagnosis or state of the condition.[18] However, one's care team reevaluates the person over time. Though the 6-month time frame is used as a threshold, there is never a guarantee that one will die. Rather a physician determines that the patient is eligible to receive hospice services based on the condition and approximate time frame.[18]

It is important for the patient, their family, their physician, or the palliative care team to discuss hospice care options. Sometimes, patients do not begin hospice care soon enough to take full advantage of the help it offers.[18] For example, some patients wait too long to begin hospice and are too close to death. Or a patient and/or the family wishes to continue treatment as one last chance for a cure. Starting hospice early provide months of meaningful care and quality time with loved ones.[12]

Hospice is an approach to care but is not defined as a specific place. Hospice is offered in two types of settings: at home or in a facility such as a nursing home, hospital, or even in a separate hospice center.[12] Hospice care consists of a team of people with special skills, including physicians, nurses, social workers, spiritual advisors, case managers, and trained volunteers. The hospice team works together with the patient, the caregiver, and/or the family to provide the medical, physical, emotional, and spiritual support needed. A member of the hospice team visits the patient on a regular scheduled basis, and a team member is available by phone at all times of day or night. Hospice may be covered by Medicare and other insurance companies, but it is important to verify if patient's insurance covers a particular situation.[12]

When a patient enters hospice, it is important to remember that stopping treatment aimed at curing an illness does not mean discontinuing all treatment. For example, the patient may not be responding to the cancer treatment, so they stop the treatment. However, other prescription medications will continue, if desired, for symptom management, such as hypertensive medication or an inhaler to ease breathing.[12] See **Table 10.2**.

Quantity of Life Versus Quality of Life

Quantity and quality may appear easy to define until the terms are applied to the life of an individual. Quantity is an amount or number of something, while quality is the degree to which an object or entity (e.g., process, product, or service) satisfies a specified set of attributes or requirements.[19]

Quantity of life refers to number of days in an individual's life. Using statistics, an individual's life-span is estimated based on the available data, including gender, age, ethnicity, geographical location, comorbidities, environmental exposures, occupation, and numerous other variables.[19] For example, when a patient is given a cancer diagnosis, the individual may ask the physician, "How long do I have to live?"[19] The physician starts this

Table 10.2 Comparison of Palliative Care and Hospice Care

Question	Palliative Care	Hospice Care
Who can be treated?	Anyone with a serious illness	Anyone with a serious illness when a physician believes the patient has less than 6 months to live
Will the symptoms be relieved?	Yes, as much as possible	Yes, as much as possible
Will the treatment to cure the illness continue?	Yes, if desired	No, only relief of symptoms will be provided to enhance quality of life
Will Medicare or private insurance pay for the services?	It depends on the plan	It depends on the plan
How long is the care available?	It depends on the insurance and the patient needs	If the patient meets the hospice criteria with a life expectancy of months
Where is care provided?	Home, assisted living facility, nursing home, or hospital	Home, assisted living facility, nursing home, hospice facility, or hospital

Data from National Institutes of Health, National Institute on Aging. What Are Palliative Care and Hospice Care? Available at https://www.nia.nih.gov/health/what-are-palliative-care-and-hospice-care. Accessed November 8, 2021.[12]

discussion by stating, "It depends on the treatment options that you select, how you respond to the treatment, and many other factors." At best, the physician can estimate length of life if the patient chooses to decline any surgery or treatment. If the patient selects any or all options, the accuracy of the estimate declines due to an increase in the response to treatment. Therefore, estimating the length of an individual's life is difficult to access with any degree of accuracy.[19–20]

Quality of life refers to the degree in which an individual is healthy, comfortable, and able to participate in or enjoy life events.[19] It refers to both the experiences and living conditions in an individual's life. Quality of life is highly subjective.[19–20]

Here are a few examples:

- An individual may have excellent education, wealth, a large home, and a beach condo. However, the person may have a low quality of life due to marital problems, health issues due to obesity, and employment stress.
- An individual had a long-term, happy marriage, sufficient money for a comfortable lifestyle, but his spouse died of cancer, his adult children made bad financial decisions thus causing him, their dad, to reduce his retirement savings. The overall situation is causing stress and health problems. To cope, he joined a grief support group and a fitness center. He reports that his quality of life is improving due to making new friends and participating in physical activity.
- An individual is a veteran from the Vietnam War. In the past, he suffered from post-traumatic stress syndrome and still has complications from injuries to his legs. Thus, he has a disability and uses a motorized scooter. Most people would think this gentleman would have a low quality of life due to his circumstances. However, he rates his quality of life as excellent. He receives adequate disability benefits for a simple lifestyle, lives in a small apartment with disability features in the kitchen and bathroom, drives a renovated car with hand controls, volunteers two days a week at the VA Hospital with his two small pet therapy dogs, teaches guitar to middle school in the afternoon program, and plays bridge at the local senior center. See **Critical Thinking 10.1**.

Critical Thinking 10.1 Quality Versus Quantity of Life

Sam is 87 years old, drinks only diet soda, and consumes mostly salty snacks. Alice, Sam's daughter, is concerned that her dad refuses to drink anything besides diet soda. Sam suffers from diabetes and deteriorating cognition due to age and his poor diet and consumption of diet soda. He tells Alice that he does not care about getting well. His exact quote is: "I am 87. I should be able to decide what I want to drink and eat." Alice tried purchasing every variety of flavored and sparkling water at the grocery store with special cups for sipping and straws, but Sam refuses to accept change. When she buys low-salt snacks, Sam throws the bag in the trash.

Alice made an appointment with the CHW at the clinic where Sam receives health care. She wants to receive some advice. Alice knows that as individuals age, their taste buds decrease, and so older adults may consume more unhealthy foods with high salt, high sugar, and high fat content. Alice wants to keep her father healthy, if possible, but her efforts are beginning to diminish due to Sam's perception on his quality of life.

Question

1. As the CHW, what advice would you give Alice?

Quality of life is perceived and defined differently by everyone.[19] Since the perception of a person's quality of life changes across the life-span due to situations and circumstances, CHWs need to be aware that there are several broad categories of quality-of-life scales to measure an individual's quality of life.[19–20]

Last, quality of life represents an important aspect of health that is different from the usual forms of physical assessment, such as blood tests, X-rays, blood tests, and clinical opinions.[19] These physical assessments dominate health care because they are objective and specifically measurable. However, quality of life measurements are subjective views of the patient. These views help the healthcare provider determine how

the patients are reacting to their diagnosis.[19–20] For example, the healthcare providers or family members may view a patient's serious disability as having a much larger impact on the person's life than it is perceived to be by the patient. Another example would be when a patient's blood tests show that the disease is stable, but the patient reports increasing pain, discomfort, and a worsening prognosis. In summary, the main purpose of health care is to improve the well-being of the patient's life. By incorporating the patient's perceptions into the treatment plan, the healthcare provider is looking at a comprehensive view of the patient.[19–20]

Aspects of End-of-Life Care Planning

This section covers the aspects of **end-of-life planning**, including diverse cultural and religious beliefs, alternative pain management, language barriers, communication and accommodation, and the conversation that occurs when determining end-of-life plans.[21] When healthcare providers explore quality and quantity of life issues, the first consideration is to determine how the individual and family decisions are influenced by one's culture and family dynamic.[21] If the healthcare provider starts any poor prognoses or end-of-life planning conversation based on his or her own cultural beliefs, the patient and family members are likely to dismiss any further conversation due to the healthcare provider's bias or assumption.[21] For example, providers need to be aware that in many cultures it is considered inappropriate and insensitive to discuss impending death.[21] Therefore, the conversation begins by asking the patient and family members about their cultural beliefs regarding pain and death prior to discussing the option of palliative care. Without knowledge and understanding about cultural beliefs, such a discussion may possibly harm the patient-provider relationship and act as a barrier to appropriate pain management.[21]

For example, globally populations have diverse cultural beliefs regarding the meaning, origin, and role of pain, which can affect how a patient interprets and perceives pain.[21] After reviewing the information in **Table 10.3**, it becomes evident that a vast number of the entire population has various ways in which their culture approaches death. The following table provides an overview of cultural influence and relative perceptions on end-of-life care, options, pain management, familiar influence, and coping. However, culture exists on a spectrum and can be subjective.[21] Descriptions of cultures may be generally correct; however, individual patients may differ based on diagnosis, access, education, personal history, rituals and traditions, gender influences, normative values, or beliefs, which dictate the patient's overall experience. As CHWs and members of the healthcare team, it is important to ask appropriate questions, listen carefully to the patient's wishes, and address family concerns.[21] It is important to avoid assumptions or generalizations regarding a specific culture. For example, a Hispanic family may identify and respect their cultural heritage, while having completely different wishes that may be described as counterculture when compared to other Hispanic families.[21]

As for pain management, the patient and families may find it advantageous to instruct and guide providers in how, when, or if the patient's pain should be treated according to their cultural beliefs.[21] Since many cultures do not accept or encourage the use of strong pain management medications (e.g., opioids), it becomes a challenging barrier for providing palliative care to those in severe pain nearing the end of life.[21] Here are a few other examples of culturally diverse options. Some cultures place a substantial value on the community, while others encourage individual independence. Some let the family make decisions, while others help each patient to make their own decision.[21] Some cultures discuss pain and end-of-life decisions as a family, while others may leave the choice to the patient and possibly a spouse. In some cultures, the decisions regarding the care of the elderly are left to the children.[21] Many countries are a melting pot of different cultures, and it becomes

necessary and difficult for the healthcare providers to develop an understanding of the various influences that guide patient and family decisions. For the healthcare provider to learn both proper pain management and cultural sensitivity goes a long way toward providing a more functional environment and better patient and family care at this most sensitive time.[21]

In addition to culture, religion may influence patients' and their families decisions regarding end-of-life care, pain management, and palliative care options.[21] For example, many individuals affiliated with or recognized as Christian Scientists, Hindus, Jehovah's Witnesses, Mormons, Muslims, or Seventh-day Adventists are reluctant to accept interventions or medications due to their organization's or church's teaching on euthanasia and the belief that some medications may hasten death.[21] Other religions and cultures believe that pain should be endured bravely to preserve their standing in the afterlife, while others may perceive death as God's will, a test of faith, or penance for past sins.[21] Recognizing how culture and religion can influence one's perception toward end-of-life issues is important to avoid undertreating pain, maintaining a value neutral stance, and tailoring clinical recommendations to a align with a patient's beliefs.[21]

Alternative Pain Management

Healthcare providers and hospitals benefit from being aware of some alternative pain relief techniques that may be used safely in conjunction with pain management medications, such as opioids.[21] For example, alternative pain management can include acupuncture, marijuana infused with CBD oil for ointments and lotions, music, art, pet therapy, mindful meditation, herbs and herbal teas, cupping, and moxibustion (traditional Chinese medicine technique during acupuncture that involves the burning a small, spongy herb to facilitate healing). Sometimes patients request a spiritual healer, pastor, or chaplain for prayer, guidance, and support.[21] Whenever possible, healthcare providers should

Table 10.3 Examples of Diverse Cultural Beliefs Surrounding End-of-Life Care

Culture	Perception of Death	Pain	Palliative Care
African American	Display grief openly alongside family and relatives.	May avoid pain management while under supervision, due to fears related to addiction. Pain scales are helpful tools.	Generally accepting of palliative care with adequate education on how to manage pain safely.
Amish	Death is deeply spiritual.	Very high pain tolerance is common.	May accept palliative care.
Arab	Discussions about death may be avoided.	Expressed in various ways.	Usually, unwilling to accept "do not resuscitate" orders (DNRs).
Cuban	Everything possible should be done to prevent death.	Individuals may be stoic regarding pain and reluctant to accept pain medication or treatment.	May be reluctant to accept palliative care.
East Asian	Reluctant to talk about death.	Stoic and poised; it is important to be aware of nonverbal signs indicating pain.	Some may believe that dying at home may bring bad luck; will accept palliative care.
East Indian	Death should be discussed with family first, who might not inform the patients.	Will accept pain medicine for severe pain.	May accept palliative care.
Filipino	A loud grieving process is typical. May avoid discussing.	Pain is often expressed as "cold" or "hot."	Will accept palliative care and pain control.
Jamaican	Maybe very emotional with crying and mourning typically.	Highly variable.	Will seek health care but may believe in a possible cure despite terminal illness. Generally, accept end-of-life care.
Japanese	May avoid discussion.	Maybe very stoic.	May take assistance, often at home.
Hispanic	Many family members may be present. The family may not want to inform the patient of the end-stage of a terminal illness.	May not complain of pain and may only provide nonverbal clues.	May have reservations regarding accepting end-of-life care.
Indigenous Tribes/ Native American	May avoid contact with dying. Verbal grieving may include wailing.	May be undertreated and only expressed privately to family or friends.	May not be willing to discuss terminal status as it is thought to hasten death.
Vietnamese	Will have a difficult time discussing death and DNR. These subjects stir deep emotions.	Maybe very stoic.	Will probably accept palliative care and pain medicine.

Givler A, Bhatt H, & Maani-Fogelmann, PA. The importance of cultural competence in pain and palliative care. Florida: *STAT PEARLS*; 2021.[21]

allow traditional remedies for pain palliation, providing they are not harmful to the patient. Pharmacists and prescribers should collaborate to ensure the safety of alternative therapies, especially when combined with prescription medications. If possible, healthcare professionals should be willing to accommodate the wishes and desires of the family and patients while maintaining their dignity and independence as much as possible.[21]

Language Barriers

One of the difficult challenges of palliative care is when the patient and family communicate in a different language.[21] When using a paid translator or computer software translation, the words, phrases, and concepts may have different meanings that cause poor decisions or communicate misconstrued information. Using a family member as a translator may be convenient, but the family member may result in miscommunications. Also, the patient may not wish to have the family know the extent of their diagnosis.[21] For instance, a family member from a culture that avoids discussing death would be reluctant to translate the words from a patient's doctor regarding a serious or terminal diagnosis. Using a professional translator is always preferred for accurate and sensitive discussions.[21]

In the case of significant pain, the patient's pain level, due to misinterpretation, may not be understood and thus results in lack of appropriate pain management. If a patient's English skills are limited, the use of professional interpreters will decrease communication errors, improve clinical outcomes, and increase patient satisfaction.[21]

Communication and Accommodation

Many patients and families are reluctant to discuss religious and cultural issues affecting their care.[21] The patient may consider it inappropriate to ask for pain medications and may rely on the pain treatment options supplied by the healthcare provider.[21] In other cases, if the patient requests pain medicine, it may be considered a sign of weakness, particularly in some cultures that believe pain is part of the dying process and must be accepted and tolerated without complaint. Many patients will rely on prayer to ease and treat pain, especially at the end of life. As a result, healthcare providers must be aware of the cultural beliefs, religious customs, and rituals near the end of life and make time and space to accommodate religious and spiritual practices.[21]

Palliative care is often underutilized by culturally diverse communities.[21] For several reasons, non-White patients are substantially less likely to receive end-of-life care and appropriate pain management. It is essential that all healthcare providers learn to feel comfortable asking patients about their personal preferences regarding pain management and end-of-life care.[21] The discussion should take place with the patient and, if desired, with the immediate family. If there is a language barrier, a trained professional translator should be used. When patients are understood by the healthcare provider, they receive care that aligns with their cultural and religious beliefs.[21] See **Box 10.1**.

Last, healthcare providers must be instructed to care for patients with compassion, especially during their final moments. Improving cultural competence and cultural humility ensures that

---

Box 10.1 Questions for the Patient with a Terminal Diagnosis

Here are a few questions that healthcare providers may ask patients regarding pain management:

1. How important is staying mentally alert to you in the final days before death?
2. What pain level are you willing to endure?
3. What type of pain medicine or alternatives should be considered?

Givler A, Bhatt H, & Maani-Fogelmann, PA. The importance of cultural competence in pain and palliative care. Florida: *STAT PEARLS*; 2021.[21]

healthcare professionals can provide pain relief and optimal palliative care to all patients regardless of their age, gender, or cultural background.[21]

The Conversation: Communicating and Navigating Difficult Decisions

Having a conversation about end-of-life decisions is difficult at any age and for most cultures.[22] However, some families may benefit from discussing options and arranging documents together as a family unit. Because death is inevitable, it is easier to engage in the conversation at a time when no one is experiencing a life-threatening diagnosis.[22] Also, the earlier the conversation takes place, the sooner everyone in the family feels a sense of relief. This relief eases the burden and stress when the time comes to act on behalf of the individual's final wishes and written decisions. This conversation allows the seniors family members to teach the next generation the valuable perspective of the family's cultural and religious beliefs as the discussion moves forward. In addition, it allows the younger generation to express their personal beliefs, which may or may not align with the thoughts presented by their elders. Everyone has the right to develop their own plans for end of life, and those plans should be respected by their loved ones.[22]

How to Start the Conversation

According to a national survey conducted by the Conversation Project, one-fifth of the surveyed individuals said they were waiting for their loved one to start the conversation about end-of-life planning, although 9 out of 10 respondents believed that having these discussions were important.[22] If starting this conversation feels awkward at a family event, another suggestion is to write a letter to invite family members to a gathering to discuss end-of-life options,

desires, and wishes. This invitation letter reduces any surprises and allows everyone to have time to gather their thoughts.[22] See **Critical Thinking 10.2**.

Critical Thinking 10.2 The Conversation Project

The Conversation Project was launched to enable more people to sit down with family and friends to talk about what will matter most at the end of their lives.[22] It will always be too early, until it's too late.

The survey results show why Americans have *not* discussed their own wishes:

- It is not something they need to worry about at this point in life. (29 percent)
- They are not sick yet. (23 percent)
- The subject makes them feel uncomfortable. (21 percent)
- They do not want to upset their loved ones. (19 percent)

Nearly half (48 percent) of Americans say that if a loved one asked them about their wishes for end-of-life care, they would welcome it and be relieved to discuss it.[22] Another 41 percent admit that while it would be a difficult discussion to have, they would be willing to do it. When the conversation begins, the experience is improved. In addition, more than half of those who have lost someone without ever discussing end-of-life wishes would admit that some aspect of the experience could have been improved if they had a conversation. Those who did have the conversation stated that they felt better knowing they were honoring the wishes of their loved ones (63 percent) while others found comfort know their loved one was able to die the way they wanted (39 percent).[22]

Question

1. What are some reasons why your family has or has not had such a conversation?

Reproduced from The Conversation Project. New Survey Reveals 'Conversational Disconnect:' 90 percent of Americans know they should have a conversation about what they want at the end of life, yet only 30 percent have done so. Available at https://theconversationproject.org/wp-content/uploads/2013/09/TCP-Survey-Release_FINAL-9-18-13.pdf. Accessed November 11, 2021.[22]

What to Say at the Family Meeting

Before the conversation begins, take a few minutes to relax and focus on the message. This conversation is not about saying good-bye but is to have a productive discussion on the end-of-life wishes for a person. It is about making sure the family members are comfortable and taking the guesswork out of complicated issues that everyone will face later in life. A good place to begin the conversation is to distribute notepads and pens to each person for taking notes and then ask each person to state their opinion regarding their choice between burial or cremation.[22] See **Box 10.2**.

Box 10.2 **Suggestions to Navigate Difficult Discussions**

The following recommendations may help one navigate difficult discussions:

- Make time.[23]
- Choose an intimate, quiet setting.[23]
- Eliminate any distractions (e.g., turn off your phone, remove any interruption).
- Reframe the discussion (this is not about saying goodbye, rather it is a gift to honor one's wishes at the end).[24]
- Start small conversations.[24]
- Discuss concepts and avoid actualities.[24]
- Listen carefully to the individual's desires, wishes, and goals.
- If the conversation becomes negative or emotionally charged, take a break and re-group when things have settled.
- Follow the conversation lead.[25]
- Focus on their needs.
- Express your thoughts, feelings, suggestions, and opinions honestly.[24-25]
- Take time to reflect on life experiences that matter to them and the entire family.[25]

The conversation may begin by recalling an example, such as, "I remember how hard it was for everyone when Grandma was dying. No one could agree if she should or should not have a feeding tube for nutrition. She died before the decision was made. When she died, no one knew what kind of memorial service she wanted. I want to make sure that those topics do not happen to the rest of us."[22-25] Ask everyone to describe a little about their wishes surrounding death and their end-of-life care.

Topics to Cover

Since participants have a notepad and pen, it is important to remind them to write down topics to reflect upon later. If a few family members have already made funeral arrangement, they should describe the process, decisions, and cost. It is thought-provoking to see how some people arrange their funeral rather than advance directives regarding their care for prior to dying.[26]

Other topics for discussion:

- Find out whether your parents or other family members have a will and a power of attorney. If your relatives become incapacitated, the POA determines who makes health and financial decisions on their behalf. When needed, assist with making an appointment with an attorney to complete such documents.[26]
- Ask about what kind of insurance and other financial resources are available for long-term care.[26]
- Request copies of all important documents, including birth certificates, wills and POAs, medical records, property records, financial documents, insurance documents, and lists of any doctors, attorneys, and financial planners.[26]
- Talk about their end-of-life desires, such as life support and organ donation.
- Discuss desires about how spend their remaining years, such a traveling or creating records of family history.[26]
- Discuss the various types of funeral and burial services.[26]
- This conversation is not a single event but rather a beginning to future conversations and updates.[26]

A Planning Guide for End of Life

Though CHWs are not directly involved with advance care planning, patients may feel more comfortable asking CHWs questions during a conversation about such a sensitive topics. In such circumstances, the CHW should have enough information to dispel myths, convey facts, and do so with empathy. It is best to have a brochure available to clarify information. See **Box 10.3**.

Approximately 37 percent of Americans have advanced directives for end-of-life care if they become seriously ill or unable to make healthcare decisions, according to a new analysis of recent research.[27] Since many Americans die in facilities such as hospitals or nursing homes receiving care that is not consistent with their wishes, it is important for adults of any age to plan and discuss their end-of-life preferences in advance with family members and healthcare providers.[12] For example, if a person wants to die at home without life support measures, receiving end-of-life care for pain and other symptoms, and makes

---

Box 10.3 A Planning Guide for End-of-Life Care and Advance Directives

Step 1: Questions to ask your healthcare provider

- Make an appointment to discuss end-of-life care and advanced directives. Medicare began reimbursing physicians for advance-care planning counseling in 2016 (Frequently Asked Questions about Billing the Physician Fee Schedule for Advance Care Planning Services at cms.gov).
- Take a list of questions to ask your healthcare provider.
- Ask for the positive and negative features of artificial life-support and other medical measures for end-of-life care:
  - Cardiopulmonary resuscitation (CPR)
  - Do not resuscitate (DNR)
  - Mechanical ventilator for breathing
  - Artificial nutrition and hydration (tube feeding)
  - Kidney dialysis

Step 2: Decide who will make health decisions for you

- Think about who you trust to follow your wishes and make difficult decisions.
- Consider who is willing and able to serve as your health advocate.
- Discuss your wishes with several individuals before making the final decision.

Step 3: Make decisions about your wishes

- What type of care would you like if you can no longer speak for yourself?
- What is most important to you regarding your end-of-life decisions?
- What personal wishes and values should your health advocate consider when making decision for your care?

Step 4: Write down your wishes

- There are websites that offer easy-to-follow directions to guide you through the process:
  - Advance Care Planning Program for Medical Practices (honormydecisions.com)
  - Free Advance Directive Forms by State from AARP
  - Thinking Ahead—My Way, My Choice, My Life at the End (mn.gov)
  - My End-of-Life Decisions: An Advance Planning Guide and Toolkit | Compassion & Choices (compassionandchoices.org)
  - Advance Care Planning: Health Care Directives | National Institute on Aging (nih.gov)
- In addition, consider making a video that clearly states your end-of-life wishes to accompany your documents.

Step 5: Share your wishes

- After completing your advance healthcare directive, it is important to share your wishes.
- Keep an original copy of your advance healthcare directive in a safe place.
- Ask your healthcare provider to upload a copy to your electronic medical record.
- Take a copy with you if you are admitted to the hospital.
- Give a copy to your healthcare advocate and discuss your wishes.
- Talk about your advance directive with any family or friends you would expect to attend to your needs if you cannot speak for yourself or if your healthcare advocate is not available.

(continues)

- End-of-life circumstances are stressful. It is possible to decrease this burden with clear, well-written advance directive health documents.
- In today's world of social media, family members may wish to decide which family member will be chosen to post the passing of a loved one on social media.

Data from Pennsylvania Medical Society. Five Steps: A Guide to Help Plan Your End-of-Life and Future Health Care. Available at https://www.pamedsoc.org/list/articles/Advanced-Directive-..Steps#:~:text=%20Five%20Steps%3A%20A%20Guide%20to%20Help%20Plan,down%20your%20decisions.%20Write%20down%20your...%20More%20. Accessed November 25, 2021.[29]

this known to healthcare providers and family, it is less likely he or she will die in a hospital receiving unwanted treatments.[12]

End-of-life conversations about values and life preferences can be difficult. However, it is easier to have such discussions prior to a medical complications or terminal illness diagnosis is causing stress and anxiety for the patient and the family.[28] See **Case Study 10.1**.

After completing the Five-Step Planning Guide for creating an advanced directive, individuals must realize that simply completing a written document is not sufficient.[29] To ensure that an individual's wishes are known and honored requires serious reflection and candid discussion with family members, other loved ones, and healthcare providers.[30] Advanced directives are more inclusive if they include features of both a living will and a power of attorney. In addition, the advance directive document must adhere to state laws when related to the provision of health care when an individual is incapacitated.[30] See **Case Study 10.2**.

Case Study 10.1 CHW Involved with End-of-Life Decisions

Frank, a CHW, has been employed for 6 years at a geriatric clinic at the large university hospital complex in the metropolitan city. He speaks fluent Spanish because his grandparents came to the United States from Spain during World War II. The health educator and senior CHW at the clinic, Nancy, realizes that Frank has excellent rapport with many of the patients. Every 3 months, Nancy offers a 3-hour patient education seminar related to advanced directives and end-of-life options. She has Frank help with the facilitation of this seminar because most patients ask specific questions. Nancy is confident that Frank has learned how to respond correctly to the participants' questions. She also knows that Frank will bring her into the conversation if he does not know how to address the question.

On Monday, Frank was at work, when he received a phone call from his mother. Frank's grandmother, Sadie, age 89, had fallen and fractured her hip. Sadie speaks English but prefers to speak Spanish. She is frail and has hearing aids but does not like wearing them. She is a devoted Catholic and attends Mass weekly. Since Frank is the oldest of Linda's three children and the only family member working in health care, Linda called him immediately. Linda has one sister, Mary. Frank's entire extended family lives within a 50-mile radius, and they consider themselves to be a close-knit family. Sadie had been taken by emergency responders to the university hospital near where Frank works and had been admitted a few hours ago. Linda was at the hospital and at her mother's bedside. Sadie has lived with Linda for the past 2 years after Sadie's husband, Sam, died. Sam died of heart failure and spent the last two weeks of his life in the intensive care unit (ICU) with a feeding tube (nutrition and fluids) and a respirator (breathing). Sadie sat by his bedside day after day. She told Frank multiple times that she did not wish to died connected to tubes in ICU. Each day she prayed that Sam would die and be relieved of his condition.

Frank notifies his supervisor, Nancy, that he must leave work and get to the hospital. Nancy agreed and told Frank to keep her posted on Sadie's condition. Frank was close enough to walk over to the hospital. When he arrived in Sadie's room, a physician was talking to Linda. Sadie had been given pain medicine and was sleeping. Dr. Williams, an internal medicine hospitalist physician, was asking questions about Sadie's advance directives and end-of-life planning documents. Linda was too upset to talk, so Frank stepped in to continue the conversation. After Frank introduced himself, Dr. Williams turned the questions to Frank, but

Linda was nearby in Sadie's room. Dr. Williams also explained to Linda and Frank that he was an internal medicine hospitalist physician. He works for the hospital and does not have a private practice. He would be Sadie's hospital physician and be consulting with other hospitalist, such as orthopedic and geriatric physicians as needed.

Frank said that he had attempted several times to engage Sadie in the conversation, but she was still grieving the death of Sam. Frank told the physicians the story about Sadie sitting at Sam's bedside. However, Frank was never able to get Sadie to put her wishes in writing. While this conversation was occurring, Linda would occasionally nod her head and say, "Yes, Frank has Sadie's wishes correct." Dr. Williams ended the conversation and said that he would order a few radiology scans to learn the extent of Sadie's fracture and some lab tests. The scans and lab tests were completed later that afternoon.

By Tuesday morning, Frank and Linda arrived at the hospital. Fortunately, they arrived about 2 minutes after Dr. Williams started talking to Sadie. She was awake and listening to Dr. Williams. He stepped over when Frank and Linda arrived. He explained that Sadie's hip joint and several areas of her pelvis were fractured. In addition, her wrist sustained a fracture when she tried to break her fall in the kitchen. Dr. Williams said that they would put her wrist in the splint. He said the orthopedic surgeon, Dr. Patel, would be in later to explain Sadie's pelvic and hip fractures. In addition, he explained that Sadie's lab tests showed that she was dehydrated, had a urinary tract infection, and her chest x-ray showed a mild form of pneumonia. He stated that he did not believe that Sadie would be an ideal candidate for surgery, but Dr. Patel could provide a thorough review of the situation.

Frank and Linda spent the day in Sadie's room. Due to the pain medication, Sadie drifted in and out of sleep. Fortunately, the Emergency Department nurse had inserted a urinary catheter, so Sadie did not have to use a bedpan for urination. She could rest moderately comfortable while receiving intravenous fluids and pain medication. During the day, Frank and Linda discussed options about how they might proceed. They kept coming back to the conversation between Frank and Sadie while Sam was

dying in the ICU. They both agreed that no heroic efforts would be permitted. On Monday evening, Frank emailed the family and scheduled a virtual meeting for Tuesday evening. He assumed that he would have updated information about Sadie's condition for the meeting.

Late on Tuesday morning, Mary, Linda's older sister, stopped by for a visit. Linda lives about 50 miles away and was never involved with Sadie's and Sam's health care due to her busy career schedule in real estate. Linda walked into Sadie's room and immediately started asking questions. She wanted to know when Sadie's surgery was scheduled. Frank and Linda tried to explain that they were waiting for Dr. Patel to provide more details. Linda was not willing to wait for Dr. Patel. She spoke to Sadie for a few minutes and left to go to a scheduled open house. She did not stay long enough to hear that there may not be any surgery and about Sadie's pneumonia, urinary infection, and fractured wrist.

Dr. Patel arrived around 2:00 p.m., after Linda left. Dr. Patel explained that Sadie was not a candidate for a hip replacement due to her pelvic fracture and her low-grade pneumonia. However, she suggested that Sadie could receive several injections of surgical glue in her hip joint and pelvis to aid in the healing. She would be lightly sedated for the procedure, would feel no pain, and would not have the risk of general anesthesia. Sadie was awake during the conversation and agreed along with Frank and Linda that this option would be optimal given the circumstances. Dr. Patel agreed and went over the consent form, so the procedure could be scheduled for the next day. She explained the customary risks and asked Sadie if she wished to be resuscitated if her heart stopped during the procedure. Sadie stated clearly, "If my heart stops or I have any medical complications, I never want to spend a day in ICU or be put on any kind of tubes or machines. Just let me pass peacefully so I can go be with my husband, Sam." Frank and Linda were pleasantly surprised at Sadie's ability to make that statement so clearly.

By 4:00 p.m., Frank had a great idea. He asked Linda if it would be a good idea to ask Nancy, his supervisor, if she would be willing to facilitate the family meeting that evening. Linda thought it was a good idea especially since Linda

(continues)

knows Nancy. Immediately, Frank contacted Nancy, and she agreed to facilitate the meeting at 7:30 p.m. Frank and Linda wanted every family member to hear the same message at the same time.

At 7:30 p.m., Frank and Linda started the meeting and gave the latest update on Sadie's condition. When the discussion started, Nancy took over the facilitation of the 90-minute family meeting.

Questions

1. What questions should Nancy expect that the family might ask?
2. How should Nancy control the conversation among the family members?
3. What questions should Nancy ask the family members participating in the virtual meeting?

Case Study 10.2 CHW Role with Grief and Assembling End-of-Life Care Documents

Ralph, 52, has been married to his husband, Steve, for 8 years. They are both employed as computer software engineers. Since their degrees are in engineering, they have a limited background in health care. Ralph had been hospitalized once for a hernia operation at age 28. He never smoked, consumes alcohol in moderation, is not overweight, and takes one pill each day for his hypertension. Lately, Ralph has noticed that he is tripping when he walks more than usual, and he feels weakness in his legs in the morning. He has been ignoring these symptoms because he does not wish to trouble Steve with such minor symptoms. However, last week at the gym, Ralph was walking on the treadmill and had to grab the sidebars to avoid falling. Steve was on the treadmill next to Ralph and noticed the near-fall incidents. On the drive home, Steve insisted that Ralph schedule an appointment with his primary care physician. Ralph was anxious about making an appointment and afraid of a possible serious diagnosis.

At the appointment, Ralph explained his symptoms. Dr. Sharon Murray, the primary care physician, conducted simple tests of strength and reflexes. She concluded that Ralph did have

muscle weakness but was not certain of the cause or diagnosis. Dr. Murray referred Ralph to Dr. James Peters, neurologist, and had her CHW make the appointment for Ralph for the following week. Of course, Ralph was afraid that the diagnosis might be serious. He insisted that Steve accompany him to the appointment.

During the first appointment, Dr. Peters was concerned but offered no conclusive diagnosis and ordered additional testing (e.g., MRI scans, nerve conduction tests, muscle tissue biopsies) over the next few weeks. Ralph complied with the additional testing in hopes of obtaining a correct diagnosis; however, the tests were exhausting and often painful.

After Dr. Peters reviewed the test results, an appointment was schedule with Ralph and Steve to discuss the diagnosis. The day before the appointment, Ralph fell at work. He did not sustain any fractures, but he realized that the unknown illness was progressing. He was ready to learn the diagnosis tomorrow.

Dr. Peters gave Ralph the conclusive diagnosis of amyotrophic lateral sclerosis (ALS), which is a progressive nervous system disease that affects nerve cells in the brain and spinal cord and causes loss of muscle control.[39] The symptoms of ALS usually start with muscle twitching and weakness in a limb, slurred speech, and then spreads to other parts of the body. Eventually, ALS affects control of the muscles needed to move, speak, eat, and breathe.[39] This fatal disease has no cure. There is generally no pain in the early stages of ALS, and pain is uncommon in the later stages.[39] According to the ALS Association, the average life expectancy of a person with ALS is 3 years.[39-40] However, it varies greatly with the typical range being 20 percent live 5 years or more, 10 percent live 10 or more years, and 5 percent will live for more than 20 years.[40] Of course, Ralph and Steve were devastated by the diagnosis and immediately had questions. Dr. Peters had planned for these questions and scheduled a two-hour appointment. By the time Ralph and Steve left his office, they had their initial questions answered.

Since Dr. Peters deals with all types of neurological diseases (e.g., ALS, Parkinson's, multiple sclerosis, and strokes), he is familiar with delivering a diagnosis of such a serious illness. As a result, he hired Jackie, a CHW, to coordinate patient appointments, phone calls, insurance eligibility referrals, general information, and community resources to assist the patients and their families throughout the disease process. As Dr. Peters walked Ralph and Steve out of his office, he introduced them to Jackie, the CHW. He explained that she would be their first point of contact for all nonclinical questions. She handed Ralph a cloth tote bag filled with brochures and community resources, a small stack of her business cards, and two bottles of water for the ride home. Ralph and Steve walked to their car, drank the water, and tried to take a few deep breathes of the new reality before attempting to drive home. Use the information provided in this chapter to answer the following questions.

Questions

1. What information would you, the CHW, include in the tote bag that was given to Ralph and Steve at their initial appointment with Dr. Peters?
2. When you first meet with Ralph and Steve next week, what information and questions would you anticipate for the appointment?
3. At what point, would you suggest that Ralph and Steve begin attending the ALS Community Support group?
4. When would you start a conversation about advance directive choices for Ralph? How did you make this decision?
5. What research would you conduct to update your knowledge and understanding about ALS since you have limited experience about the progression of this disease?

Burial Options

This section describes burial options, including embalming, cemetery burial, cremation, green burial, and other available burial options. State laws determine what options are available.

Embalming. States have varying laws about embalming, such as if the body is cremated, it may or may not need to be embalmed in all situations. Funeral directors will know the laws in their state.

Cemetery Burial. The traditional form of burial is a formal casket with the embalmed body sealed within the casket. Some states allow a viewing of the embalmed body during the service prior to sealing the casket. Most cemeteries require that the casket be placed in a concrete vault in the ground. The purpose of the sealed vault is so the ground stays level on top for the groundskeeper maintenance and so the cemetery may place the graves closer together without side-to-side collapse of the ground. Most cemeteries have strict rules about the size and material of the headstones to maintain a uniform appearance across the cemetery grounds.

Cremation. Some, but not all, mortuaries have the capability for cremation. They may move the body to an appropriate facility and return the cremains (ashes) back to the mortuary for the service. States have varying laws about where cremains may be scattered or buried. The mortuary will know the state laws. Mortuaries package the cremains in a sealed and labeled box for the family to transport in the box via car, airplane, bus, or train across state borders to the final resting place. The Neptune Society offers low-cost cremation services and legal scattering of the ashes at sea if the family selects that option.[26]

Green Burial. Green cemeteries are available in some states, such as Prairie Creek Conversation Cemetery in Gainesville, Florida.[31] Their website offers an excellent video showing an actual green burial service. Most traditional cemeteries do not offer green burial options. A green burial takes place within about 24 hours after the loved one dies, and there is no embalming. The family wraps the loved one's body in a shroud and places it in an eco-friendly basket.[31] The green cemetery provides the transportation services to move the body from the location of the death to the grave site. The groundskeepers who work for the green cemetery services dig the grave, and there is no concrete vault. The body is placed in the grave when the family gathers at the grave site. Green cemeteries put a three-inch brass maker at the grave site and name and date is recorded. Headstones are usually not allowed for environmental reasons.[31]

Other Available Burial Options. Other burial options include donating the loved one's body to universities for research,[32] medical colleges for teaching,[33] whole body burial at sea,[34] sending a cremains into space,[35] and making art and jewelry from cremains.[36]

Bereavement and Grief

Bereavement and grief have similar definitions. **Bereavement** is defined as the period after loss and includes the time where grief is experienced and mourning occurs.[37] Bereavement is not always tied to the suffering of a loss due to death. Bereavement may be attached to other types of significant losses in life, including loss of a spouse due to divorce, loss of property due to natural disaster, losing a job, friend, or even a pet. Loss of any type can have a lasting effect on an individual's emotional and psychological well-being.[37] **Grief** is experienced in many ways and affects everyone differently. Depending on the circumstances surrounding an individual's experiences, there can be variability between emotional and psychological well-being due to cultural beliefs, relationship to the deceased, or attachment to the loss. The level of suffering due to grief is subjective and unique to the experiences of the individual.[38] Although two people may experience the same loss, their experiences, feelings, and emotions will differ. In addition, grief is a strong, overwhelming emotion for individuals, regardless of whether the sadness stems from the loss of a loved one or is related to the loss of function from a terminal diagnosis. The

individual may feel numb and removed from daily life and unable to continue with regular duties due to the sense of loss. Because grief is a natural experience that accompanies loss, it is important to remember that grief is both a universal and a personal experience. Individual experiences of grief vary and are influenced by the nature of the loss.[38]

Chapter Summary

This chapter begins with an explanation of the descriptive U.S. landmark cases that involved three different women under the age of 30 and the intricacies associated with making end-of-life decisions after tragic circumstances. The next section describes and defines the terminology associated with the legal terms used in end-of-life planning and explains the differences between palliative care and hospice care. After exploring the differences between quality of life and quantity of life, the focus changes to the aspects of end-of-life planning, including diverse cultural and religious beliefs, alternative pain management, language barriers, communication, and accommodation, and ends with providing information on how to navigate the sensitive conversation on end-of-life care or wishes. The next topic describes burial options, including embalming, cemetery burial, cremation, green burial, and other available burial options. Last, there is a discussion about differences between grief and bereavement.

References

1. Give peace of mind: advance care planning. Centers for Disease Control and Prevention Web site. https://www.cdc.gov/aging/advancecareplanning/index.htm. Accessed November 4, 2021.
2. Karen Ann Quinlan biography. Who2Biographies Web site. https://www.who2.com/bio/karen-ann-quinlan/. Accessed November 4, 2021.
3. The Karen Ann Quinlan case. Centers for Disease Control and Prevention Web site. https://www.cdc.gov/training/ACP/page33994.html. Accessed November 4, 2021.
4. The Nancy Cruzan case. Centers for Disease Control and Prevention Web site. https://www.cdc.gov/training/ACP/page42985.html. Accessed November 4, 2021.

5. The Terri Schiavo case. Centers for Disease Control and Prevention Web site. https://www.cdc.gov/training/ACP/page52792.html. Accessed November 4, 2021.
6. Grimminck R. 10 heartbreaking right-to-die cases. https://listverse.com/2014/11/15/10-heartbreaking-right-to-die-cases/. Accessed November 4, 2021.
7. Johnstone JM. Quality versus quantity of life: Who should decide? *Aust J Adv Nurs.* 1988;6(1):30–37.
8. Transition to module 3. Centers for Disease Control and Prevention Web site. https://www.cdc.gov/training/ACP/page34655.html. Accessed November 4, 2021.
9. Living wills and advance directives for medical decisions. Mayo Clinic Web site. https://www.mayoclinic.org/healthy

-lifestyle/consumer-health/in-depth/living-wills/art -20046303/. Accessed November 6, 2021.

10. The proxy. Centers for Disease Control and Prevention Web site. https://www.cdc.gov/training/ACP/page34181 .html. Accessed November 6, 2021.

11. Palliative care. Mayo Clinic Web site. https://www .mayoclinic.org/tests-procedures/palliative-care/about /pac-20384637. Accessed November 8, 2021.

12. What are palliative care and hospice care? National Institutes of Health, National Institute on Aging Web site. https://www.nia.nih.gov/health/what-are -palliative-care-and-hospice-care. Accessed November 8, 2021.

13. Hui TJ. Palliative care 101: all you need to know about end-of-life care. Homage Web site. https://www .homage.sg/health/palliative-care/. Accessed November 19, 2021.

14. Is palliative care right for you? Get Palliative Care Web site. https://getpalliativecare.org/rightforyou/. Accessed November 8, 2021.

15. Ellison N. Mental health and palliative care: Literature review. *Mental Health Foundation.* https://www .mentalhealth.org.uk/sites/default/files/mental_health _palliative_care.pdf. Accessed March 7, 2022.

16. Sheridan AJ. Palliative care for people with serious mental illnesses. *The Lancet.* 2019;4(11):545–546.

17. O'Malley K, Blakley L, Ramos K, Torrence N, Sager Z. Mental healthcare and palliative care: Barriers. *BMJ Support Palliat Care.* 2021;11(2):138–144.

18. Hospice care is not a death sentence. Blanchard Valley Health System Web site. https://www.bvhealthsystem .org/expert-health-articles/hospice-care-is-not-a-death -sentence. Accessed November 9, 2021.

19. Diaz E. What is your definition of quality? https://www .gbnews.ch/what-is-your-definition-of-quality/. Accessed November 9, 2021.

20. Quality of life. Britannica Encyclopedia Web site. https://www.britannica.com/topic/quality-of-life. Accessed November 11, 2021.

21. Givler A, Bhatt H, & Maani-Fogelmann, PA. *The importance of cultural competence in pain and palliative care.* Florida: STAT PEARLS; 2021.

22. New survey reveals "conversational disconnect": 90 percent of Americans know they should have a conversation about what they want at the end of life, yet only 30 percent have done so. The Conversation Project Web site. https://theconversationproject.org/wp-content /uploads/2013/09/TCP-Survey-Release_FINAL-9-18-13. pdf. Accessed November 11, 2021.

23. Old JL. Discussing end-of-life care with your patients. AAFP Web site. https://www.aafp.org/fpm/2008/0300 /p18.html. Accessed November 23, 2021.

24. Rogers JD. What to say when someone doesn't want to talk to you? https://beforeigosolutions.com/talking-about -death/what-to-say-when-someone-doesnt-want-to-talk -to-you/. Accessed November 24, 2021.

25. 10 tips for talking to someone who is dying: how to find the right words. Agapé Hospice & Palliative Care Web site. https://agapehospicepc.org/blog-post/10-tips-for-talking -to-someone-who-is-dying-how-to-find-the-right-words/. Accessed November 24, 2021.

26. How to talk to your aging parents about end-of-life planning. Neptune Society Web site. https://www.neptunesociety. com/cremation-planning-for-caregivers/how-to-talk-to -your-aging-parents-about-end-of-life-planning?utm _ad=&utm_campaign=&adgroup=&keyword=end%20 of%20life&device=c&network=o&placement=&u tm_source=bing&utm_term=end%20of%20life&utm _content=&utm_medium=cpc&msclkid=df0fd6d966ec 1f5c46a0b7e866ce28c1. Accessed November 24, 2021.

27. Crist C. Over one third of U.S. adults have advanced medical directors. https://www.reuters.com/article/us-health -usa-advance-directives-idUSKBN19W2NO. Accessed November 24, 2021.

28. Module 2—the essential elements. Centers for Disease Control and Prevention Web site. https://www.cdc.gov /training/ACP/page43022.html. Accessed November 24, 2021.

29. Five steps: a guide to help plan your end-of-life and future health care. Pennsylvania Medical Society Web site. https://www.pamedsoc.org/list/articles/Advanced -Directive-Steps#:~:text=%20Five%20Steps%3A%20 A%20Guide%20to%20Help%20Plan,down%20your%20 decisions.%20Write%20down%20your...%20More%20. Accessed November 25, 2021.

30. The realities. Centers for Disease Control and Prevention Web site. https://www.cdc.gov/training/ACP/page34059. html. Accessed November 25, 2021.

31. Prairie Creek Conservatory: the natural choice. Prairie Creek Conservatory Cemetery Web site. https://www .prairiecreekconservationcemetery.org/. Accessed November 26, 2021.

32. Cremation at no cost through whole body donation to science. Science Care Web site. https://www.sciencecare.com/landing /cremation-body-donation-b?utm_source=bing&utm _medium=cpc&utm_keyword=%2Bcremation%20 %2Bservices&utm_device=c&matchtype=p&location=7199 9&utm_campaign=Nonbrand_Cremation_FL&msclkid=a5 70db951d281fe03d0cbac30485e9b0. Accessed November 26, 2021.

33. The Willed Body Program. Florida State University College of Medicine Web site. https://med.fsu.edu/giving /willed-body-program. Accessed November 26, 2021.

34. Full body burials at sea. Teraloom Web site. https://www .nationwideburialatsea.com/full-body-burials#: ~:text=In%20recent%20history%2C%20whole%20 body%20burials%20at%20sea,assure%20the%20 body%20sank%20to%20the%20ocean%20floor Accessed November 28, 2021.

35. SpaceX will take your ashes to space for $2,490. Inverse Web site. https://www.inverse.com/article/31722-spacex -elysium-space-ashes. Accessed November 28, 2021.

36. Top selling memorials for pets and people. Spirit Pieces Web site. https://www.spiritpieces.com/?msclkid=bd653f62e4e61a8c02765e34ffeafd46&utm_source=bing&utm_medium=cpc&utm_campaign=Bing%20Ads%20III&utm_term=cremation%20orbs&utm_content=Primary. Accessed November 28, 2021.

37. Vasquez A. Is bereavement the same as grief? 3 key differences. https://www.joincake.com/blog/bereavement-vs-grief/. Accessed November 28, 2021.

38. What is grief? Mayo Clinic Web site. https://www.mayoclinic.org/patient-visitor-guide/support-groups/what-is-grief. Accessed November 28, 2021.

39. Amyotrophic lateral sclerosis (ALS). Mayo Clinic Web site. https://www.mayoclinic.org/diseases-conditions/amyotrophic-lateral-sclerosis/symptoms-causes/syc-20354022. Accessed November 29, 2021.

40. Stages of ALS. ALS Association Web site. https://www.als.org/understanding-als/stages. Accessed November 29, 2021.

Health Care, Ethics, and Professionalism

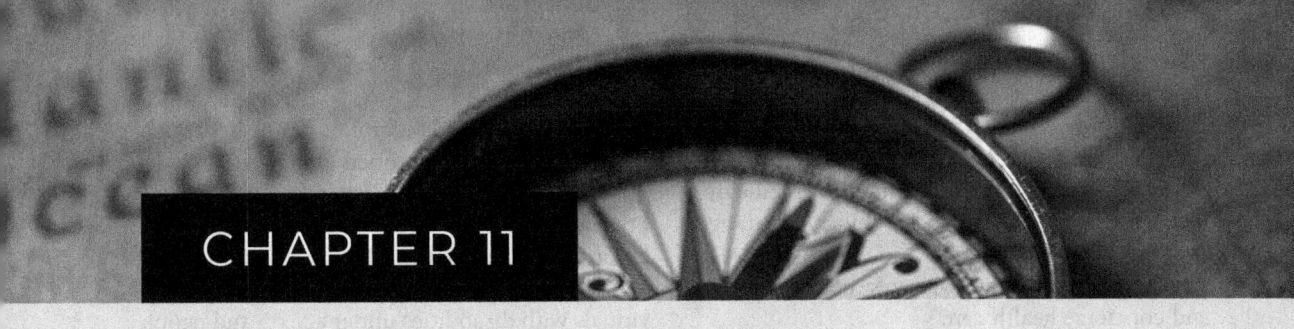

CHAPTER 11

Health Insurance

LEARNING OBJECTIVES

1. Discuss the history of health insurance in the United States.
2. Explain an overview of the various types of health insurance in the United States.
3. Describe the reasons for the uneven coverage of health insurance in the United States.
4. Define the most common terms used in health insurance.
5. Identify and define the most common types of U.S. health insurance.

KEY WORDS

single-payer system
all-payer system
coinsurance
copayment
deductible
flexible spending accounts (FSA)
health maintenance organization
  (HMO)
lifetime maximum dollar limit

managed care plans
preadmission certification
preadmission testing
preferred provider organization
  (PPO)
primary care physician (PCP)
second opinion
usual, customary, and reasonable
  (UCR) charges

utilization review
employer-based health insurance
Social Security Disability Insurance
  (SSDI)
Supplemental Security Income (SSI)
calendar quarter
workers' compensation
fee for service
medical tourism

Introduction

This chapter begins by providing a historical summary of health insurance in the United States followed by presenting a current overview of how health insurance has evolved today. While there are many reasons for the uneven coverage of health insurance in the United States, the next section describes the most prominent reasons for the disproportionate coverage among the

American population. The following sections define the most common terms used in health insurance. Because health insurance in the United States is complex and filled with numerous terms, community health workers (CHWs) are encouraged to have a general understanding of the outlined terminology to deliver excellent health care to diverse populations. Thus, the next section provides a description of the most common types of health insurance available in the

United States along with some alternative methods, including the Affordable Care Act (ACA), employer-based health insurance, Medicare, Medicaid, Social Security Disability Insurance and Supplemental Security Income, TRICARE and Veteran Benefits, worker's compensation, and concierge health care .

History of Health Insurance in the United States

The history of U.S. health insurance began in Washington state around the time it became the 42nd state, November 11, 1889.[1] By the 1890s, Washington lumber companies paid physicians to care for their workers. In the early 1900s, President Theodore Roosevelt introduced social health insurance as a prototype for states to follow. By 1915, the American Association for Labor Legislation proposed a bill for compulsory health insurance.[2] Baylor University Hospital became the first to implement this bill by providing health care to local teachers by charging a $6 monthly fee for hospital services in 1929. This concept was the beginning of Blue Cross health insurance plans.[2] Blue Shield was introduced in the 1930s by the lumber and mining industries as a health insurance plan that covered physician services. Over time the Blue Cross and Blue Shield insurance plans merged to create the National Association of Blue Shield Plans of today, which covers physician and hospital services.[3]

In 1939, the federal government created the Department of Health and Human Services (DHHS) to focus on health, welfare, and social insurance. By 1945, President Truman proposed a universal health insurance program,[4] and in 1948 the National Health Assembly issued a report that endorsed voluntary health insurance and emphasized the need for universal coverage.[2]

In 1954, President Dwight Eisenhower proposed a federal insurance fund for private insurance companies to help expand the availability of health coverage.[2] In 1956, the government enacted a program that provided health insurance for military families.[5] By the 1960s, President Kennedy outlined the need for adequate health insurance to cover seniors. In 1964, President Lyndon B. Johnson signed the legislation that created the Medicare (elderly) and Medicaid (low income) system.[6] In 1972, individuals with disabilities under age 65 and people with end-stage renal disease became eligible for Medicare benefits.[6]

During the 1990s, there were several attempts to create a national single-payer insurance, but none of the efforts were successful.[2] It was not until 2010, when President Barack Obama changed American healthcare history by signing the ACA, that significant changes were introduced to American health care, including protections for people with pre-existing health conditions and allowing children to remain covered by a parent's plan until age 25. Additionally, the ACA has helped lower U.S. uninsured rates.[7]

Overview of Health Insurance in the United States

The U.S. healthcare system is unique compared to other advanced industrialized countries. The U.S. does not have a uniform health system, has no universal healthcare coverage, and only recently enacted legislation mandating healthcare coverage for almost everyone.[8] Rather than operating a national health service, a single-payer national health insurance system, or a multi-payer universal health insurance fund, the U.S. health care system can best be described as a hybrid system.[8]

It is important to begin the overview by comparing the United States with other developed countries. The Organization for Economic Co-operation and Development (OECD) is an international group that compares the 34 member countries to improve the economic and social well-being around the world.[8] Out of the 34 countries, the United States pays the most per capita for health care.[9] See **Figure 11.1**.

It is important to understand and identify how the American population pays significantly

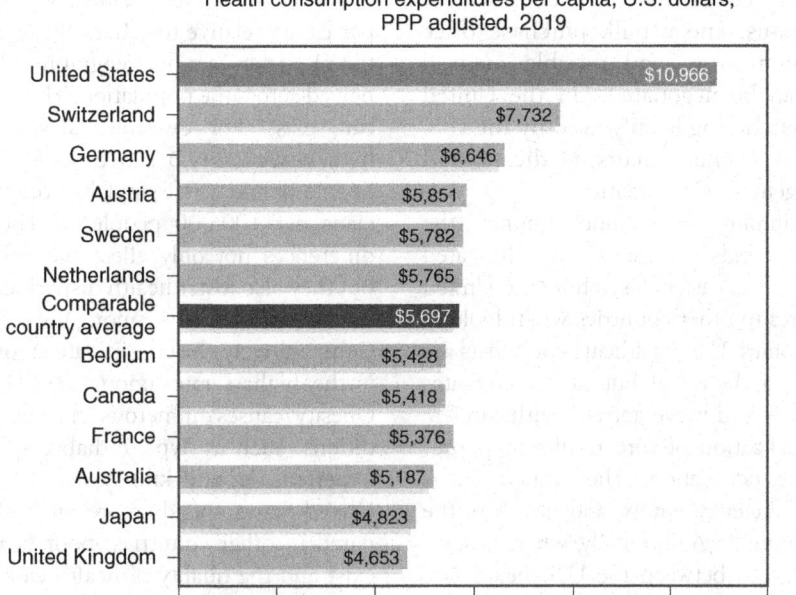

Health consumption expenditures per capita, U.S. dollars, PPP adjusted, 2019

United States	$10,966
Switzerland	$7,732
Germany	$6,646
Austria	$5,851
Sweden	$5,782
Netherlands	$5,765
Comparable country average	$5,697
Belgium	$5,428
Canada	$5,418
France	$5,376
Australia	$5,187
Japan	$4,823
United Kingdom	$4,653

Notes: U.S. value obtained from National Health Expenditure data.
Health consumption does not include investments in structures, equipment, or research.

Figure 11.1 Health Consumption Expenditures per Capita

Reproduced from Kamal R, Ramirez G, Cox C. How does health spending in the U.S. compare to other countries? Available at https://www.healthsystemtracker.org/chart-collection/health-spending-u-s-compare-countries/#item-spendingcomparison_health-consumption-expenditures-per-capita-2019. Accessed December 6, 2021.[9]

more for their health care when compared to similar countries. Since the other OECD countries have more effective and equitable healthcare systems, they can control healthcare costs and protect vulnerable segments of the population from falling through the cracks. Compared to the United States, the other countries have three main types of health insurance programs.

National Health Services. Taxes are collected by the government to finance medical services. The government owns and operates the hospitals and clinics. The medical services are delivered by government employees. This system is available in the United Kingdom, Spain, and New Zealand.[9]

National Health Insurance System. This **single-payer system** is defined as the government acting as the single administrator to collect all healthcare fees and pays out all associated healthcare costs. Healthcare services are publicly financed through taxes. This system is available in Canada, Denmark, Taiwan, and Sweden.[9]

Multi-Payer Health Insurance System. This **all-payer system** is defined as providing a universal health insurance. The insurance fees collected are used to pay physicians and hospital services at constant and uniform rates. This system eliminates the administrator costs for billing services. This system is available in Germany, Japan, and France.[9]

In addition, mandated universal healthcare coverage reduces healthcare costs by eliminating the need for the uninsured to pay higher costs. Reducing these costs helps reduces the usage of emergency services that are due to the lack of preventative care. Under this system, health care cost funding is linked to people's medical history rather than their employment or income status, and a bulk purchase price for prescription drugs and durable medical equipment can be negotiated.[9] In the United States bulk purchasing is only used by the U.S. Department of Veterans Affairs, Medicaid, and Health Management Organizations.[9]

After examining how much money the United States spends on health care, illustrated in Figure 11.1, it is easier to see how the United States compares to other countries when looking at health outcomes. U.S. healthcare specialists are among the best in the world, but the United States neglects primary and preventative health care.[9–10] The overspecialization of care results in poorer health for the population. The United States ranks low in efficiency, equity, and health of the entire population.[9–10] Additionally, when observing the differences between the U.S. healthcare system and the healthcare systems in other OECD

countries, the United States has fewer physicians per capita relative to other OECD countries, and the physicians are not geographically equally dispersed across the population. Thus, gaps in health care exist. For example, Massachusetts ranks highest with 349.5 active doctors per 100,000 people, while Mississippi has only 170.3 physicians per 100,000 people.[9–10] These significant differences not only affect the delivery of care, but they also foster health disparities and increase the burden of disease among the U.S. population. Comparatively, the obesity rate among U.S. adults is the highest rate among OECD countries.[9–10] Obesity causes numerous chronic medical conditions, such as Type 2 diabetes, heart disease, hypertension, and kidney disease. Although the United States spends more on health care compared to other countries, poor health outcomes exist and the quality of health care decreases.[9–10] See **Figure 11.2**.

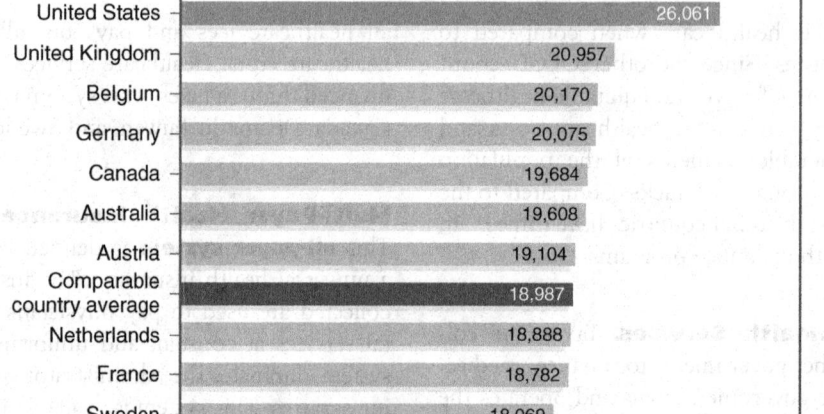

Figure 11.2 Overall Health Rankings

Uneven Coverage of Health Insurance in the United States

Universal healthcare coverage in countries like the United Kingdom, Switzerland, Japan, and Germany makes the number of bankruptcies related to medical expenses minor.[8] Conversely, three U.S. surveys found that (1) medical bills are the single largest cause of consumer bankruptcy; (2) 56 million Americans under the age of 65 had trouble paying medical bills; and (3) 10 million individuals have medical bills they are unable to pay despite having year-round insurance.[8] While most U.S. citizens have some form of health insurance, premiums continue to increase while the quality of insurance policies are failing to cover the burden of the cost, leaving many with significant healthcare debt.[8]

From 2005 to 2015, the average annual health insurance premium for family coverage increased by 61 percent, while worker contributions to those plans increased 83 percent in the same period. This rate of increase outpaces both inflation and the increases in workers' wages.[8] Health insurance deductibles are rising even faster.[8] Health insurance coverage is uneven and often minorities and those at or below the poverty line are underserved. Approximately, 40 million workers or nearly two out of five individuals, do not have access to paid sick leave. Experts suggest that the economic pressure to go to work even when sick can prolong pandemics, reduce productivity, and increase healthcare costs overall.[8]

In 2014, the ACA allowed young adults (19–25) to remain on their parents' health plans and banned the practice of denying insurance coverage for pre-existing health conditions.[8] Coverage by employer-provided insurance varies considerably by wage level. Among all small workplaces (3–199 workers) in 2015, only 56 percent offered healthcare coverage, compared to 98 percent of large workplace institutions that offered health insurance.[8]

Furthermore, minority populations and children are disproportionately uninsured. In 2014, 7.6 percent of non-Hispanic Whites were uninsured, 11.8 percent of Blacks were uninsured, 9.3 percent of Asians, and 19.9 percent of people of Hispanic origin were uninsured.[8] The Kaiser Family Foundation has found that approximately 80 percent of the uninsured are U.S. citizens.[8] Uninsured children are 10 times more likely than insured children to have unmet medical needs and are five times as likely as an insured child to go more than two years without seeing a doctor.[8] Lastly, there are significant disparities in both the availability and the cost of healthcare coverage across the states including Medicare reimbursements per enrollee and annual premium costs that are similarly unequal.[8] For example, companies in the South compared to companies in the Northeast are less likely to provide adequate insurance coverage for an employee's domestic partner.[8] Additionally, not all policies adequately cover individuals and their same-sex partner.[8]

Terms Used in Health Insurance (Alphabetical Order)

This section provides many of the common terms and definitions related to health insurance. Given the complexity of the health insurance industry, CHWs benefit from maintaining a list of such terms to avoid the need to search the internet while talking to patients and their families.

Coinsurance: The *percentage of costs* of a covered healthcare service that the insured pays after paying the deductible.[11] For example, assume a health insurance plan will pay $100 for an office visit, and the coinsurance is 20 percent. After paying the full deductible, the insured would pay 20 percent of $100, or $20. The insurance company pays the cost of $80 for the office visit.[11-12]

Copayment: A form of medical cost sharing in a health insurance plan that requires the insured person to pay a *fixed dollar amount* when a medical service is received.[12] The insurance company is responsible for the rest of the reimbursement. For example, if the neighborhood urgent care clinic charges $128 for a chest x-ray, the insured's health insurance requires a fixed cost for medical services. The fixed cost may be $35 for all urgent care services. Keep in mind that coinsurance is a percentage of costs and copayment is a fixed dollar amount.[12]

Deductible: A fixed dollar amount during the annual benefit period that the insured pays before the insurer starts to make payments for covered medical services. Plans may have both per individual and family deductibles.[12]

Flexible spending accounts (FSA): These accounts are offered and administered by employers and provide a way for employees to set aside, out of their paychecks, pretax dollars to pay for the employee's share of insurance premiums or medical expenses not covered by the employer's health plan, such as eyeglasses, dental expenses, and medical products not covered by the health insurance policy.[12] Some employers provide contributions to the employee's FSA. Typically, benefits or cash must be used within the given benefit year, or the employee loses the money. Lastly, some FSA policies pay a portion of childcare expenses.[12]

Health maintenance organization (HMO): HMOs are health insurance plans that typically cost the least but offer a limited number of providers and facilities.[12] Also, the individual's primary care physician must give the patient a referral for any specialist visits or needed tests. HMOs assume both the financial risks associated with providing comprehensive medical services and the responsibility for healthcare delivery in a particular geographic area to HMO members. The individuals pay a fixed, prepaid fee without any addition costs.

Financial risk may be shared with the providers participating in the HMO.[12–13]

Lifetime maximum dollar limit: Some health insurance policies have an annual or lifetime maximum dollar limit.[12] The most typical of maximums is a lifetime amount of $1 million per individual. An amount of $1 million may sound like a generous dollar limit, but keep in mind that health care is extremely expensive, and many long-term hospitalizations can reach that limit in a few months. For example, during the COVID-19 pandemic, it was not unusual for patients to stay in the intensive care unit for several months.[12]

Managed care plans: Managed care plans generally provide comprehensive health services to their members and offer financial incentives for patients to use the providers under the plan.[12] With such plans, facilities and physicians have negotiated contracts with the insurance company to provide lower rates for member's plan. If an individual selects a physician or hospital that is not in the managed care plan network, the expenses will likely not be paid. This arrangement leaves the individual with the responsibility of paying the full cost of the medical services or hospital stay.[12–13]

Preadmission certification: An authorization for hospital admission given by a healthcare provider to a group member prior to their hospitalization.[12] Failure to obtain a preadmission certification in nonemergency situations reduces or eliminates the healthcare provider's obligation to pay for services rendered.[12]

Preadmission testing: A requirement designed to encourage patients to obtain necessary diagnostic services on an outpatient basis prior to nonemergency hospital admission. The testing is designed to reduce the length of a hospital stay.[12]

Preferred provider organization (PPO): A health insurance plan where coverage is provided to participants through a network of selected health-care providers, such as hospitals and physicians.[12] The premiums tend to be higher in return for the choice option. Unlike HMOs, insured participants does not need referrals to go to a specialist. Insured participants may go outside the network for healthcare services but would incur larger costs in the form of higher deductibles, higher coinsurance rates, or nondiscounted charges from the providers.[12]

Primary care physician (PCP): A physician who serves as a group member's primary contact within the health plan.[12] In a managed care plan, the PCP provides basic medical services as well as coordinates and, if required by the plan, authorizes referrals to specialists and hospitals. A PCP is usually a board-certified internal medicine physician.[12]

Second opinion: As a cost-management strategy, health insurance companies encourage or require patients to obtain the opinion of another physician after a physician has recommended that a nonemergency or elective surgery be performed.[12] Programs may be voluntary or mandatory in that reimbursement is reduced or denied if the participant does not obtain the second opinion. Plans usually require that such opinions be obtained from board-certified specialists with no personal or financial interest in the outcome.[12]

Usual, customary, and reasonable (UCR) charges: UCR charges are defined as a physician's usual fee for a service that does not exceed the customary fee in that geographic area and is reasonable based on the circumstances.[12] Instead of UCR charges, PPO plans often operate based on a negotiated (fixed) schedule of fees that recognize charges for covered services up to a negotiated fixed dollar amount.[12]

Utilization review: The process of reviewing the appropriateness and quality of care provided to patients. Utilization reviews may take place before, during, or after services are rendered.[12]

Types of U.S. Health Insurance

U.S. health insurance is complex and filled with numerous terms that need to be understood by CHWs working in health care. This section provides a description of the most common types of health insurance available in the United States along with some alternative methods to acquire health care, including the ACA, employer-based health insurance, Medicare, Medicaid, Social Security Disability Insurance and Supplemental Security Income, Tricare and veteran benefits, worker's compensation, concierge health care, and alternative health care.

Affordable Care Act

On March 23, 2010, the Patient Protection and Affordable Care Act was signed into law. The ACA is a comprehensive health care reform law that addresses health insurance coverage, healthcare costs, and preventive care.[7] Before the ACA, healthcare insurance costs were too expensive for many individuals and families to afford. In addition, many insurance companies denied coverage due of pre-existing medical conditions. The ACA made health care more affordable and universally available without any concerns about pre-existing health conditions.[7] The ACA has four tiers: Bronze, Silver, Gold, and Platinum. The last plan is called the Catastrophic Plan because it is very low cost and is meant to guard against worst-case medical scenarios, such as accidents or injuries. Any of the five plans provide the same quality of coverage along with the same level of care and medical treatment.[7] See **Critical Thinking 11.1**.

Critical Thinking 11.1 Selecting an ACA Plan

As a CHW, it is likely that individuals will ask you questions about the ACA Plan to obtain health insurance. Use **Table 11.1** to assist people in selecting an ACA Plan option that best fits their income.

Table 11.1 Cost Comparison for Charles

Plan Type	*Hypothetical* Monthly Costs of Plan for Charles	Percentage of Medical Costs Paid Monthly by Plan for $1,483 Prescription	Percentage of Medical Costs Paid Monthly Out of Pocket for $1,483 Prescription	Total of Monthly Costs
Bronze	$200	60% = $889	40% = $594	$200 + 594 = $794
Silver	$400	70% = $1,038	30% = $445	$400 + 445 = $845
Gold	$600	80% = $1,186	20% = $297	$600 + 297 = $897
Platinum	$800	90% = $1,334	10% = $149	$800 + 149 = $949

Charles is 58 years old, single, and currently employed in a large lumber warehouse. His employer does not offer any health insurance benefits for the employees. In the past, Charles was healthy and did not go to the doctor for any major health issues. Though he has gained weight over the years, he mostly felt fine. However, this year he was diagnosed with high blood pressure and type 2 diabetes. He was unable to control his blood glucose (sugar) levels, so his physician stated that he needed to start taking three prescription medications: one to control his blood pressure and the other two for his diabetes. The physician told Charles that if the prescription pills did not control his blood glucose, Charles would have to start using insulin each day.

Charles was not too concerned about the cost of the three prescriptions even though he did not have health insurance. The last time that he needed a prescription, it was for an antibiotic for bronchitis. The cost was only $7. He thought that he would qualify for Medicare in a few years, so why should he bother with buying health insurance now? He earns $30 per hour (40 hours per week times 52 weeks), which equals $62,400 annually. After income taxes, his take-home pay is $49,920 or $4,160 per month. After paying his major monthly expenses of $1,600 mortgage and $300 car payment, he has $2,260 for all other expenses.

He took the prescriptions to the pharmacy to get filled. When he went back the next day, Charles was shocked at the price of the medications. The cost of the three prescriptions was $1,483. Charles did a quick calculation on his phone ($1,483 times 12 months = $17,796). He was shocked to learn the percentage of his monthly income that would be spent on three prescription drugs. He asked the pharmacist if there was any way to reduce the cost of his prescriptions. The pharmacist suggested enrolling in an ACA Plan and handed Charles a brochure with a website for enrolling in an ACA Plan. Charles asked the pharmacist how long he would hold the prescription. The pharmacist said, "I can hold your prescriptions for 30 days."

Charles went home and immediately explored the ACA website. Charles may decide not to buy health insurance. However, if that is his decision, it is likely that Charles will soon decide not to purchase the three prescriptions. If left untreated, Charles' high blood pressure and type 2 diabetes will become more serious, and he will develop complications.

Questions

1. As a CHW, which plan would you recommend and why? Use Table 11.1 and Table 11.2 to help make this decision and compare the available ACA plans.
2. As a CHW, show the calculations based on your recommendations.

Data from Obamacare USA.org. Which Obamacare Plan Is Right for Me? Available at https://www.obamacareusa.org/obamacare-plans.html?_d=c;vGelPE3UjenQ QHswtz5SyGXY 4RR3hPnBLWugwObrxkKP3H1I8qZ5R2FMda9n4OKG_qt5G879LRQwfk3cxIRTjakYZyCtvg:;&msclkid=82213b3fe25611cd296a5a60c02a0653. Accessed December 7, 2021.

Table 11.2 ACA Obamacare Plans

Plan Type	Percentage of Medical Costs Paid by Plan	Percentage of Medical Costs Paid Out of Pocket	Can Subsidy/Tax Credit Be Applied If You Qualify?	Comparative Monthly or Yearly Rate	Recommended for People Who
Bronze	60%	40%	Yes	Low	Rarely see a physician and rarely take prescription medication
Silver	70%	30%	Yes	Medium	Sometimes see a physician and sometimes take prescription medication
Gold	80%	20%	Yes	High	Regularly see a physician and regularly take prescription medication
Platinum	90%	10%	Yes	Premium	Frequently see a physician and take multiple prescription medications
Catastrophic (available only if under 30 or have a hardship exemption)	Less than 60%	More than 40%	No (Already priced low)	Lowest	Must meet plan's eligibility requirements. The plan protects from worst-case medical scenarios, like serious illness or accidents.

Data from Obamacare USA.org. Which Obamacare Plan Is Right for Me? Available at https://www.obamacareusa.org/obamacare-plans.html?_d=c;vGelPE3UjenQ QHswtz5SyGXY4RR3hPnBLWugwObrxkKP3H1I8qZ5R2FMda9n4OKG_qt5G879LRQwfk3cxIRTjakYZyCtvg;;&msclkid=82213b3fe25611cd296a5a60c02a0653. Accessed December 7, 2021.[14]

The cost of each plan is based on the individual's annual income and the number of people in the household. It is possible to go to www.ObamacareUSA.org to calculate the cost based on the information that the individual enters on the website.[14] See **Table 11.2**.

Employer-Based Health Insurance

Employer-based health insurance is defined as health insurance that is contracted by employers for their employees. In the United States, most employed individuals have the option to purchase health insurance through their employers.[15] In larger companies, the employer pays a percentage of the health insurance costs, and the employee pays the remaining percent. Larger companies negotiate lower insurance rates due to the large number of employees. However, small businesses have less power to negotiate the cheaper rates due to their smaller number of employees. Unfortunately, individuals who are employed by small businesses (under 100 employees) usually pay the total cost for their health insurance. Also, many small businesses do not offer any health insurance and encourage their employees to purchase health insurance through the ACA options.[15]

Some employees choose not to enroll in their employer's health insurance benefits because they think the cost of the monthly health insurance premium is too expensive. Since the monthly insurance premium costs are deducted from their paychecks, they would rather have the extra money in their paychecks.[16] Such employees need to consider that there are many money-saving benefits connected with enrollment in employer-based health insurance. For example, when individuals are unable to afford their employer's health insurance, they most likely cannot afford to pay out-of-pocket health expenses either. As a result, they put off seeking health care and have no place to turn except the emergency department when they experience a health challenge. By paying for health insurance each month, it possible to seek preventative care and receive treatment when something is wrong. Purchasing health insurance helps individuals protect their health and reduces the financial burden should a health concern arise. Additionally, employer-based group health insurance plans often cost less when compared to the health insurance plans sold individually. Insurance companies provide discounted lower-cost rates for employer group insurance because the large number of employees paying regular premiums significantly offsets the insurer's risk of losing money.[16] Finally, employer-based plans are limited, therefore the employees are not overwhelmed with the task of finding their own individual insurance. Most employers have a company representative to assist employees in this process, ensure a thorough understanding of their options, and select the plan suits the employee's health and financial needs.[16]

Medicare

Under the Centers for Medicare and Medicaid Services (CMS), Medicare is the federal health insurance program for people who are 65 or older, certain younger people with disabilities, and people with end-stage renal disease that requires kidney dialysis treatment or a transplant.[17] If the individual receives a monthly Social Security check, Medicare costs are deducted out of the monthly check. Medicare covers four specific services:

Medicare Part A (Hospital Insurance). Part A covers inpatient hospital stays, care in a skilled nursing facility, hospice care, and some home health care. Most people do not pay a monthly premium for Part A.[17]

Medicare Part B (Medical Insurance). Part B covers certain doctors services, outpatient care, medical supplies, and preventive services, such as mammograms and bone density scans. Everyone pays a monthly premium for Part B.[17]

Medicare Part C (Advantage Plans). Advantage Plans and Medigap provide additional premiums with numerous options and choices depending on the individual's desires.[17] Medicare recipients may enroll or change their advantage plans during open enrollment in October through December every year. Medigap is Medicare Supplement Insurance that helps fill "gaps" in original Medicare and is sold by private companies. Original Medicare pays for much, but not all, of the cost for covered healthcare services and supplies. A Medicare Supplement Insurance (Medigap) policy can help pay some of the remaining healthcare costs, including copayments, coinsurance, and deductibles.[18] To purchased Medigap policies, people must have Medicare Parts A and B. A Medigap policy only covers one person rather than married couples. Any standard Medigap policy is guaranteed renewable even if the individual develops health problems as long as the monthly premiums have been paid.[18] Like all types of health insurance policies, the policy should be read carefully, experts should be asked pertinent questions, and answers should be understood.

Medicare Part D (Prescription Drug Coverage). Part D helps cover the cost of prescription drugs, including many recommended shots or vaccines. To get Medicare drug coverage, individuals must join a Medicare-approved plan that offers drug coverage.[17] See **Figure 11.3**.

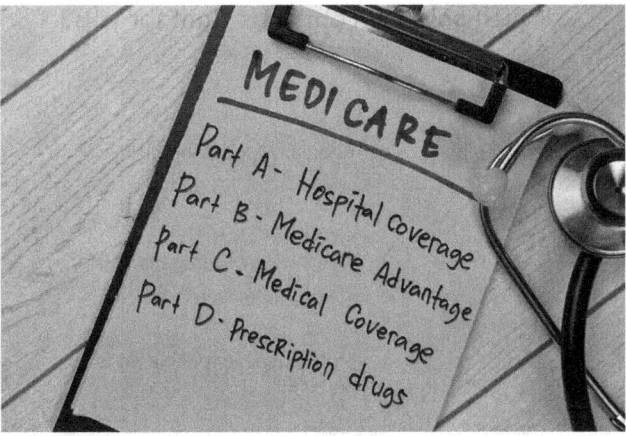

Figure 11.3 The Four Parts of Medicare
© bangoland/Shutterstock

Medicaid

Medicaid was signed into law in 1965 by President Lyndon B. Johnson and authorized by Title XIX of the Social Security Act, which also created Medicare.[20] Medicaid is a government-sponsored health insurance program for individuals of any age with insufficient income and resources to pay for health care. Medicaid covers the cost of physician office visits, hospital stays, long-term medical care, some nursing home care, and other health-related costs.[20]

Under the CMS, Medicaid is available nationwide, but each state independently manages and determines the criteria for Medicaid coverage, including eligibility, the type of coverage, and the process for paying healthcare workers and hospitals. The Medicaid program is jointly run by federal and state governments. However, each state uniquely defines Medicaid criteria and eligibility, thus Medicaid is not consistent across states nationwide. Depending on the state's criteria and policies, some physicians, hospitals, and eldercare facilities do not accept Medicaid. These patients often have a difficult time locating healthcare services. In contrast, Medicare (not Medicaid) is fully funded by the federal government and thus consistent across states nationwide.[21] Seniors and individuals with disabilities who have limited financial assets may qualify for enrollment in both Medicare and Medicaid.[21] See **Figure 11.4**.

Social Security Disability Insurance and Supplemental Security Income

The **Social Security Disability Insurance (SSDI)** and **Supplemental Security Income (SSI)** disability programs are the largest of several federal programs that aid persons with disabilities.[23] While these two programs are different in many ways, both are administered by the Social Security Administration and only individuals who have a disability and meet medical criteria may qualify for benefits under either program.[23] For a useful website, see https://www.usa.gov/disability-services[23] and explore the different types of benefits by beginning the questionnaire at https://ssabest.benefits.gov/.[24] See **Figure 11.5**.

Here are a few definitions to better explain additional complex federal programs that are important to understand as a CHW:

SSDI pays benefits to the individual and certain members of the family if the individual

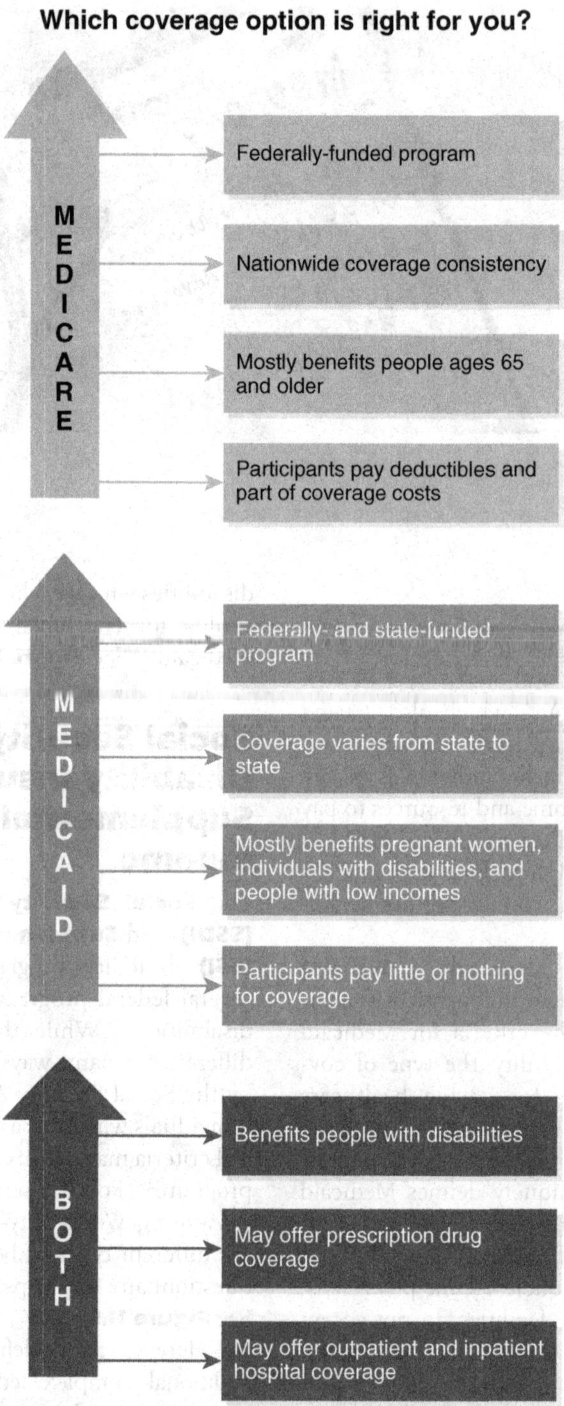

Which coverage option is right for you?

Figure 11.4 Medicare and Medicaid Coverage Options

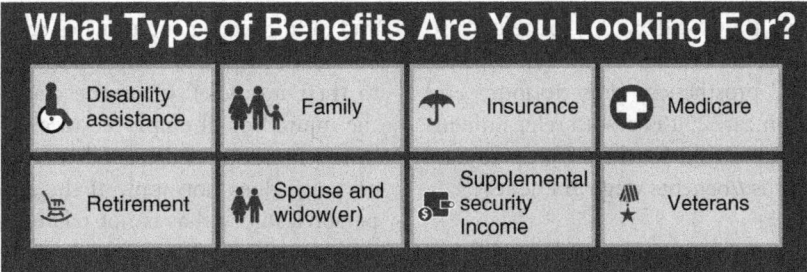

Figure 11.5 What Type of Benefits Are You Looking For?

Figure from Social Security Administration Benefits Eligibility Screening Tool. What Is SSA BEST? Available at https://ssabest.benefits.gov/. Accessed December 14, 2021.[24]

meets the eligibility requirements to receive Social Security retirement benefits. The eligibility requirements are that a worker has accumulated an overall total of 40 calendar quarters of work in their lifetime.[25] The **calendar quarter** is defined as the three calendar months ending on March 31, June 30, September 30, or December 31.[26] Workers do not need to work a consecutive 40 quarters over the 10 year period, but rather workers must accumulate 40 quarters of employment over their lifetime. In addition, there are requirements related to how much an individual must earn in each quarter. For example, in 2021, workers must earn at least $1,470 in a quarter, and in 2022, workers must earn $1,510 in a quarter to count toward their Social Security retirement benefits.[26–27]

It is important to remember that in the context of the American Disability Act (ADA), "disability" is a legal term rather than a medical term. Because it has a legal definition, the ADA's definition of disability is different from how disability is defined under some other laws, such as for Social Security Disability related benefits. The ADA defines a person with a disability as a person who has a physical or mental impairment that substantially limits one or more major life activity.[28]

SSI pays benefits based on financial need.[29] In 2019, SSI paid a monthly average in disability benefits of approximately $1,234 ($14,808 annually) to individuals with a disability, which is slightly above the poverty level of $12,140 annually.[30] These modest payments make a difference

in meeting basic needs when an individual is unable to work.[30] SSI may or may not be a lifetime benefit. If a person recovers from the injury and can obtain gainful employment, the benefit would not continue.[29–30]

TRICARE and Veteran Benefits

TRICARE is the health insurance provided by the U.S. Department of Defense for military personnel and their families, covering both active and retired members of all branches of the military services. Additional recipients of TRICARE benefits are members of the Public Health Service, National Oceanic and Atmospheric Administration, and dependents of military personnel killed on active duty.[31] TRICARE offers a variety of healthcare plans and coverage options, including vision and dental care, pharmacy services, and cancer treatment and hospice care. In some cases, TRICARE benefits can be used in conjunction with other insurance.[32] Not all members of the armed forces qualify for every type of TRICARE coverage. In general, only limited TRICARE benefits are available to National Guard and Reserve members who are not on active duty or do not have orders to activate.[32]

Veteran Administration (VA) Health Care Benefits are extensive and complex. For example, eligible individuals receive benefits for regular checkups with their PCP and appointments with specialists, such as cardiologists, gynecologists, and mental health providers. VA benefits also allow access to home health, geriatric care, medical equipment, prosthetics, prescriptions, and dental and vision care.[33] It is best to refer individuals to the official website for the most up-to-date information: https://benefits.va.gov/benefits/.[34]

Workers' Compensation

Workers' compensation is defined as a system of insurance that reimburses an employer for damages that must be paid to an employee for injury occurring in the course of employment.[35] The U.S. Department of Labor's Office of Workers' Compensation Programs (OWCP) administers four major disability compensation programs that provide support to federal workers or their dependents and other specific groups who are injured at work or acquire an occupational disease: wage replacement benefits, medical treatment, vocational rehabilitation, and other benefits.[36] Other specific groups that are covered include Federal Employees' Compensation Program, Longshore and Harbor Workers' Compensation Program, Federal Black Lung Program, and Energy Employees Occupational Illness Compensation Program.[36]

Nonfederal employees injured on the job while employed by private companies or state and local government agencies contact their state workers' compensation board to file claims related to their injuries.[36] Once the claim is approved, the injured or ill employee receives weekly payments to cover medical bills or lost wages. This coverage does not apply if the employee gets a personal injury that is not related to their work, such as falling off a ladder at home after work hours. Workers' compensation benefits provide employees a percentage of their average weekly wage based on their type of injury or illness.[36] If an employee is partially or totally disabled, the benefits are different than for an employee with a temporary injury. Each state has a maximum weekly rate or other procedures to file claims.[36–37] See **Figure 11.6**.

Concierge Health Care

There are two kinds of concierge health care.

Concierge Medicine. Concierge medicine started in the 1990s but gained popularity in the last 5 years among healthcare consumers in upper-middle class metropolitan and suburban areas. Concierge medicine is not healthcare insurance, but it is a healthcare model that provides quick access to doctors and shorter wait times for

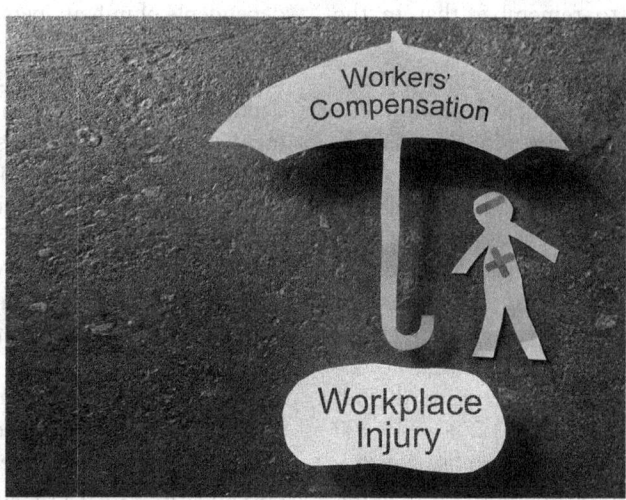

Figure 11.6 Workers' Compensation
© zimmytws/Shutterstock

a set monthly or annual fee. A typical monthly fee to subscribe to most concierge medicine practices range from $1,500 to $2,500.[39] Concierge medicine allows the patient to call or see the physician whenever desired without additional fees or co-payments. Doctors in concierge medicine groups typically have fewer patients than physicians who are in traditional medical practices. In traditional medical model, the patient pays a co-payment for each scheduled appointment, exam, test, or service. If a PCP in a concierge practice refers the patient to a specialist in the same concierge practice, the patient pays no additional costs. If the patient is referred out of the concierge practice for a special appointment, second opinion, or treatment, the patient would use his or her health insurance to cover the cost.[40]

Concierge Nursing.

Concierge nursing services were founded on the observation that clients are in urgent need of private nursing services in their home or place of business.[41] This is an opportunity to not only offer the community quality nursing services outside of the traditional hospital setting, but it also provides reassurance to patients, their family, and their healthcare providers that patients are receiving optimal health care.[41] Concierge nursing services consist of a team of experienced registered nurses, licensed professional nurses, and certified nursing assistants. The services offered include intravenous infusion therapy, postoperative services, companion and accompanying services, wellness and disease counseling, education, and special services as needed. The goal is to become the individual's healthcare advocate, while providing care and health recovery needs.[41] The costs for concierge nursing range from monthly fee plan contracts to fee-for-service for a specific short-term need.[41]

Alternative Methods to Health Care

Fee for Service. **Fee for service** means the doctor and other healthcare providers are paid for each service performed.[42] Services may include tests and office visits. This model usually does not involve traditional health insurance coverage. Patients pay out-of-pocket instead of filing a claim with their health insurance company.[42]

Medical Tourism. **Medical tourism** is defined as international travel for the purpose of receiving medical care. Medical tourists may pursue medical care abroad for a variety of reasons, including decreased costs, a recommendation from friends or family, the opportunity to combine medical care with a vacation destination, preference of receiving care from providers who share the traveler's culture, or to receive a procedure or therapy not available in their country of residence. Medical tourism is a worldwide, multibillion-dollar market that continues to grow. According to the Centers for Disease Control and Prevention (CDC) surveillance data, millions of U.S. residents travel internationally for medical care each year. However, medical tourism is not without risks, such as the possibility of acquiring infections and other adverse events.[43] Furthermore, regardless of the country, all medical and surgical procedures carry risk, and complications can occur regardless of where treatment is received. Since medical or surgical complications may require follow-up care from a healthcare provider in the United States, medical tourists should request a copy of their medical records to provide their U.S. healthcare providers for any follow-up care. Medical tourists should be aware that the drugs, medical products, and devices used in foreign countries might not be subject to the same regulations, protocol, and oversight as followed in the United States.[43] In addition, some drugs may be counterfeit or otherwise ineffective, such as expired, contaminated, or improperly stored.[43]

Before traveling, medical tourists should communicate with their PCP to discuss their plan to seek medical care outside the United States and discuss any concerns that the patient or the PCP might have.[43] Preferably 4–6 weeks before travel, medical tourists should consult a travel medicine specialist for advice related to their specific health needs. Any current medical conditions should be well controlled, and medical tourists should make sure they have enough medication for the duration of their trip.[43] All medical tourists should be up-to-date on all routine vaccinations, immunized against hepatitis B, and receive the vaccines recommended by the CDC *2020 Yellow Book* for the destination country.[44] Additionally, most medical tourists pay for their care at the time of service and often rely on private companies or medical concierge services to identify foreign healthcare facilities.[43] The following website may be a helpful resource to individuals as they prepare for travel: https://wwwnc.cdc.gov/travel/page/yellowbook-home-2020.[44]

Chapter Summary

This chapter opens with a broad historical overview of health insurance in the United States followed by a current overview of health insurance today. Since there are numerous reasons for the uneven coverage of U.S. health insurance, the next section describes the most prominent reasons for the disproportionate coverage among the American population. The next sections define the most common terms used in health insurance. Although, U.S. health insurance is complex and filled with numerous terms, the defined terminology will broaden the CHW's medical vocabulary and provide additional understanding as CHWs assist diverse patients receiving health care. The next section provides a description of the most common types of health insurance available in the United States, along with showcasing the alternative methods to acquire health care, such as the ACA, employer-based health insurance, Medicare, Medicaid, SSDI and SSI, TRICARE and VA benefits, worker's compensation, concierge medicine and health care. The chapter includes case studies throughout the text to provide CHW examples to illustrate the content of the chapter.

CASE STUDY

Retirement Years for Alice and Robert

Alice is 60 years old, and Robert is 61 years old. Both taught high school for most of their careers. After they got married, they lived in Colorado for their entire teaching careers but moved within Colorado to several different cities. They remain avid skiers, stayed in excellent physical shape, and chose not to have any children. Alice was an only child, and Robert had an older brother, Dave, who resides in Denver, Colorado. They joined the state retirement pension program within the first year of teaching. When they signed up for the Colorado state retirement pension program as a married couple, they had to make a choice between two options: (1) Each spouse would receive 100 percent of their pension, and when that spouse died, the pension would stop; (2) upon retirement, each spouse would receive 75 percent of their pension, and when a spouse died, the survivor would receive their 75 percent plus 50 percent of deceased spouse's pension. See examples:

Option 1: At retirement, Alice receives $4,000 per month, and Robert receives $4,000 per month. If Alice dies first, Robert receives only his pension of $4,000 per month for the rest of his life.

Option 2: At retirement, Alice receives $3,000 (75 percent of $4,000) and Robert receives $3,000 (75 percent of $4,000). If Alice dies first, Robert receives his pension of $3,000 (75 percent of $4,000) and $2,000 (50 percent of Alice's full retirement pension) for a total of $5,000 per month for the rest of his life.

Alice and Robert choose Option 1 because they expect to live into their 80s like their parents. They prefer to enjoy the extra retirement pension money now and not be concerned about having enough money later in life. Also, Alice was aware of the statistic that indicate that women live longer.

Alice and Robert received their health care at the University of Colorado Health Sciences in Colorado Springs. Before they retired, they scheduled their annual physicals and lab work. In addition, they met with Gracie, the CHW, to discuss ACA options. Since Alice and Robert were not old enough to qualify for Medicare, they decided to go with the ACA Bronze Plan because of its lower cost. Since they were both healthy and active, they were not concerned about healthcare costs or prescription medications. While meeting with Gracie, they asked questions about available services and volunteer opportunities for the retirement community. After learning about the community programs (e.g., gardening, book clubs, biking groups, and exercise classes) and numerous discounts on a variety of products, they were thrilled about taking the time to meet with Gracie.

Soon after they retired, Alice and Robert decided to remodel their 25-year-old home and make it more appropriate for retirement, such as step-in showers with grab bars, better lighting, expand and close in the patio, replace the roof, painting the exterior, and updating kitchen. The house was paid-off, so they were approved for a $350,000 home equity loan to pay for the remodeling project. They assumed that they would live in this house for at least another 20 years. They hired a contractor to manage the project. Robert did some of the work because he enjoyed working on their home. It took about 9 months to complete the entire project. It was summer, and they were tired of living in noise and dust from the construction. Alice hired a professional cleaning crew to scrub and polish the entire house. They shopped for new indoor and outdoor furniture, mirrors, and lighting fixtures.

In July, they decided to host a big pre-Fourth of July party a few days before the holiday to celebrate their newly renovated home. Even though the party was not scheduled until the weekend, after a late breakfast, Alice went shopping for decorations, food, drinks, and a few fireworks. Around 11:00 a.m., Robert started working on arranging the patio furniture, getting the gas grill set-up, and hanging a few large flower baskets in front of the house to add some color. Robert noticed some bent gutters over the front windows while he was hanging the baskets. He assumed that the roofing company ladders caused damage to the gutters, but he wanted to explore the damage before reporting the damage. Robert is the type of gentleman that likes to get things done rather than delay. Even though Robert had breakfast, he felt a bit hungry when he got the ladder out of the garage. He figured that he would check on the gutters on the north side of the house, then go inside and make a sandwich.

Alice got home and unpacked the car. She called for Robert while she put away the groceries, but he did not answer. She figured that he was upstairs or out in the backyard. As she ate a banana, she walked outside through the garage. She got to the north side of the house and her life changed forever. Robert had fallen off the ladder. She immediately called 911. She felt a pulse and started to perform CPR. The ambulance arrived, continued CPR, and transported Robert to the university hospital. Alice drove to the hospital. She entered the Emergency Department (ED), identified herself, and was told to take a seat and the nurse would come get her in a few minutes. While she waited in a panic, she called Dave, Robert's brother in Denver, and said, "Come quickly. Robert fell off the ladder. I am in the ED waiting room at university hospital. I have no information yet." The rest of the day was a total blur. Robert was stabilized in the ED, had several CT scans to determine his condition, and was moved to the trauma intensive care unit (ICU). Alice was escorted to the ICU waiting room and was told that the physician would come out and talk to her shortly. While Alice was waiting, Dave arrived from Denver. Dr. Weiss, the ICU physician, talked to both Alice and Dave about Robert's condition. Dr. Weiss said that Robert fell from the ladder because he experienced a serious myocardial infarction, also known as a heart attack. When he fell, he hit his head on the stones and sustained a serious brain concussion. Robert was in a coma, and the next few days would determine his level of recovery. Dr. Weiss brought in Dr. Patel, a cardiologist (heart surgeon), to assess Robert's cardiac condition. Dr. Patel determined that Robert needed cardiac surgery to repair the blood flow to his heart, but Robert's condition was too serious to perform surgery until he was out of the coma from the concussion.

The following day, Robert was taken to surgery to drain an accumulation of fluid around his brain. He seemed to recover a bit, was breathing on his own, and was no longer in a coma. He could squeeze Alice's hand, but he could not speak or swallow. Dr. Patel was getting anxious because Robert's cardiac condition was declining each day. By the fourth day in ICU, Dr. Patel told Alice that Robert needed cardiac surgery the following day, but the surgery would come with multiple risks. Robert's heart was unable to move enough oxygenated blood to Robert's brain and other vital organs. Alice signed the consent for Robert's surgery.

Alice called Dave, and he arrived that next morning. Dave's wife had died a few years previous, so he completely understood the stress that Alice was experiencing. The next morning, they spoke to Dr. Patel briefly prior to Robert's surgery. Dr. Patel said that the surgery would take about 6 hours. They stayed in the surgery waiting room to watch the screen for updates about Robert.

Robert's surgery was successful. He stayed in the ICU, was transferred to a cardiac floor, and then moved to the hospital rehabilitation center where he stayed for 4 weeks. The case manager told Alice that Robert's insurance for rehabilitation had expired, and he was being discharged tomorrow. Since the case manager offered no solutions, Alice remembered Gracie at the clinic. She called Gracie immediately. Gracie started investigating where Robert could go since he was too weak to go home. Alice was in a panic. She wanted Robert to come home because she knew that they were unable to afford residential assisted living and rehabilitation. She told the hospital case manager that Robert should come home because she could take care of him with home health and physical therapy at home. The case manager was reluctant, but Dr. Patel agreed to sign the discharge-to-home agreement along with several prescriptions for home health and physical therapy. Gracie ordered a hospital bed, walker, wheelchair, and bedside commode for delivery that afternoon.

After 4 days at home, Alice was exhausted caring for Robert 16 hours each day. The home health aide worked 8 hours each day and physical therapy came twice per week. Robert was not improving. Alice called Dr. Patel, and he told her that Robert needed 24-hour care in a facility. Alice called Gracie and asked for help. By the end of the day, Gracie had located a rehabilitation facility that had a bed available for Robert. Unfortunately, the facility was located about 25 miles from Alice's home. The facility came to transport Robert the next morning, and Alice followed behind in her car. While Robert was getting settled, Alice met with the financial counselor. She left their office with the information that the monthly cost would be approximately $8,000, and it was expected that Robert would be there 4 to 6 weeks. Alice and Robert's health insurance covers 28 days annually for rehabilitation, but that was used for the hospital rehabilitation costs. Alice had no idea how she was going to pay their bills. She called Gracie to schedule an appointment for advice.

Questions

1. How should Gracie prepare for the appointment with Alice?
2. As a new CHW, what type of training would you like to receive to be prepared for this situation?

References

1. Statehood. Washington State Legislature Web site. https://apps.leg.wa.gov/oralhistory/timeline_event.aspx?e=8. Accessed December 5, 2021.
2. American healthcare history: a timeline on the evolution of coverage. Health Markets Web site. https://www.healthmarkets.com/content/american-healthcare-history. Accessed December 5, 2021.
3. A brief history of private insurance in the United States. Academic HealthPlans Web site. https://www.ahpcare.com/a-brief-history-of-private-insurance-in-the-united-states/. Accessed December 5, 2021.
4. Tru blog. Truman Library Institute Web site. https://www.trumanlibraryinstitute.org/health-care/. Accessed December 5, 2021.
5. Timeline: history of health reform in the U.S. Kaiser Family Foundation Website. https://www.kff.org/wp-content/uploads/2011/03/5-02-13-history-of-health-reform.pdf. Accessed December 5, 2021.
6. History. CMS.gov. https://www.cms.gov/About-CMS/Agency-Information/History. Accessed December 5, 2021.
7. What is the Affordable Care Act? HHS.gov. https://www.hhs.gov/answers/health-insurance-reform/what-is-the-affordable-care-act/index.html. Accessed December 6, 2021.
8. The U.S. health care system: an international perspective. Department for Professional Employees Web site. https://www.dpeaflcio.org/factsheets/the-us-health-care-system-an-international-perspective#_edn1. Accessed December 6, 2021.
9. Kamal R, Ramirez G, Cox C. How does health spending in the U.S. compare to other countries? https://www.healthsystemtracker.org/chart-collection/health-spending-u-s-compare-countries/#item-spendingcomparison_health-consumption-expenditures-per-capita-2019. Accessed December 6, 2021.
10. Kurani N, Wager E. How does the quality of the U.S. health system compare to other countries? https://www.healthsystemtracker.org/chart-collection/quality-u-s-healthcare-system-compare-countries/. Accessed December 6, 2021.
11. Coinsurance. HealthCare.gov. https://www.healthcare.gov/glossary/co-insurance/. Accessed December 6, 2021.
12. Definitions of health insurance terms. U.S. Bureau of Labor Statistics Web site. https://www.bls.gov/ncs/ebs/sp/healthterms.pdf. Accessed December 6, 2021.
13. History of health insurance and 2019 & beyond projections. Health for California Web site. https://www.healthforcalifornia.com/blog/history-of-health-insurance. Accessed December 6, 2021.
14. Which Obamacare plan is right for me? Obamacare USA.org. https://www.obamacareusa.org/obamacare-plans.html?_d=c;vGelPE3UjenQQHswtz5SyGXY4RR3hPnBLWugwObrxkKP3H1I8qZ5R2FMda9n40KG_qt5G879LRQwfk3cxIRTjakYZyCtvg;;&msclkid=82213b3fe25611cd296a5a60c02a0653. Accessed December 7, 2021.
15. Wallen J, Williams SR. Employer-based health insurance. *J Health Polit Policy Law.* 1982;7(2):366–379.
16. How to choose a health insurance plan. Health Resource Now Web site. https://healthresourcenow.com/health-insurance/get-insured/choosing-a-health-insurance-plan/. Accessed December 7, 2021.

17. What's Medicare? Medicare.org. https://www.medicare.gov/what-medicare-covers/your-medicare-coverage-choices/whats-medicare. Accessed December 8, 2021.

18. What's Medicare Supplement Insurance (Medigap)? Medicare.org. https://www.medicare.gov/supplements-other-insurance/whats-medicare-supplement-insurance-medigap. Accessed December 9, 2021.

19. Know all types of primary Medicare coverage. KMC University Website. https://www.kmcuniversity.com/know-all-types-primary-medicare-coverage. Accessed December 10, 2021.

20. Program history. Medicaid.gov. https://www.medicaid.gov/about-us/program-history/index.html. Accessed December 11, 2021.

21. What is Medicaid? Health Insurance.org. https://www.healthinsurance.org/glossary/medicaid/. Accessed December 13, 2021.

22. The primary differences between Medicare and Medicaid. Healthtian Web site. https://healthtian.com/the-primary-differences-between-medicare-and-medicaid/. Accessed December 13, 2021.

23. Benefits and insurance for people with disabilities. USA.gov. https://www.usa.gov/disability-benefits-insurance#:~:text=Benefits%20and%20Insurance%20for%20People%20with%20Disabilities%201,Disabilities.%20...%204%20VA%20Disability%20Compensation%20Benefits.%20. Accessed December 14, 2021.

24. What is SSA BEST? Social Security Administration Benefits Eligibility Screening Tool. https://ssabest.benefits.gov/. Accessed December 14, 2021.

25. Who is eligible for Social Security retirement benefits? Elder Law Answers Web site. https://www.elderlawanswers.com/who-is-eligible-for-social-security-retirement-benefits-12052. Accessed December 14, 2021.

26. Quarter and quarter of coverage. SSA.gov. https://www.ssa.gov/OP_Home/ssact/title02/0213.htm. Accessed December 14, 2021.

27. Korbey M. Social Security's definition of disability. https://blog.ssa.gov/social-securitys-definition-of-disability/. Accessed December 14, 2021.

28. What is the definition of disability under the ADA? National Network Web site. https://adata.org/faq/what-definition-disability-under-ada. Accessed December 14, 2021.

29. Benefits for people with disabilities. SSA.gov. https://www.ssa.gov/disability/. Accessed December 14, 2021.

30. The faces and facts of disability. SSA.gov. https://www.ssa.gov/disabilityfacts/facts.html. Accessed December 14, 2021.

31. Tricare. The Free Dictionary by Farlex. https://medical-dictionary.thefreedictionary.com/TRICARE. Accessed December 14, 2021.

32. Eligibility. TRICARE Web site. https://eligibility.com/tricare. Accessed December 14, 2021.

33. About VA health benefits. U.S. Department of Veteran's Affairs Web site. https://www.va.gov/health-care/about-va-health-benefits/. Accessed December 14, 2021.

34. Veteran Benefits Administration. U.S. Department of Veteran's Affairs Web site. https://benefits.va.gov/benefits/. Accessed December 14, 2021.

35. Worker's compensation. Merriam-Webster Web site. https://www.merriam-webster.com/dictionary/workers'%20compensation. Accessed December 14, 2021.

36. Workers' compensation. U.S. Department of Labor Web site. https://www.dol.gov/general/topic/workcomp. Accessed December 14, 2021.

37. How is workers' comp calculated? The Hartford Web site. https://www.thehartford.com/workers-compensation/how-to-calculate-cost. Accessed December 14, 2021.

38. What qualifies as a workers' compensation injury? Core Medical Center Web site. https://www.coremedcenter.com/2021/07/09/what-qualifies-as-a-workers-compensation-injury/. Accessed December 14, 2021.

39. Smith Z. Concierge medicine: costs, factors, and considerations. https://www.partnermd.com/blog/concierge-medicine-costs-factors-considerations. Accessed December 14, 2021.

40. Castaneda R. What is concierge medicine? https://health.usnews.com/wellness/articles/what-is-concierge-medicine. Accessed January 2, 2022.

41. About concierge nursing services. Concierge Nursing Services Web site. https://www.conciergenurseservice.com/. Accessed January 4, 2022.

42. Fee for services. HealthCare.gov. https://www.healthcare.gov/glossary/fee-for-service/. Accessed January 6, 2022.

43. Benowitz I, Gaines J. Chapter 9 travel for work & other reasons: medical tourism. *CDC Yellow Book 2020*. Atlanta GA: Centers for Disease Control and Prevention; 2020. https://wwwnc.cdc.gov/travel/yellowbook/2020/travel-for-work-other-reasons/medical-tourism. Accessed January 6, 2022.

44. *CDC Yellow Book 2020*. Atlanta, GA: Centers for Disease Control and Prevention; 2020. https://wwwnc.cdc.gov/travel/page/yellowbook-home-2020. Accessed January 6, 2022.

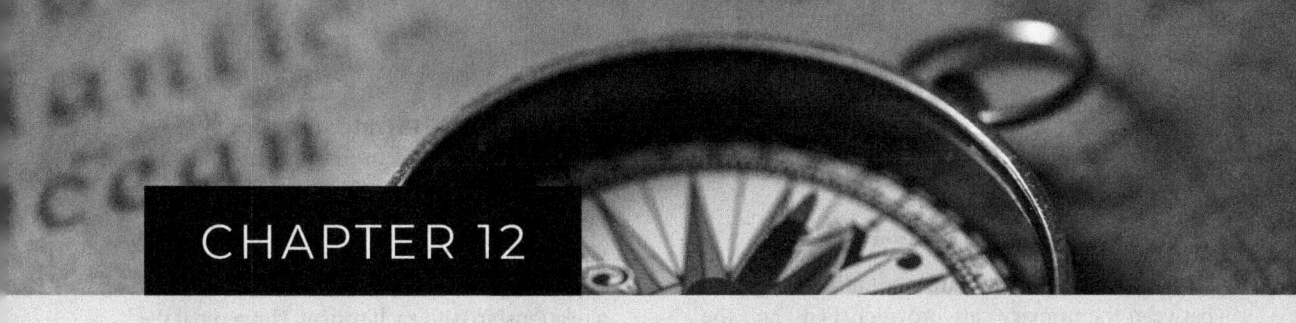

CHAPTER 12

Health Care Facilities

LEARNING OBJECTIVES

1. Describe the difference between an urgent care clinic and the emergency department in a hospital.
2. Identify four types of physician practices.
3. Define federally funded nonprofit health centers (FQHC). What services do FQHCs offer?
4. Describe six types of integrative therapies including the benefits of each therapy.
5. Identify practical ways for seniors to age in place.
6. Explain the difference between assisted living facilities and nursing home/skilled nursing facilities.
7. Describe the five signs when family members may wish to begin the process of exploring memory care centers.

KEY WORDS

urgent care clinics	birth centers	registered dietitian nutritionists (RDN)
private practice	dialysis	
group practice	dialysis centers	Tai chi
health maintenance organization (HMO)	employee health programs	yoga
	infusion centers	radiation therapy center
hospitalists	acupuncture	rehabilitation center
locum tenens	art therapy	travel clinics
federally qualified health centers (FQHC)	chiropractic care	wound care center
	functional medicine	aging in place
local health departments (LHDs)	mindful meditation	memory care centers
ambulatory surgery centers (ASCs)		hospice

Introduction

This chapter explores the wide spectrum of healthcare facilities ranging from urgent care clinics to end-of-life hospice care. As the role of community health workers (CHWs) expands, the choices of employment have increased across the United States. The first section describes outpatient healthcare services, including numerous types of medical facilities, outpatient services, and centers. The second section defines inpatient healthcare facilities, including various types of hospitals, choices of residency for seniors, and hospice services.

Outpatient Facilities

Medical Facilities

Urgent Care Clinics

Urgent care clinics are the middle ground between the primary care provider (PCP) and the Emergency Department (ED). If the individual has a minor injury (sprain or cut), urgent care is appropriate. Also, urgent care is a good option for people who have an illness without other symptoms, such as a sore throat or cough, and no major underlying medical conditions.[1] Typically, urgent care clinics are staffed with physician assistants, nurse practitioners, and nurses, although some urgent care clinics have physicians on staff as well.[1] Urgent care providers can order basic labs and imaging tests, such as X-rays, to provide diagnoses and develop treatment plans. Urgent care clinics have set hours and an established list of conditions treated. As a result, urgent care clinics often are less expensive and have shorter wait times than EDs.[1]

Hospital Emergency Departments

Hospital EDs treat life- or limb-threatening health conditions in people of all ages. It is the best option when the individual requires immediate medical attention. EDs are staffed 24/7 with physicians, physician assistants, nurse practitioners, and nurses trained in delivering emergency care.[1] The team has quick access to expert providers in advanced specialties such as cardiology, neurology, and orthopedics. EDs also have advanced imaging and laboratory resources needed to diagnose and deliver care for severe and life-threatening situations. Always call 911 if the person is having difficulty breathing, shortness of breath, life threatening symptoms, limb injury, or signs of stroke or heart attack.[1]

Patient Choices from Types of Physician Practices

There are several types of medical practices for physicians. It is useful to understand each type of physician practice prior to choosing a physician. Additionally, it is important to be familiar with the following options as a CHW to better serve patients.

- Private Practice: **Private practice** is also called a solo practice. In this practice, the physician practices medicine alone with a small office staff. When seeking health care at a private practice, the patient may wait longer for appointments, but the physician is able to form a relationship with each patient. However, if the physician becomes ill or is away on vacation, the office is likely closed. When the office closes, the patients are referred to another physician who is not familiar with the patient's medical history. This situation may also occur during nights and weekends. It is up to the patient to ask questions about what type of health insurance is accepted and how coverage of care is handled when a solo practitioner is away prior to agreeing to receive care at this location.

- Group Practice: A **group practice** involves several physicians with usually the same specialty that practice in the same building. The physicians share the office staff. The physicians' income is based upon contracts that were signed when the group was started. The patients benefit because the office staff is larger and there are generally more appointments available. It is important for patients to ask about types of health insurance the group practice accepts.

- Large Health Maintenance Organizations: A **health maintenance organization (HMO)** employees a large number of physicians who form networks. The patients join the specific physician networks and receive lower medical costs as the benefit. The patients benefit from scheduling faster appointments with their primary care physician and with specialty physicians within the network. Physicians get paid based on their productivity and patient satisfaction. Since the physicians are paid by how many patients they see each day, the patients receive less time with the physician at every visit.

- Hospital Based: **Hospitalists** are physicians who are employed by the hospital. They are assigned to care for a specific specialty of medicine. The hospitalized patients may or may not have contact with their primary care physician while in the hospital. Since the hospitalists are employed by the hospital, they are assigned a routine schedule each week. For example, they may work three 12-hour shifts per week. While this schedule is advantageous for the physician, it causes confusion for the patients and their families in terms of attempting to talk to the hospitalist.

- Locum Tenens: Physicians employed as **locum tenens** travel to geographical locations that are in need of healthcare professionals including physicians, nurses, lab technicians, physical therapists, pharmacists, and a variety of other health workers. The salary is higher than the other steady healthcare workers in the same location because they are filling a desperate need such as during a pandemic or a natural disaster. Locum tenen workers ease the burden of short staffing during a time of need. The patients benefit by receiving care during dire times in the hospital. The hospital does not pay benefits (e.g., sick leave and vacation days), but it may pay for malpractice insurance.

Federally Qualified Health Centers

Federally funded nonprofit health centers or clinics serve medically underserved areas and populations. **Federally qualified health centers (FQHC)** provide primary care services to these populations using a sliding scale model where the fee is based on the individual's ability to pay.[3] According to the Health Resources and Services Administration (HRSA), FQHCs provide comprehensive services (either on-site or by arrangement with another provider), including preventive health services, dental services, mental health and substance abuse services, transportation services necessary for adequate patient care, and hospital and specialty care services.[4]

Local Health Departments

All **local health departments (LHDs)** are governmental entities and obtain their authority and responsibility from the state and local laws.[5] LHDs exist for the common good and are responsible for demonstrating strong leadership in the promotion of physical, behavioral, environmental, social, and economic conditions that improve health and well-being. Additionally, LHDs are committed to the prevention of illness, disease, injury, and premature death and work to eliminate health disparities.[5] In addition, the LHDs do the following:

1. Monitor health status and understand health issues facing the community
2. Protect people from health problems and health hazards
3. Give people information they need to make healthy choices
4. Engage the community to identify and solve health problems
5. Develop public health policies and plans
6. Enforce public health laws and regulations
7. Help people receive health services
8. Maintain a competent public health workforce
9. Evaluate and improve programs and interventions
10. Contribute to and apply the evidence base of public health[5]

Outpatient Services, Centers, and Facilities (Alphabetical Order)
Ambulatory Surgery Centers

Ambulatory surgery centers (ASCs) perform surgeries and medical procedures that do not require a hospital admission after the procedure. ASCs provide cost-saving services in a less stressful environment that is often located near a hospital in case of unforeseen events. Prior to outpatient surgery or procedures, the patients are examined by a specialty surgeon to determine if the ASC procedure is appropriate for an outpatient and will not require a hospital admission. Patients arrive the day of the procedure, have the surgery or procedure, recover, and are discharged to home the same day. The patient's family benefits from a more comfortable environment while they wait. The physicians and nurses working in ASCs have the identical training and knowledge of hospital employees. ASCs are equipped with the same safety measures and equipment that is required in hospital operating rooms. Some ASCs are owned by hospitals, healthcare organizations, and physician groups. During the process of establishing an ASC, the accrediting agency works with the invested hospital and physicians to establish policies, procedures, equipment, and staff needed for safety and positive outcomes. See **Figure 12.1** and **Figure 12.2**.

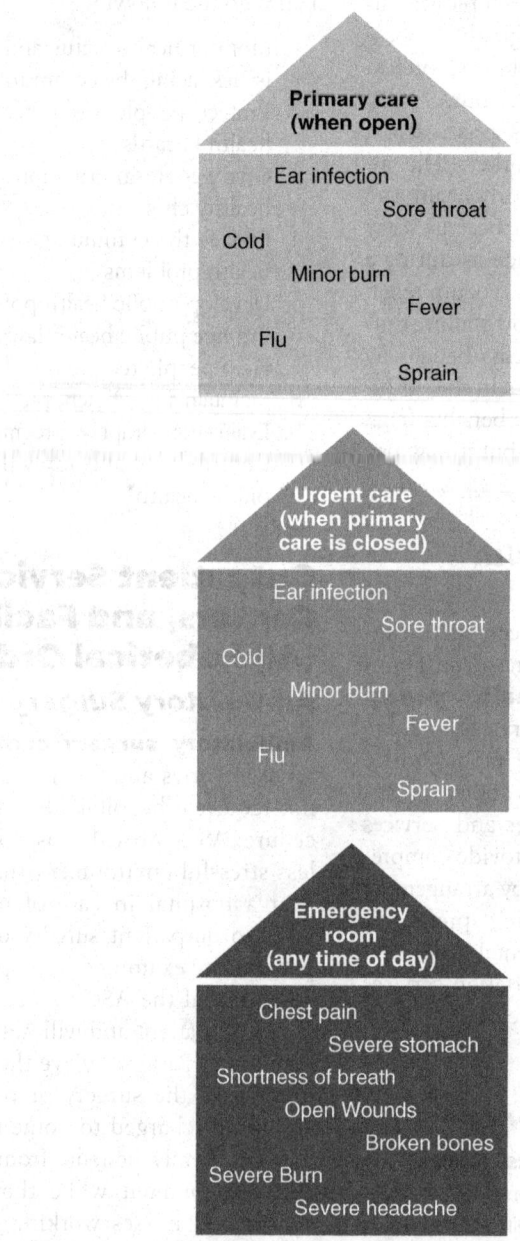

Figure 12.1 Receiving Appropriate Care at the Right Facility

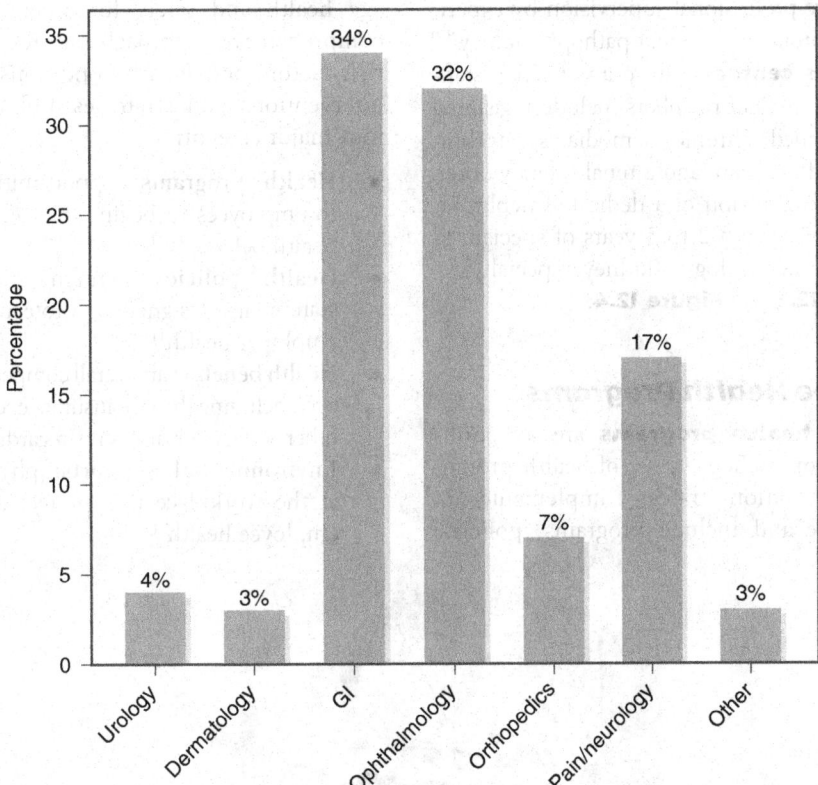

Specialties served in ASCs

Figure 12.2 Top Specialties Served in Ambulatory Surgery Centers

Birth Centers

The American Association of Birth Centers (AABC) defines a **birth center** as a home-like facility existing within a healthcare system with a program of care designed in the wellness model of pregnancy and birth.[6] Birth centers are guided by the principles of prevention, sensitivity, safety, appropriate medical intervention, and cost effectiveness. Birth centers provide family-centered care for healthy women before, during, and after a normal, uncomplicated pregnancy, labor, and birth.[6] Birth center mothers and babies have minimal analgesia, receive no general or regional anesthesia, and are capable of ambulation, even in second-stage labor. The birth center is freestanding, or distinctly separate from acute care services within a hospital.[6]

Dialysis Centers

Dialysis is defined as a type of renal replacement therapy which is used to provide an artificial replacement for inadequate or lost kidney function.[7] Dialysis may be used for very sick patients who have recently lost kidney functions (acute renal failure) or for stable patients who have permanently lost kidney functions (chronic or end-stage renal failure).[7] There are two types of dialysis: hemodialysis (only performed at a dialysis center) and peritoneal dialysis (self-administered by patient at home). Both forms of dialysis are defined as supportive care treatment. Dialysis does not treat kidney diseases.[7–8] Dialysis centers offer highly specialized services to provide treatment to patients with irreversible renal insufficiencies (kidney failure). Treatment procedures require professional supervision by experienced staff proficient in renal pathophysiology.[8–9] The **dialysis centers** feature an effective staff-to-patient ratio. Staff members include registered nurses, certified chronic hemodialysis technicians, a renal dietitian, and a renal social worker, all under the direction of a dedicated nephrologist, a physician with 2 to 3 years of specialized training in nephrology (kidney specialty).[7–9] See **Figure 12.3** and **Figure 12.4**.

Employee Health Programs

Employee health programs are a coordinated and comprehensive set of health promotion and protection strategies implemented at the worksite and include programs, policies, benefits, and environmental supports to encourage health and safety for all employees.[11] A comprehensive approach addresses multiple risk factors and health conditions along with interventions and strategies and includes the four major categories:

- **Health programs:** opportunities available to employees to begin, change, or maintain health behaviors[11]
- **Health policies:** written and approved statements designed to protect or promote employee health[11]
- **Health benefits:** an overall compensation package including health insurance coverage and other services or discounts regarding health[11]
- **Environmental supports:** physical factors at the workplace that protect and enhance employee health[11]

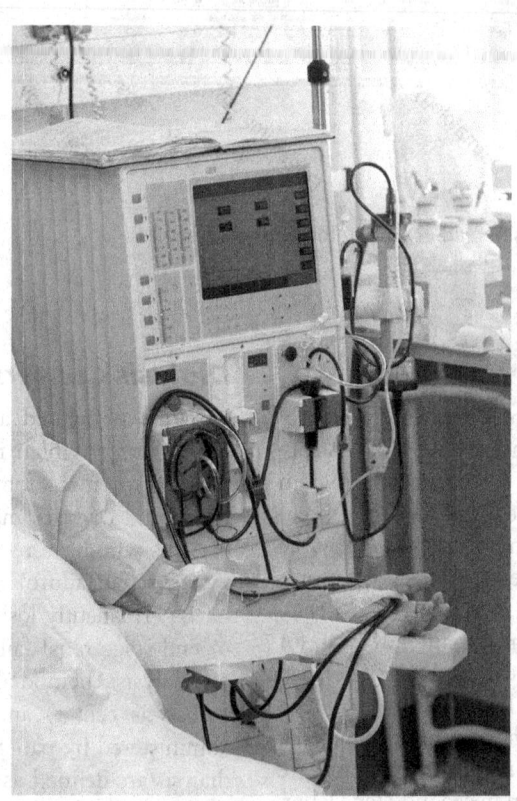

Figure 12.3 Patient Receiving Dialysis
© Pics five/Shutterstock.

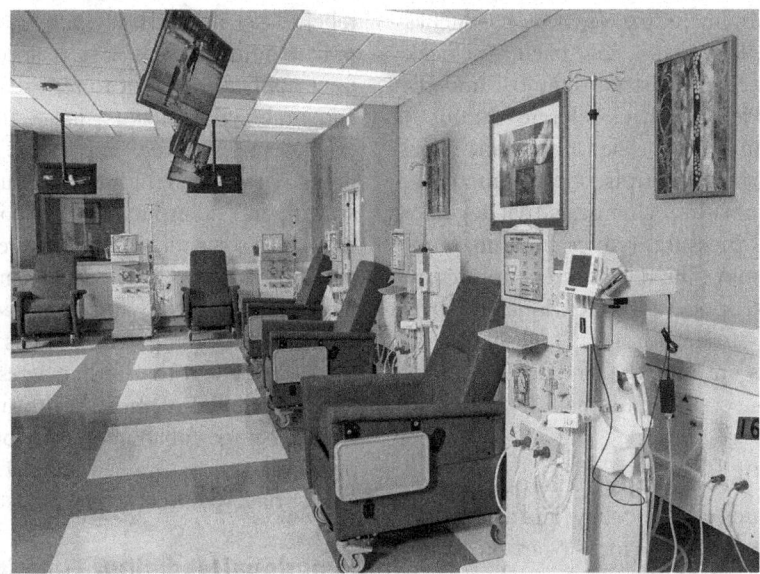

Figure 12.4 Dialysis Center Treatment Area

Reproduced from United Dialysis Center. Receiving Dialysis. Available at http://www.pompanodialysis.com/. Accessed January 2, 2022.[19]

Additionally, employee health programs benefit from community partnerships to offer health-related programs and services to employees when the employer does not have the capacity to provide support for healthy lifestyles to employees when not at the workplace.[11] For example, community program may address specific health risks (e.g., physical inactivity, poor nutrition, tobacco use, stress), conditions (e.g., obesity, musculoskeletal disorders, mental health), and diseases (e.g., heart disease and stroke, diabetes, cancer, arthritis).[11]

Infusion Centers

Infusion centers are outpatient facilities located in a freestanding location, in a medical clinic complex, or in an outpatient area of a hospital. Infusion therapy is prescribed for patients with diseases or conditions where oral medications are not effective, such sepsis, wound care, burns, and cancer treatment. The medication is administered through an intravenous (IV) port. The patients find infusion centers are more convenient and cost less than in-patient hospital care. Infusion centers are staffed by registered nurses with specific training. Comfortable reclining chairs make the

experience relaxing for the patients. The length of infusions varies from one hour to up to several hours depending on how fast the medication can be infused and the volume of each infusion. Some infusion centers administer chemotherapy prescriptions depending on the physician's orders.

Integrative Therapies

Acupuncture. Traditional Chinese medicine explains **acupuncture** as a technique for balancing the flow of energy through pathways (meridians) in the body.[12] By inserting tiny, thin needles into specific points along these meridians, acupuncture practitioners rebalance the energy flow. In contrast, many Western practitioners view the acupuncture points as places to stimulate nerves, muscles, and connective tissue to stimulate the body's natural painkillers.[12] A key component of acupuncture is to treat pain. Increasingly, it is being used for overall wellness, including stress management.[12] Acupuncture is used mainly to relieve discomfort associated with a variety of diseases and conditions, including chemotherapy-induced and postoperative nausea and vomiting, dental pain, headaches, including tension headaches and migraines, labor pain, low back and neck pain, osteoarthritis, menstrual cramps, and respiratory disorders, such as allergic rhinitis.[12] Acupuncture influences the autonomic nervous system (which controls bodily functions) and releases the natural chemicals that regulate blood flow and pressure, reduce inflammation, and calm the brain. The risks from acupuncture are low if the acupuncture practitioner is certified and using sterile needles. Single-use, disposable needles are now the practice standard, so the risk of infection is minimal.[12]

Art Therapy. Art therapy includes drawing, painting, sculpture, clay modeling, and a variety of other creative outlets.[13] The focus of art therapy is to work with individuals through creating artwork as an addition to existing care to further promote successful rehabilitation.[13,14] This type of therapy is thought to be especially helpful for people who have difficulty articulating feelings, including children and those on the autism spectrum, individuals with complex medical conditions, those with emotional disorders, persons with cognitive impairment related to dementia or Alzheimer's disease, and individuals who have had strokes or have post-traumatic stress disorder.[13–14]

Chiropractic Care. Chiropractic care is a healthcare profession that focuses on the spine, various joints of the body, and the connection to the nervous system.[15] Certain diagnoses related to the spine and joints may benefit from manipulative treatment to prevent the onset of additional disorders that would affect nerves, muscles, and organs. The focus is on prevention, diagnosis, and conservative care of spine-related disorders and other painful joint issues.[15] Additionally, chiropractors also provide various therapies to treat soft-tissue injuries, make lifestyle recommendations, and give fitness and nutritional advice. Prior to receiving any manipulations, it is crucial for patients to first discuss the nature of their injury or related symptoms with their medical healthcare team prior to seeking chiropractic care. Depending on the nature of the injury, manipulations may harm the patient rather than provide modest

relief to benefit the body holistically. Each chiropractic adjustment is a safe, specific, controlled force applied to a joint to restore proper function and mobility. Accidents, falls, stress, or overexertion can negatively impact the spine or other joints. These changes impact tissues, the nervous system, and other areas of the body.[15] Left unresolved, this type of injury may result in chronic problems. Chiropractic adjustments reduce pain, increase movement, and improve performance. The cost of chiropractic care is approximately the same or less than other types of health care and is included in most health insurance plans. Chiropractors collaborate with other healthcare providers and are trained to refer patients to the appropriate specialist when needed.[15]

Functional Medicine. Functional medicine is a systems biology–based approach that focuses on identifying and addressing the root cause of disease.[16] Each symptom or differential diagnosis may be one of many contributing to an individual's illness. Functional medicine is an individualized, patient-centered, science-based approach to health care that looks beyond symptom resolution to identify why illness occurs and address those root causes to restore health.[16] **Figure 12.5** illustrates how one diagnosis can be the result of more than one cause, contributing to a cascade of symptoms. For example, depression can be caused by many different factors, such as stress, which can then produce inflammation. The precise manifestation of each cause is often difficult to determine because of factors including people's genetics, their surrounding environment, lifestyle, access to preventative care, mental well-being, and various other reasons. By isolating the appropriate cause, treatments can be recommended to provide holistic benefits beyond symptom suppression.[16]

Massage Therapy. A massage therapist is a trained, certified medical professional that manipulates the soft tissues of the body which includes muscles, connective tissues, tendons, ligaments, and the skin.[18] The massage therapist uses varying degrees of techniques, pressure, and movements tailored to the patient's needs. Massage therapy have been found to reduce stress, lessen pain, decrease muscle tension,

One condition, many causes

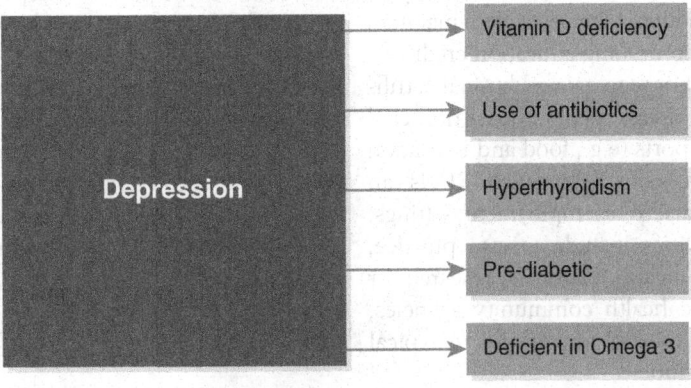

One cause, many conditions

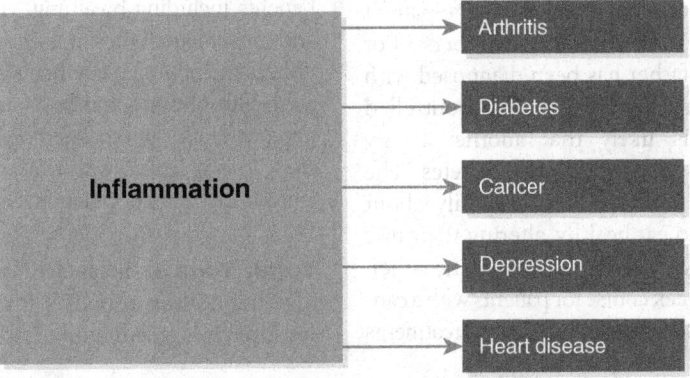

Figure 12.5 Example of Functional Medicine

increase relaxation, and improve overall immune function. Medical professionals may recommend massage therapy to help individuals cope with the pain and stress of various conditions, such as cancer, heart disease, stomach problems or fibromyalgia.[18]

Mindful Meditation. Mindfulness is the basic human ability to be fully present, aware of location and actions.[19] Intentional awareness combined with deep breathing helps one to not overreact. The goal of mindfulness is to wake up to the inner workings of the mind, emotions, and physical processes. Mindfulness is available in every moment, whether through meditations and body scans or mindful moment practices.[19] Research shows how individuals can train their brain to be mindful.[20] Meditation is the process of

awakening the body's senses by focusing on deep breathing and relaxation to produce mental clarity and improve concentration over time.[20] **Mindful meditation** asks the participant to suspend judgment and unleash the natural curiosity about the workings of the mind and approach the experience with warmth, gratitude, and kindness.[19–20]

Registered Dietitian Nutritionists (RDNs). **Registered dietitian nutritionists (RDN)** are food and nutrition experts. They are licensed by the Accreditation Council for Education in Nutrition and Dietetics (ACEND) of the Academy of Nutrition and Dietetics. After completing the bachelorette degree courses, the students must complete a supervised minimum six month practice program at a healthcare facility, community agency, or foodservice corporation. Upon completion of the practicum, the students must pass a national examination to receive and maintain their license with continuing education credits.

Some RDNs choose to gain additional certification in specialty areas, such as pediatric, renal (kidney) disease, sports (e.g., food and hydration needs, training), or diabetes education. RDNs can work in a wide variety of employment settings. The job opportunities include private practice, corporations (e.g., health insurance, research, or businesses), public health community agencies, government agencies, and universities. A typical workday might include:

- Meeting with individuals and their families to teach everyone involved about how food affects the disease progression for the patient but also the other family members. For example, the father has been diagnosed with chronic kidney failure due to uncontrolled diabetes. It is likely that another family member(s) is diagnosed with diabetes. The RDN would advise the entire family about simple ways to eat healthy, altering their diet instead of only changing the diet of the father.
- Teaching a 2-week course for patients with a cancer diagnosis starting chemotherapy treatments

in a few weeks. The patient and caregivers need to understand how to cope with the side effects while attempting to eat healthy foods.

- Serve as an advisor for agency committees on topics, such as governmental nutrition programs and food stamps.
- Advise corporations about healthy foods in on-site cafeterias or vending machines so workers have nutritious meal options instead of foods with high sugar and salt content.

The RDN employment opportunities are expected to increase due to the increase in chronic disease and the rising number of elderly.

Tai Chi. Tai Chi, once a form of martial arts, is now a whole body exercise that provides many health benefits including breathing, visualization, balance, and movement of most muscle groups in the body. It utilizes the natural movements and breathing to create health of mind and body and improve posture, longevity, and internal strength. This low-impact exercise is practiced with relaxed muscles and excellent for the aging population. See **Figure 12.6**.

Yoga. Yoga is an ancient practice that brings together mind and body.[22] It incorporates breathing exercises, meditation, and poses designed to

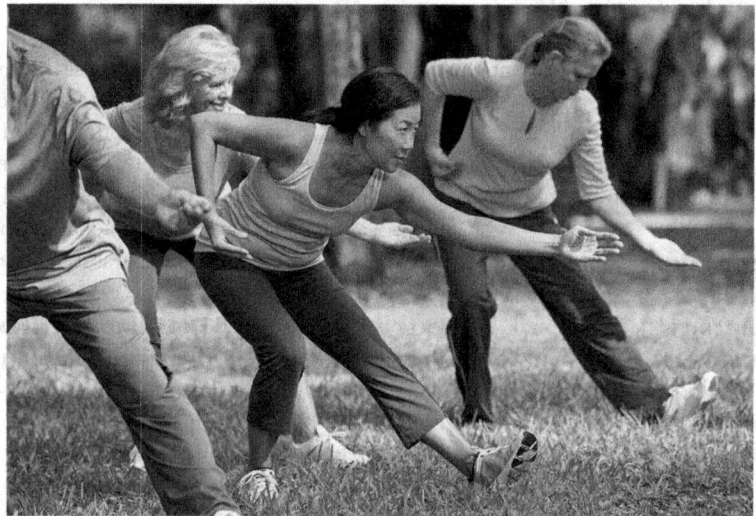

Figure 12.6 Adults Participating in a Tai Chi Class
© Kali9/ E+/Getty Images.

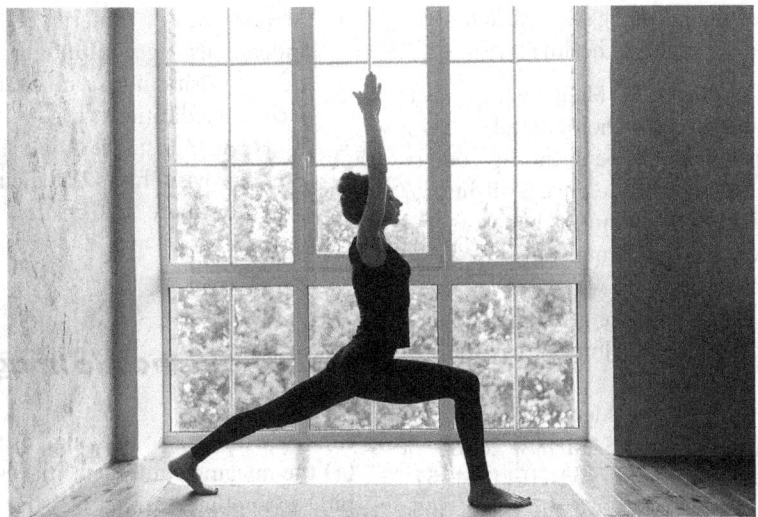

Figure 12.7 Example of a Yoga Pose
© MestoSveta/Shutterstock

encourage relaxation and reduce stress. The health benefits of yoga include improvement of flexibility, strength building, increased muscle tone, improved balance, better joint health, and prevention of back pain and injury.[22] Additionally, yoga teaches better breathing, fosters mental calmness, reduces stress, increases self-confidence, and improves sleep.[22-23] See **Figure 12.7**.

Mental Health Services

Many individuals do not have adequate funds or the insurance to pay for mental health services. As a CHW, following is a list of helpful ways to locate care despite one's lack of insurance or money.

Hotlines

- National Suicide Prevention Lifeline: 1-800-273-8255 or TTY: 1-800-799-4889. Visit https://suicidepreventionlifeline.org/[25]
- http://suicide.org/[26] has a 24-hour email support for those who are feeling suicidal. Additionally, http://suicide.org/[26] has additional cost-effective recommendations to support individuals in need of mental health services.

Obstacles to Receiving Mental Health Services

Mental health services in the United States are insufficient despite more than half of Americans (56 percent) seeking help.[27] Limited options, lack of insurance coverage, costs, and long wait times are the norm; however, 76 percent of Americans are now beginning to recognize how mental health is just as important of physical health.[27] This message is central to increasing access, dismantling stigma, and opening conversations about the importance of seeking services. The demand for mental health services is now strong, with nearly 6 out of 10 (56 percent) Americans seeking or wanting to seek mental health services either for themselves or for a loved one.[27] Studies have indicated that these individuals are younger and are more likely to be of lower income and have a military background.[27] Despite the demand and growing societal awareness of the importance of mental health, the research revealed that most Americans (74 percent) do not believe such services are accessible for everyone, and almost half (47 percent) believe options are limited.[27] These beliefs are driven by several perceived barriers in Americans' ability to seek mental health treatment, including high cost, insufficient insurance coverage, limited options, long waits, lack of awareness about finding services, and social stigma around seeking mental health services.[27]

- Finding a Therapist or Mental Health Services: The website Psychology Today has a free Therapist finder. Type in the zip code or state to find clinics in the area. Visit https://www.psychologytoday.com/us/therapists.[28]
- National Alliance on Mental Illness (NAMI) provides information on where to find mental health treatment in the geographical location at https://nami.org/Home or call toll free at 1-800-950-NAMI.[29]
- Substance Abuse and Mental Health Services Administration (SAMHSA) offers a national helpline: 1-800-662-HELP (4357) is a confidential, free, 24-hour-a-day, 365-day-a-year, information service, in English and Spanish, for individuals and family members. This service provides referrals to local treatment facilities, support groups, and community-based organizations. Additionally, a list of mental health services or facilities can be located by using the online locator at https://findtreatment.samhsa.gov/.[30]
- If a nearby university offers graduate training programs in psychology, psychiatry, social work, or counseling, they may provide mental health services to the community for reduced fees. Also, students in training under the direct supervision of a licensed faculty member may offer therapy at a reduced cost.
- Some therapists offer group therapy as a more affordable alternative to one-on-one sessions. Find a certified group therapist by using American Group Psychotherapy Association's locator: https://member.agpa.org/cgpdirectory.[31]
- Contacting the state licensing boards for referrals for providers who offer sliding fee structures that are determined by the patient's level of income or arrange for a payment plan.

Financial Help for Prescription Medications

- Needy Meds is an organization that may provide aid in obtaining medications. Visit https://www.needymeds.org/.[32]

- Mental Health America help low-income individuals get funding for medications. Visit https://mhanational.org/issues/access-medications.[33]
- Medicine Assistance Tool: Call 1-571-350-8643 or visit https://medicineassistancetool.org/ for more information on medication payment assistance.[34]

See **Figure 12.8**.

Mobile Diagnostic Imaging Center

A mobile diagnostic imaging has two definitions: (1) the imaging equipment moves from one hospital to another hospital; (2) the imaging equipment is installed in a bus, and the bus travels to different communities to provide services.[36] For example, the mammogram imaging equipment is installed in a bus to offer breast screening services to rural areas in the county.[36]

Radiation Therapy Center

A **radiation therapy center** is a freestanding facility or linked to a clinic or hospital. It provides radiation therapy services to patients. Most commonly the patients are receiving radiation treatment for a cancer diagnosis.[37]

Rehabilitation Center

A **rehabilitation center** is a facility that exists to help individuals recover from a variety of diseases, post-surgical instances, mental conditions, injuries, and ailments.[38] Rehabilitation center treatments range from physical therapy, speech therapy, occupational therapy, substance abuse, eating disorders, and mental illness, such as depression, suicide ideation, and anxiety. Some centers treat specific health conditions, such as eating disorders, while other centers focus on physical therapy, such as cardiac recovery or joint replacement rehabilitation.[38] Some centers offer residential areas where those being treated may stay overnight for short-term or extended treatment needs, while others are strictly outpatient facilities.[38]

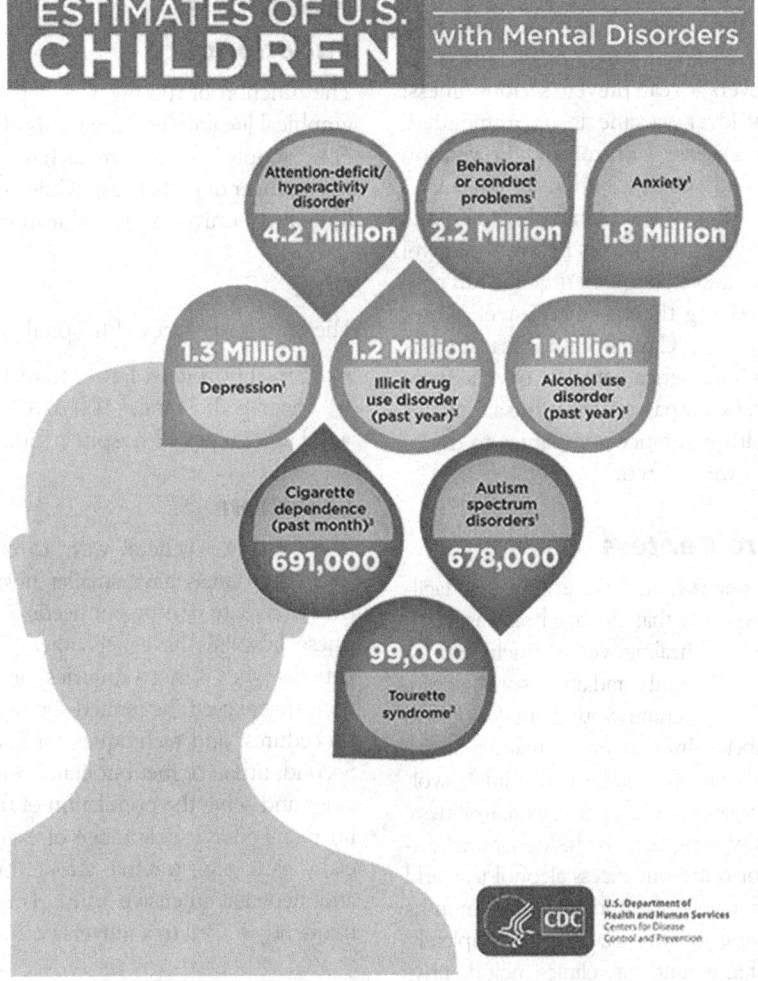

Figure 12.8 Top 10 Most Common Mental Disorders

Courtesy of CDC. Reference to specific commercial products, manufacturers, companies, or trademarks does not constitute its endorsement or recommendation by the U.S. Government, Department of Health and Human Services, or Centers for Disease Control and Prevention.

Travel Clinics

Travel clinics educate travelers about the known health risks associated with traveling abroad.[39] Knowing how to prevent illness and having the necessary medical supplies when traveling helps protect travelers from illness and prevents any disruption during the trip. A reputable travel clinic provides specialized care tailored to individual medical profiles and offers tips on how to stay healthy in the destination country.[39] Travel clinics go beyond offering vaccinations. Patients receive consultations on reducing risks from food, water, parasitic diseases, and insect-transmitted illnesses, such as malaria and dengue fever. They provide information on how to adequately fight jet lag and prevent altitude sickness and increase the traveler's knowledge on how to pack an emergency medical kit.

A traveler clinic is especially important for people with high-risk medical conditions, such as HIV, organ transplant recipients, or other serious conditions.[39] Some clinics offer a review of food- and water-borne disease prevention for travelers' diarrhea, for instance, as well as insect-borne disease prevention for malaria. When traveling to countries in the tropical zone, knowing how to avoid parasites, prevent insect bites, and safely drink canned beverages can prevent serious illness.

If a yellow fever vaccine is recommended, the Centers for Disease Control and Prevention (CDC) recommends going to an authorized vaccine center.[39] Travelers should schedule their clinic appointment preferably 8 weeks before the travel departure date to allow adequate time for full protection after receiving the vaccine. Travel clinics may be found at Travel Clinics of America (https://www.travelclinicsofamerica.com/)[39] or Passport Health (https://www.passporthealthusa.com/).[40] Check with health insurance companies to determine if the costs are covered.[39]

Wound Care Centers

A **wound care center**, or clinic, is a medical facility for treating wounds that do not heal easily.[41 42] Common types of nonhealing wounds include pressure sores, surgical wounds, radiation sores, severe burns, or foot ulcers. Certain wounds may not heal well due to diabetes from poor circulation, nerve damage, chronic bone infection (osteomyelitis), swollen legs, inactivity, or immobility (e.g., due to illness, paralysis, disability, long-term bedridden or wheelchair usage), poor nutrition, excess alcohol use, and smoking.[41-42] Nonhealing wounds may take months to heal, while some wounds never heal completely. The medical staff at wound care clinics include physicians who oversee the care, nurses who clean the wound, apply bandages, and teach the patients and caregivers how to care for the wound at home, and physical therapists who work with the patients to help them stay mobile. The providers keep the patient's PCP up to date on the progress and treatment.[41-42]

In-patient Facilities

This section explores the hospitals based on functionality, size, location, ownership, and specialization. The next section provides the categories of the most common types of hospitals. The discussion ends with residential healthcare facilities focus on elderly care.

Hospitals
Functionality

The function of the hospital depends on the geographical location and the needs of the community. For example, some hospitals have a specialty focus (e.g., cancer or pediatrics), while other hospitals are linked to a university for education and training.

Size

There are three sizes of hospitals:

- Small hospitals: Fewer than 100 beds
- Average hospitals: 100 to 499 beds
- Large, regional hospitals: 500 or more beds

Location

There are two general ways to classify hospitals. First, rural areas have smaller hospitals that serve the immediate non-urgent needs of the community. These hospitals have helicopter pads to transport patients with serious injuries or medical conditions that exceed the limited specialized equipment, procedures, and techniques for such emergencies. Second, urban or metropolitan hospitals are in large cities and serve the population of the region. These hospitals offer a wide range of excellence and specialty care (e.g., trauma, stroke, burns, and adult and neonatal intensive care). These hospitals are frequently linked to a university.

Types

There are numerous types of hospitals. This alphabetical list of hospitals provides a brief description.

- **Children's hospitals** provide specialty care for newborn infants through adolescents. The training of the staff includes specialized services and care for children but also for the parents and siblings of the young patient. Besides medical and surgical treatment services, the medical staff is trained in the psychological, social, emotional, and spiritual care for the patients and their extended family whether the hospitalization is in outpatient services or a long-term stay.

- **Community hospitals** are in urban and rural communities and serve the needs of the population. These hospitals are not linked to universities and do not receive federal funding. Emergencies and critical care patients are transferred to regional hospitals for specialized care.
- **For-profit hospitals** are for-profit and owned by investors or large corporations (e.g., Hospital Corporation of America or HCA). The profits are linked to the shareholders rather than back to the hospital for medical and treatment improvements. Decisions are made by shareholders for the corporation rather than one hospital at a time.
- **General service hospitals** provide basic care for the community including surgery, mom and baby care, pediatrics, elderly care, and general outpatient and inpatient medical services. These hospitals do not provide long-term care and rehabilitation services.
- **Government-funded hospitals** are funded by federal and state government grants or public funding for business expenses. Veterans' hospitals and Indian Health Service hospitals are examples of this type of hospital.
- **Hospitals in a network** connect with the other affiliated hospitals. The benefits allow shared services and treatment facilities while minimizing duplicative services, equipment, and treatment. The shared services are cost saving for the hospitals as well as the patients. For example, a hospital network may include a general hospital with additional facilities, such as a trauma center, a pediatric center, cancer treatment specialties, and mom and baby facilities.
- **Long-term care hospitals** offer long-term services for patients with chronic, long-term care needs, such as psychiatric care, rehabilitation for patients after accidents, injuries, burns, or strokes. Some such hospitals offer care for cancer patients needing long-term bone marrow transplant procedures. Another type of long-term care hospitals is long-term acute care (LTAC) hospitals. LTAC hospitals specialize in therapy to improve the chances of living without being on a ventilator. This treatment may take months of in-patient therapy prior to being able to manage an injury or illness at home. These patients are dependent on a ventilator due to brain and spinal cord injuries, stroke, lung disorders, or infectious diseases, such as COVID.
- **Not-for-profit hospitals** are among about two-thirds of hospitals in urban locations. These hospitals are not linked to profits and shareholders. These facilities operate on an annual budget and often rely on foundations, grants, and generous philanthropic donations for capital improvement campaigns.
- **Private hospitals** are operated by owners and administrators who manage finances, compliance, policies, codes, and regulations. Private hospitals are for-profit, so the care may be more expensive, but they offer increased amenities and services with a better physician-to-patient ratio.
- **Psychiatric hospitals** offer mental health, addiction, eating disorders, and other services to serve the needs of the patients. The staff is trained to offer prescription therapy, individual and group psychotherapy, and behavioral therapy (e.g., art, music, meditation, or exercise). Some hospitals offer long-term, short-term, and outpatient services for a continuum of care to recovery and maintenance.
- **Rehabilitation Hospitals** service the needs of patients recovering from injuries or illness. Some facilities are attached to a hospital and others are free-standing centers. These centers offer a wide array of services including long-term inpatient care, outpatient services and in-home physical therapy.
- **Research Hospitals** focus on researching cures for a specific condition or disease. In addition, they offer treatment for the specific condition. Here are two examples: a) National Cancer Institutions (NCI), such MD Anderson, Sloan Kettering, and Dana Farber for the research of cancer; b) Shriners' Hospitals for children with orthopedic conditions or the Shriners' Burn Hospitals.
- **Specialty Hospitals** are usually connected to large hospitals or healthcare networks to

offer specific treatment or services. Examples of specialty hospitals include children's hospital, women's hospital, burn care, trauma, behavioral health treatment, and cancer treatment.

- **Teaching Hospitals** are affiliated with universities and colleges. These hospitals offer teaching and training both in the classroom and at the hospital. Qualified and licensed faculty instruct the students in medicine, nursing, pharmacy, physical therapy, occupational therapy, dietetics and nutrition, along with non-clinical degrees such as master's degree in hospital administration of Finance.

- **Trauma Center Hospitals** are usually linked to a larger hospital and have use specific, high-tech equipment related to serious injuries, trauma, strokes, burns, gunshot wounds, amputations, and care of numerous individuals involved in a mass shooting event. Trauma Hospitals employ physicians, nurses, and support staff with specialized life-saving treatment and triage skills. Most trauma hospitals have helicopter pads to receive the injured patients rapidly.

Choices of Residency for Seniors

This section explores various residency choices that seniors chose from as they grow older. The types of housing start with aging in place through skilled nursing facilities.

Aging in Place

Aging in place refers to an individual being able to live in the place of their choice without losing their quality of life when they reach senior age.[45] It is important that individuals plan for retirement as early in their younger years as possible with an emphasis on financial saving.[45] These plans will be changed, revised, and adjusted according to changing needs and requirements.

Aging in place is challenging and is not as simple as staying in the same location.[45] Individuals will experience inevitable physical, mental, and emotional changes as they age. Some individuals experience subtle changes at 50 years of age, while others encounter sudden or major changes after age 75.[45] These slight changes occur slowly and include poorer eyesight, reduced muscle mass and hence less strength, diminished endurance both physical and mental, higher risk of accidents due to bone fragility, less balance while walking, reduced hearing capacity, diminished mobility and agility, and decreased flexibility.[45] When individuals plan for a future residence with these changes in mind, they will be better prepared to cope with their health challenges and the additional changes that accompany age. Without proper planning, individuals may be forced to make quick decisions that are out of their control.[45]

Aging in place correctly is defined as planning in advance for any future changes. As individuals age, they will encounter physical, mental, and emotional changes that will affect their activities of daily living (ADLs).[45] See **Box 12.1**.

Box 12.1 Examples of Activities of Daily Living (ADLs)

Common examples of ADL include the following:
- **Positioning and turning:** self-positioning in a chair and/or in a bed for posture and comfort
- Bathing: taking a shower or tub bath with no or limited assistance
- Hygiene: maintaining personal cleanliness, using deodorant, oral hygiene, and nail care
- Grooming: shampooing and combing hair, shaving, beard trimming, and applying lotion
- Dressing: selecting appropriate clean clothing for occasion and temperature, putting on clothing correctly
- Toileting: self-care for bladder and bowel elimination
- Transferring: moving from laying to sitting; sitting to standing; getting in and out of a car
- Eating: selecting appropriate food; using utensils correctly; cutting food as needed; wiping mouth as needed
- Drinking: holding a cup or glass of liquid to drink; appropriately drinking with a straw; not spilling liquid

Many seniors age in place at home and live alone without family in proximity.[45] Their personal challenges and changes typically become more difficult, such as redesigning the existing home for easier accessibility or moving to an easier, smaller home to comfortably maintain.[45] There are many choices when deciding the level of aging in place choices, such smaller independent houses, independent housing in senior communities, care homes but with minimal assistance, and many other choices to suit the needs, preferences, and budgets of the senior individual.[45] The first step in making such a decision is to answer the following questions:

- What is the ideal way to spend your retired years?[45]
- What type of home environment is desired, such as buying a home or condo; renting an apartment; forming a communal living arrangement with others; moving in with family members; living in an over-55 retirement community with no communal dining or health services; an all-inclusive retirement community that includes dining, recreation, independent, assisted living; skilled nursing; or rehabilitation facilities?[45]
- What special health care is required or desired for the future, such as transportation, dining, and health services?[45]
- What other types of supplementary services are desired, such a recreation and house-cleaning services?[45]
- What options are in place such as long-term care insurance, in case of emergencies or life changing events?[45]

Aging in place is defined as making plans about the future years before an event becomes urgent and life changing.[45] It is advantageous to communicate plans and preferences with family and friends. Aging in place does not mean that individuals must achieve ADLs without assistance.[45] Individuals can pay for services needed, including house cleaning services, grocery delivery services, drivers, home visitors, and caregivers. In addition, technology resources, such as medical alert systems, allow seniors to live at home safely for longer periods of time.[45] In conclusion, aging in place is commonly viewed as the ideal situation, but remember it does not occur without early and detailed planning to remain safe at home.[45]

Options for Aging in Place

- Continue to live in a home or condo in their established neighborhood.[45]
- Communal living with like-minded friends and neighbors.
- Government-funded low-income senior housing.[45]
- Senior living communities offer options of progression from independent living, assisted living, rehabilitation, skilled nursing facilities, and hospice.
  - Buy-in apartments with monthly fees that cover three meals every day, housekeeping, maintenance, transportation, and light laundry service.[45]
  - Rental apartments with monthly fees including three meals every day, housekeeping, maintenance, transportation, and light laundry service.[45]

Assisted Living

Assisted living consists of a residential community equipped to help individuals with daily life and routine self-maintenance when needed. However, these facilities do not provide extensive or round-the-clock medical care.[46] Some assisted-living facilities have onsite clinics and resident nurses who oversee medical services like offering medication administration and management.[46] The facilities also take care of other things like grocery shopping, transportation, and finance management. Aging individuals who opt to reside in assisted living homes can also receive medical services through regular channels, such as going to doctor's appointments or with on-site or visiting nurses.[46] In assisted living, individuals have a choice of a private or shared room or apartments. The residents gather in common areas for dining and recreation. The cost of most facilities include room, meals, medication management, and housekeeping.[46] Some provide bathing and bathroom assistance, social and leisure activities, and emergency care. Different facilities offer different levels of service, benefits, and expertise, depending on the cost. Assisted-living facilities are approximately $3,628 per month.[46] Most assisted-living facilities require out-of-pocket payment.[46] Medicare and Medicaid do not cover the costs. However, other payment options are available, including veteran's benefits and long-term care insurance. Some facilities have created a hybrid model so the individual can start in independent apartments and move to assisted living easily when more services are needed.[46] This type of model makes the transition simple because the residents are familiar with the facility, staff, food, and other residents.[46] See **Box 12.2**.

Nursing Homes and Skilled Nursing Facilities

Skilled Nursing Facilities (SNF): **Skilled Nursing Facilities (SNF)** are also known as Nursing Homes. For this section, the term Skilled Nursing Facilities (SNF) is used.

SNFs require a licensed nurse in the facility for a portion of each day. There are not physicians on staff for specialized care. The care provided includes bathing, dressing, eating, using the toilet or change of adult diapers, medication management (ordering refill prescriptions and giving correct dose at the correct time), transferring from bed to chair and sitting to standing, onsite therapy (physical, occupational, and respiratory, 24-supervision and emergency care, and social activities.

Individuals admitted to a SNF are usually transferred from hospitals where they received care, but they have not recovered enough to return home. Being admitted to a SNF for recovery and physical therapy does not mean that they will never leave to go back home. For example, after Joe (age 86) fell, broke his hip, and was admitted to the hospital for surgery, he was discharged to a SNF for a few weeks to receive care

Box 12.2 **Considerations for Assisted Living**

A few benefits to consider when exploring assisted living:

- **Increasing independence:** Assisted living provides the help needed to remain independent by receiving a small amount of assistance as needed to help the individual remain active and safe in their living environment.

- **Socialization:** Individuals living in an assisted living community enjoy activities and exercise classes along with community bus trips and other opportunities.

- **Food:** Community meals in an assisted living facility allow individuals to eat with other residents instead of eating alone in their residence. There is likely more variety of food in a facility and the individual no longer needs to purchase, store, prepare, and clean after each meal.

- **Injuries and Falls:** When an individual is living alone and experiencing injuries and falls more frequently, it is time to begin thinking about moving to an assisted living facility or paying for increased hours of home health care services.

- **Chronic Health Conditions:** When chronic health conditions become worse, the individual may need help managing self-care, keeping track of medication lists, scheduling medical appointments, and arranging transportation.

- **Cleanliness:** As individuals age, they may have trouble maintaining a clean home environment, personal hygiene along with doing laundry, changing bed linens, and paying bills.

- **Loneliness:** When individuals live alone, they may be at a greater risk of depression and isolation. This loneliness may also cause the individual to withdraw from activities.

and physical therapy. His wife, Elaine (age 84) was suffering from several chronic diseases, and she did not feel comfortable being Joe's caregiver at home. She knew that she could not manage his personal of toileting and transferring in and out of the bed. Joe recovered at the SNF near their home and Elaine was able to visit and have meals with him each day. It worked out flawlessly. Joe was safe and Elaine was not worried about being his caregiver. Other individuals have SNF short-term stays for wound care, intravenous medication administration, respiratory therapy, physical therapy, and nutrition management. Unlike assisted living facilities, SNF offer fewer activities and bus excursions because the residents are less mobile, need close medical attention, and supervision due to cognitive and physical conditions.

There are no age restrictions for care in SNFs. Long-term residents are provided medical assistance for as long as it is needed. For example, a newly admitted residents may have advanced and progressive e neurological conditions, such a Parkinson's, ALS, multiple sclerosis, or may have had a several stroke. In most cases, SNF residents share a room to reduce the monthly costs. If the roommates are incompatible, a more compatible roommate might be found. Depending on the geographical locations, the average cost of a SNF ranges from $6,800 to $10,000 per month with additional costs depending on the types of therapy required. Each individual and their family need to explore the cost prior to admission. Medicare, Medicaid, and most health insurance policies only cover a fraction of the costs. Some individuals purchase long-term care insurance policies, however, these policies can be expensive and may never be needed.

Memory Care Centers

Memory care centers are designed in retirement communities or stand-alone facilities for individuals with dementia, Alzheimer's, or other memory-related diseases. If the memory care center is in a retirement community, it is in a unit that is separated from the independent living facilities, assisted living, and skilled nursing areas. The main purpose for admission into a memory care center is for security and safety. The services and amenities focus on quality of life. All staff (e.g.,

nursing, activity directors, housekeeping, food preparers, and servers) are trained for the special needs of the residents. The activities provided are to reconnect the residents with the activities (e.g., music, arts and crafts, dance, and gardening) that they enjoyed years ago.

The design layout of the memory care center is generally circular for lack of confusion and with plenty of light. Most memory care centers have doors that open into an enclosed garden so residents may enjoy the fresh air and sunshine without risk of wandering away and getting lost. The garden has tables with chairs, lounge chairs, and maybe a garden swing. Families and visitors may take their friend or relative to the garden for a visit. Memory care centers have locks on all entryways for the safety and security of the residents. The community rooms have a large screen television, comfortable chairs, and tables with chairs for playing simple card games or completing a jigsaw puzzle. The hallways are painted with bright light colors with large windows. Pet therapy is always welcome in memory care centers. Most residents have memories of their childhood or more recent pet, especially dogs and cats.

The resident rooms are like the rooms in skilled nursing facilities. Some residents have a roommate to lower the cost, though private rooms are available. The bathroom is large, and the shower has safety grab bars. Mirrors are frequently removed from the bath and bedroom. Mirrors may be frightening for the residents who no longer recognize themselves in the mirror. The dining room offers family-style meals for socialization. The meals are specifically designed for patients who are no longer able to use utensils. For example, small sandwiches are served with finger foods such as fruit cubes. Soup is served in cups with handles on both sides to prevent spilling and provide ease of holding the cup. Meat is cut in bite-size pieces and served as finger food with crackers or bread cubes.

It is important for the resident's family to explore all options to cover the cost of the memory care center. Trained staff in the finance office at the center will be able to provide all options before the resident moves in the center and again after all assets have been spent for memory care. The cost for memory care is similar to the cost of skilled nursing facilities, which is about $7,000 to $10,000 per month depending on the geographical location, services, and amenities available.

See **Box 12.3**.

Box 12.3 **Five Signs When Memory Care Is Needed**

With age-related cognitive decline, such as Alzheimer's disease and dementia, the signs and symptoms display over time, making it difficult to know when memory care is needed.

1. Once a diagnosis is given, it is time to begin having conversations about memory care. This is the best opportunity to visit licensed memory care facilities. Transitioning earlier allows the individual to make choices, allows for adjustment time, and allows the individual to become familiar with surroundings, residents, and staff.
2. Caregiving for an individual with memory care needs is a 24/7 commitment. Without engaging in regular respite care, it becomes impossible to sustain quality of life. When caregiving becomes all-consuming, it is time to consider memory care.
3. A decline in overall health includes the following physical and mental signs:
   - Rapid weight loss
   - Lack of food in the refrigerator or cabinets
   - Evidence of medication not taken (or taken too much)
   - Neglected personal hygiene
   - Hunched or sunken posture
   - Inexplicable bruises or injuries
   - Unpaid bills and missed appointments
   - The inability to remember how to get home or where one is going puts patients at risk for injury, getting lost, or becoming victims of scams and potentially crimes
4. The social life of someone with dementia shrinks considerably and may even accelerate the condition. Memory care facilities offer daily activities with positive benefits.
5. Spouses and family members find themselves at a loss once the tipping point is reached,

which is often a fall or injury. The choices of memory care centers are diminished due to lack of time to visit and evaluate. The research begins before the individual needs it to eliminate hasty decisions.

Reproduced from The Memory Center Atlanta. How to Know It's Time for Memory Care. Available at https://www.thememorycenter.com/how-to-know-its-time-for-memory-care/. Accessed January 12, 2022.[47]

Hospice

Hospice includes specialized care for patients who are in the late phase of an incurable illness and wish to receive end-of-life care at home or in a specialized care setting.[48] Hospice facilities value the patient and family's choice and is dedicated to minimizing pain and discomfort caused by the advanced or terminal disease. Hospice includes the following components:

- Ongoing communication among patients, families, and providers[48]
- Aggressive pain control and management of symptoms such as nausea, fatigue, anxiety, shortness of breath, and tissue breakdown[48]
- Medication monitoring and maintenance[48]
- Assistance with limited ADLs, such as bathing[48]
- Advance care planning[48]
- Psychosocial and spiritual care[48]
- Grief and bereavement counseling for the patient and family[48]

Chapter Summary

This chapter explores the wide spectrum of healthcare facilities ranging from urgent care clinics to end-of-life hospice care. As the role of the CHWs expands, the choices of employment will continue to increase across the United States. The first section described the outpatient healthcare facilities, including numerous types of medical facilities and outpatient services, centers, and facilities. The second section defined inpatient healthcare facilities, including various types of hospitals, choices of residency for seniors, and hospice.

CASE STUDY

CHW Career Options

After graduating from a community college, Joan started working as a CHW in an FQHC located in a rural area in Georgia. She has enjoyed her 7 years of employment, while gaining a vast amount of experience related to serving the elderly population. However, after visiting her mom, Joan and her husband, Jose, decided that they need to move closer to help Joan's sister with their mom's needs. Louise is 78, lives alone, and can drive safely during the day. She is involved with her church community, so she likes to attend evening activities. Louise has been a widow for about 10 years, owns her home, and has a reasonable amount of money from her pension and Social Security. At this point, she hires a driver for evening activities since her other daughter is a nurse and works the evening shift at the hospital. Louise is thinking about moving into a retirement community and living in an independent apartment so that she has a larger selection of friends, activities, dining options, and health services.

Jose obtained an excellent sales position. Before seeking employment, Joan decided to get their home arranged and help her sister by taking Louise to visit several retirement communities.

Questions

1. What questions should Louise ask when she visits the retirement communities?
2. With Joan's employment experience at the FQHC, where would be a good location for Joan to seek employment in her new city?

References

1. Emergency vs. urgent care: What's the difference? Mayo Clinic Web site. https://www.mayoclinichealthsystem.org/hometown-health/speaking-of-health/emergency-vs-urgent-care-whats-the-difference. Accessed January 1, 2022.
2. Right care. Right place. Right Time. Mercy Health Web site. https://www.mercy.com/health-care-services/emergency-urgent-care. Accessed January 12, 2022.
3. Federally Qualified Health Center (FQHC). HealthCare.gov. https://www.healthcare.gov/glossary/federally-qualified-health-center-FQHC/. Accessed January 2, 2022.
4. What is an FQHC? FQHC.org. https://www.fqhc.org/what-is-an-fqhc/. Accessed January 2, 2022.
5. Operational definition of a functional local health department. National Association of County & City Health Officials Web site. https://www.naccho.org/uploads/downloadable-resources/Operational-Definition-of-a-Functional-Local-Health-Department.pdf. Accessed January 2, 2022.
6. Birth center definitions. American Association of Birth Centers Web site. https://cdn.ymaws.com/www.birthcenters.org/resource/resmgr/about_aabc_-_documents/Birth_Center_Definitions-12..pdf. Accessed January 2, 2022.
7. Chapter 316: Dialysis center. U.S. Department of Veterans Affairs Web site. https://www.cfm.va.gov/til/space/spChapter316.pdf#:~:text=Dialysis%20Center%3A%20A%20highly%20specialized%20program%20which%20provides,professional%20supervision%20by%20staff%20experienced%20in%20renal%20pathophysiology. Accessed January 2, 2022.
8. Dialysis services. Mayo Clinic. https://www.mayoclinic.org/departments-centers/dialysis-programs/overview/ovc-20464948. Accessed January 2, 2022.
9. Dialysis centers—what to expect. MedlinePlus Web site. https://medlineplus.gov/ency/patientinstructions/000706.htm. Accessed January 2, 2022.
10. Receiving dialysis. United Dialysis Center Web site. http://www.pompanodialysis.com/. Accessed January 2, 2022.
11. Workplace health program definition and description. Centers for Disease Control and Prevention Web site. https://www.cdc.gov/workplacehealthpromotion/pdf/workplace-health-program-definition-and-description.pdf. Accessed January 2, 2022.

12. Wong C. The benefits and side effects of acupuncture. https://www.verywellhealth.com/acupuncture-health-uses-88407#:~:text=Acupuncture%20is%20said,Sinus%20congestion. Accessed January 4, 2022.

13. Art Therapy. Jefferson Health, Magee Rehabilitation Web site. https://mageerehab.jeffersonhealth.org/about-us/care-team/art-therapy/. Accessed January 4, 2022.

14. Definition of art therapy. Merriam-Webster Web site. https://www.merriam-webster.com/dictionary/art%20therapy. Accessed January 5, 2022.

15. What is chiropractic? Palmer College of Chiropractic Web site. https://www.palmer.edu/about-us/what-is-chiropractic/. Accessed January 5, 2022.

16. What is functional medicine? Functional Medicine Coaching Academy, Inc. Web site. https://functionalmedicinecoaching.org/about/what-is-functional-medicine/#:~:text=Functional%20Medicine%20is%20an%20individualized%2C%20patient-centered%2C%20science-based%20approach,and%20address%20those%20root%20causes%20to%20restore%20health. Accessed January 5, 2022.

17. The functional medicine approach. The Institute for Functional Medicine Web site. https://www.ifm.org/functional-medicine/what-is-functional-medicine/. Accessed January 5, 2022.

18. Massage Therapy. Mayo Clinic Web site. https://www.mayoclinic.org/tests-procedures/massage-therapy/about/pac-20384595#:~:text=Massage%20is%20a%20type%20of%20integrative%20medicine%20in,therapist%20uses%20varying%20degrees%20of%20pressure%20and%20movement. Accessed January 6, 2022.

19. What is mindfulness? Mindful.org. https://www.mindful.org/meditation/mindfulness-getting-started/. Accessed January 6, 2022.

20. Mindfulness and meditation. Harvard Medicine Web site. https://www.harvard.edu/in-focus/mindfulness-meditation/. Accessed January 6, 2022.

21. Weil R. What is Tai Chi? https://www.medicinenet.com/tai_chi/article.htm. Accessed January 6, 2022.

22. Ezrin S. 16 benefits of yoga that are supported by science. https://www.healthline.com/nutrition/13-benefits-of-yoga. Accessed January 6, 2022.

23. Pizer A. 11 benefits of yoga. https://www.verywellfit.com/top-health-benefits-of-yoga-3566733. Accessed January 6, 2022.

24. Pizer A. 30 must-know yoga poses for beginners. https://www.verywellfit.com/essential-yoga-poses-for-beginners-3566747. Accessed January 7, 2022.

25. The lifeline. National Suicide Prevention Lifeline Web site. https://suicidepreventionlifeline.org/. Accessed January 7, 2022.

26. Suicide.org Information. Suicide.org. http://suicide.org/. Accessed January 7, 2022.

27. Wood P, Burwell J, Rawlett K. New study reveals lack of access as root cause for mental health crisis in America. National Council Web site. https://www.thenationalcouncil.org/press-releases/new-study-reveals-lack-of-access-as-root-cause-for-mental-health-crisis-in-america/#:~:text=Mental%20health%20services%20in%20the%20U.S.%20are%20insufficient,seeing%20mental%20health%20as%20important%20as%20physical%20health. Accessed March 9, 2022.

28. Find a therapist. Psychology Today Web site. https://www.psychologytoday.com/us/therapists. Accessed January 7, 2022.

29. Find your local NAMI. National Alliance on Mental Illness Web site. https://nami.org/Home. Accessed January 7, 2022.

30. Behavioral health treatment services locator. U.S. Department of Health and Human Services, Substance Abuse and Mental Health Services Administration Web site. https://findtreatment.samhsa.gov/. Accessed January 8, 2022.

31. Find a certified group psychotherapist. International Board for Certification of Group Psychotherapists Web site. https://member.agpa.org/cgpdirectory. Accessed January 8, 2021.

32. Find help with the cost of medicine. NeedyMeds Web site. https://www.needymeds.org/. Accessed January 8, 2022.

33. Access to medications. Mental Health America Web site. https://mhanational.org/issues/access-medications. Accessed January 8, 2022.

34. Worried about affording your medicine? MAT is here to help. MedicineAssistanceTool.org. https://medicineassistancetool.org/. Accessed January 8, 2022.

35. Top ten most common mental disorders in America. My Anxiety Companion Web site. http://www.myanxietycompanion.com/. Accessed January 8, 2022.

36. How does mobile diagnostic imaging work? Alpha 1 Imaging Web site. https://www.alphaoneimaging.com/how-does-mobile-diagnostic-imaging-work/. Accessed January 8, 2022.

37. Rule 3701-83-43: Definitions—freestanding radiation therapy centers. Ohio Laws and Administrative Rules, Legislative Service Commission Web site. https://codes.ohio.gov/ohio-administrative-code/rule-3701-83-43. Accessed January 8, 2022.

38. Black K. What is a rehabilitation center? https://www.thehealthboard.com/what-is-a-rehabilitation-center.htm#:~:text=A%20rehabilitation%20center%20is%20a%20facility%20that%20seeks,will%20stay%20overnight.%20Others%20are%20strictly%20outpatient%20facilities. Accessed January 8, 2022.

39. Eagle Creek. Adventure healthy: Everything you need to know about travel clinics. https://www.eaglecreek.com/blog/adventure-healthy-everything-you-need-know-about-travel-clinics.html. Accessed January 9, 2022.

40. Travel with confidence. Travel Clinics of America Web site. https://www.travelclinicsofamerica.com/. Accessed January 9, 2022.

41. Travel immunizations, travel health. Passport Health Web site. https://www.passporthealthusa.com/. Accessed January 9, 2022.

42. De Leon J, Bohn GA, DiDomenico L, et al. Would care centers: critical thinking and treatment strategies for wounds. *Wounds*. 2016;28(10):1–23.

43. Wound Care Centers. Medline Plus Web site. https://medlineplus.gov/ency/patientinstructions/000739.htm. Accessed January 9, 2022.

44. Prolonged mechanical ventilation. Kindred Hospitals Web site. https://www.kindredhealthcare.com/our-services/ltac/types-of-care/prolonged-mechanical-ventilation. Accessed January 9, 2022.

45. Witt S. Aging in place—What does aging in place really mean? https://www.seniorliving.org/aging-in-place/. Accessed January 9, 2022.

46. Witt S. Assisted living vs. nursing home. https://www.seniorliving.org/compare/assisted-living-vs-nursing-home/. Accessed January 9, 2022.

47. How to know it's time for memory care. The Memory Center Atlanta Web site. https://www.thememorycenter.com/how-to-know-its-time-for-memory-care/. Accessed January 12, 2022.

48. A definition of hospice care. Centers for Disease Control and Prevention Web site. https://www.cdc.gov/training/ACP/page35093.html. Accessed January 12, 2022.

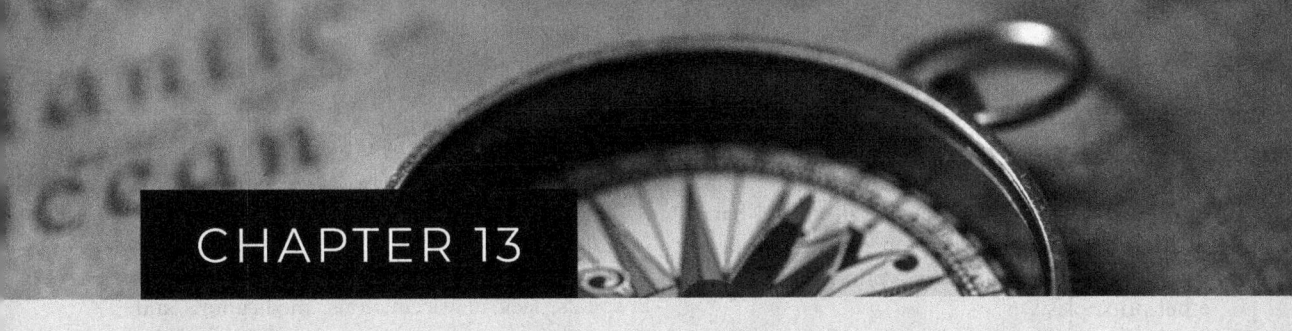

CHAPTER 13

Ethics, Rights, and Responsibilities

LEARNING OBJECTIVES

1. List and define the four main principles of healthcare ethics.
2. Define the Health Insurance Portability and Accountability Act (HIPAA) and explain the purpose of protecting patient health information.
3. Explain three professional rights and responsibilities for community health workers.

KEY WORDS

healthcare ethics
autonomy
beneficence
nonmaleficence

justice
electronic health records (EHRs)
Health Insurance Portability and
   Accountability Act (HIPAA)

electronic medical records (EMR)
core values
code of ethics

Introduction

This chapter begins with a discussion about healthcare ethics including the four main principles: autonomy, beneficence, nonmaleficence, and justice. The next section explains three commonly used acronyms by health providers: Health Insurance Portability and Accountability Act (HIPAA), **electronic medical records (EMR)**, and electronic health records (EHR). Each term is described to enhance understanding and to teach appropriate use of these terms for community health workers (CHWs). Furthermore, Patient and Health Care Providers Rights and Responsibilities are examined in further detail. Last, the discussion turns to the role of CHWs including values, code of ethics, rights, responsibilities, and resources.

Healthcare Ethics

Healthcare ethics are also known as medical ethics or bioethics. In the United States, healthcare professionals owe patients four main ethical duties:

- **Autonomy**: respect and honor the patients right to make their own decision
- **Beneficence**: do good

- **Nonmaleficence**: do no harm
- **Justice**: be fair and treat all persons alike

All four principles are always in affect and have equal importance. However, in practice, respect for patient autonomy takes priority over the other principles.[1]

The common features of ethical conflicts include uncertainty regarding the right action or decision, stress and disagreement between the patient, family, and staff, and determining the decision-maker.[2] When such ethical conflicts occurs, the healthcare provider has an ethical obligation to the patient to return to the four basic ethical principles. First, the provider must respect patients' right to decide what is to be done to their bodies after receiving the information needed to make an informed decision and an absolute right to refuse unwanted treatment (autonomy).[2] Prior to patients making informed decisions, providers must disclose their willingness to help patients advance their own good (beneficence), not harm patients intentionally or indirectly (nonmaleficence), and finally, treat each patient with the same fair distribution of medical benefits (justice).[2]

Healthcare ethics and quality care are important and are commonly stated in the healthcare organization's mission and vision statement. These common values serve as the foundation for health care: respect the patient, and act in the patient's best interest. When the hospital administration and the healthcare professionals fail to provide patient-centered care, overall quality of care is diminished.[2]

Last, the discussion includes the relationship between healthcare ethics and the law. Ethics are the foundation of the law. Law sets minimally acceptable conduct and provides minimum conclusive guidance to ethics conflicts.[2] The law informs, conducts compliance programs, and monitors staff adherence to a specific set of established regulations. Despite the differences, ethical decision-making in health care works closely with the hospital attorneys.[2]

Now the conversation moves to investigating six critical thinking examples related to healthcare ethics. Note: each example is followed with a few questions for thoughtful deliberation rather than providing possible responses.

Critical Thinking Example 1: Do No Harm

"Do not harm" appears to be a simple concept in health care. But with overcrowded clinics and hospitals, lack of vaccinations, medications and personal protective equipment (PPE), lack of trained physicians, nurses, and staff, and populations most in need of care strain the health care systems. With the increased need for research to cure diseases and pandemics, the researchers are put under stress to work faster and with more productivity. This stress among health care workers, hospital staff, researchers, and many others become prone to mistakes even though the intentions remain "do no harm".

Possible Questions for Discussion

1. How should the resources be divided equally among the community population?
2. Who should decide which patients receive care and which patients do not receive care when the hospital is beyond capacity?

Critical Thinking Example 2: Who Owns Stored Medical Data's

In today's health care, there are laws and policies, such as HIPAA, to protect the privacy of the patients' personal information. However, to move research forward it is important for researchers to have access to tissue and blood samples. For example, if a physician removes a sample of a cancerous tumor for a biopsy to determine the type of treatment needed to cure the cancer for that patient. After this tissue sample was examined, it is given to researchers to be cataloged for present and future cancer research. The patient may have given permission for the tissue to be once. However, the tissue is stored, it is likely to be used in cancer research multiple times in the future.

Possible Questions for Discussion

1. Would you object to having a sample of your tissue used in research in the future? Why? Why not?
2. Should current regulations and policies be changed to protect patient's privacy related to their biospecimens? Would it be possible years later to locate the patients to receive their consent?

Critical Thinking Example 3: Patient Privacy in Electronic Health Records (EHR)

Electronic health records (EHRs) are common for most medical offices, clinics, and hospitals. Patients create portals and passwords without much thought in today's world. Large data banks are at risk of being hacked or privacy violations, even though federal law restricts the release of patient data. However, by analyzing the relationships in large datasets, researchers discover relationships between lifestyle, environmental factors, occupations, and diseases. For example, researchers were able to determine the link between lead paint and pipes with children acquiring lead poisoning at an early age. When the large data research predicts health outcomes of the population, there is a possibility for negative impacts, such as health insurance companies denying health insurance policies based on zip code or occupation or companies denying employment to a person with a history of cancer or diabetes.

Possible Questions for Discussion

1. Is it possible for patients to be protected from negative effects when population health researchers discover links between lifestyle (employment, unhealthy habits, geographical location) and risk of disease? How should this topic be addressed?
2. Is it possible for an individual to keep their health data out of large public health databases?

Critical Thinking Example 4: Access to Health Care

In the United States, health care is a privilege rather than a right. This statement means that only certain individuals have equal access to health care, while others have moderate or limited access to health care including the elderly, individuals with disabilities, and specific ethnic groups. Also, health care is not equality distributed across geographical locations. Some rural communities have limited access the same as overcrowded low-income neighborhoods in large metropolitan areas.

Possible Questions for Discussion

1. If you were given an unlimited budget and a team of health care experts, how would you provide equal access to the entire population of one U.S. city to make the health care system available for all individuals?
2. Do you think the current healthcare system provides equal access in the U.S.? Why or why not?

Critical Thinking Example 5: Financial Management Within Hospitals

For hospitals to stay in business, they must charge fees for their services. They collect the fees by billing health insurance companies for the cost of the services provided to the patients. The patients are billed for the costs that were not covered by their health insurance policy. When patients do not have health insurance, they are asked to pay for the services. If the patients do not have enough money, the hospital is forced to eliminate the unpaid debt by spreading the unpaid debt by increasing the cost of services. This is called "cost sharing". The technique of cost sharing means that hospital administrators are forced to decide which patients get the newest and most expensive treatment or procedure, while other patients may receive routine treatment or procedures that yield a lower cost. Such decisions are never easy but are necessary for the hospital to stay in business and never go into bankruptcy to serve the community. Sometimes the administrators and physicians consult the hospital bioethics committee to get advice regarding these difficult decisions.

Possible Questions for Discussion

1. Which of the four ethical principles represent how hospitals balance the financial decisions along with providing standard of care for all patients?
2. As a consumer of healthcare services, what is your opinion of the term "cost sharing" since it means that you get charged more for healthcare services to help pay for services for patients without health insurance or money?

Critical Thinking Example 6: Ethical Responses to Widespread Pandemics and Medical Emergencies

During the COVID pandemic, many hospitals had severe staff shortages, lack of adequate personal protective equipment to keep the staff safe, insufficient number of beds, and a significant scarcity of ventilators for the most critical patients. When the Emergency Departments are overwhelmed, the physicians and nurses access each patient quickly to determine which patients

are most critical and most likely to live. This system is called triage. In other words, if the patient is critically ill or injured and has a slight chance of surviving, the trauma team must focus their staffing and resources on patients that have a better chance of surviving if treated quickly. This scenario happened during COVID. Hospitals provided the best treatment for the most patients but that does not mean that everyone survived due to lack of staff, resources, and ventilators.

Possible Questions for Discussion

1. Which of the four ethical principles represent how Emergency Departments make decisions during the time when patients are being triaged.
2. If two patients are considered to be equally sick with COVID and both need the last available ventilator, what criteria would you use to make this decision?

Health Provider Accountability: HIPAA, EMR, and EHR

This section explains three commonly used acronyms by health care providers and medical staff: Health Insurance Portability and Accountability Act (HIPAA), electronic medical records (EMR), and electronic health records (EHR). Each term is described for greater understanding and clarifies the application for CHWs.

Health Insurance Portability and Accountability Act of 1996 (HIPAA)

The **Health Insurance Portability and Accountability Act (HIPAA)** of 1996 is a federal law that required the creation of national standards to protect patient health information from being disclosed without the patient's consent or knowledge via the Privacy Rule. As a CHW, it is important to understand the HIPAA rules. CHWs may be asked to transfer a patient's medical records

Table 13.1 HIPAA Rules

HIPAA	Who Must Comply?	Protected Information	Permitted Disclosures
A federal law that protects sensitive patient health information from being disclosed without the patient's consent or knowledge. The main goal of the Privacy Rule is to ensure that individuals' health information is properly protected while allowing the flow of health information needed to provide and promote high quality health care and to protect the public's health and well-being.	Every healthcare provider who electronically transmits health information in connection with certain transactions must comply: health plans: health, dental, vision, and prescription drug insurers; health maintenance organizations (HMOs); Medicare, Medicaid, Medicare supplement insurers, and long-term care insurers; healthcare clearing houses; and business associates that act on behalf of a covered entity, including claims processing, data analysis, utilization review, and billing.	Individually identifiable health information that is transmitted or maintained in any form or medium (electronic, oral, or paper) by a covered entity or its business associates, excluding certain educational and employment records	To the individual Treatment, payment, and healthcare operations Uses and disclosures with opportunity to agree or object by asking the individual or giving opportunity to agree or object Incident to an otherwise permitted use and disclosure Public interest and benefit activities (e.g., public health activities, victims of abuse or neglect, decedent, research, law enforcement purposes, serious threat to health and safety) Limited dataset for the purpose of research, public health, or healthcare operations

Centers for Disease Control and Prevention. HIPPA vs. FERPA Infographic 2018. Available at https://www.cdc.gov/phlp/docs/hipaa-ferpa-infographic-508.pdf. Accessed February 5, 2022. Reference to specific commercial products, manufacturers, companies, or trademarks does not constitute its endorsement or recommendation by the U.S. Government, Department of Health and Human Services, or Centers for Disease Control and Prevention.[3]

to another medical office or hospital. HIPAA may be confusing in some situations, so it is important to ask questions rather than assume the procedure is correct. See **Table 13.1**.

It is likely that CHWs will be asked to describe HIPAA to patients and families, since healthcare organizations are now required by law to give patients a notice of their privacy practices and receive a signature from patients to confirm acknowledgement and receipt of the document.[4] A good practice to adopt is to put all relevant information in the Notice of Privacy Practices and then give patients a summary of what the policy contains.[4] For example, the CHW would explain the following to the patient:

- They may request their medical records whenever desired.[4]
- They may request that their medical records be amended to correct errors.[4]

- They can limit who has access to their personal health information (PHI).[4]
- They can choose how providers communicate with them, such as email, voicemail, or phone calls.[4]
- They have right to complain about the unauthorized disclosure of their PHI and suspected HIPAA violations.[4]

Electronic Medical Records (EMR) and Electronic Health Records (EHR)

EMR and EHR are similar terms but have different meaning

First, EMRs are a digital version of the paper charts in the clinician's office. An EMR contains the medical and treatment history of the patients in one practice. EMRs have advantages over paper records. However, the EMR information does not travel across various medical offices. In fact, the patient's record might even have to be printed out and delivered by mail to specialists and other members of the care team. In that regard, EMRs are not much better than a paper record.

EHRs, however, focus on the total health of the patient.[5] EHRs are inclusive and are built to share information with other healthcare providers, such as laboratories, specialists, medical imaging facilities, pharmacies, emergency facilities, and school and workplace clinics. EHRs contain real-time information from all the clinicians involved in the patient's care, including the specialist, the hospital, or the nursing home in the next state or even across the country.[5] EHRs contain a patient's medical history, diagnoses, medications, treatment plans, immunization dates, allergies, radiology images, and laboratory and test results.[5] The benefits of EHRs are improved patient care, increased patient participation, improved care coordination, improved diagnostics, enhanced patient outcomes, improved medical practice efficiencies, and cost savings. Because health care is a team effort, health information becomes more powerful when shared in a secure way.[6] Last, patients can log in to their own record and see their lab results over the last year, which can help motivate them to take medications and maintain the recommended lifestyle changes to achieve improved laboratories.

Patients' Rights and Responsibilities

This section discusses patients' rights and responsibilities. Some patient rights are guaranteed by federal law. For example, HIPAA guarantees that patients have the right to get a copy of their medical records and the right to have their records kept private.[7] In addition, patients have the right of informed consent that is defined as the process in which a healthcare provider educates a patient about the risks, benefits, and alternatives of a given procedure, treatment, surgery, or intervention. The patient must be competent to make a voluntary decision about whether to undergo the procedure or intervention. Informed consent is both an ethical and legal obligation of medical practitioners in the United States and originates from patients' right to decide what happens to their bodies.[8] The healthcare provider must assess the patient's ability to understand, decide how to proceed based on the information given, and document the process, such as signing the document or offer a verbal consent. The verbal and written information must be provided in the language and literacy level of the patient.[8] Informed consent requires five requires elements:[8]

1. The nature and description of the treatment or procedure
2. The risks and benefits of the treatment or procedure
3. Reasonable alternatives, including no treatment or procedure
4. Risks and benefits of alternatives, including no treatment or procedure
5. Assessment of the patient's understanding of the first four elements[8]

Many hospitals have patient advocates who can help individual and families with specific issues or problems. Many states have an ombudsman office for problems with long-term care. State departments of health may also be able to help.[7]

Now the discussion moves to the responsibilities of the patient. Successful health care requires ongoing collaboration between patients and their providers.[7] Their partnership requires both to take an active role in the health process. Competent patients control the decisions related to their health care and with those decisions come responsibilities.[7] Patients contribute to the collaboration by doing the following:

- Providing a complete medical history, including providing information about past illnesses, medications, hospitalizations, family history of illness, and other matters relating to present health.[9–10]
- Being truthful and express concerns clearly to the healthcare providers.[10] Patients should request information or clarification when the information is not fully understood related to

health status or treatment. Physicians should encourage patients to raise questions or concerns.

- Cooperating with agreed-upon treatment plans and appointments. Patients should adhere to treatment and disclose if the treatment was not followed or when the plan needs to be reconsidered.[10]
- Taking personal responsibility, when possible, to prevent the development of disease. Patients should recognize that a healthy lifestyle can prevent or reduce illness.[10] Patients should adopt health-enhancing behaviors such as the following:
  - Maximize healthy habits such as exercising, not smoking, and eating a healthy diet.[9-10]
  - Prevent the spread of disease.[10]
  - Work with healthcare providers to make healthcare decisions and carry out upon treatment plans.[10]
  - Understand the risks and limits of the science of medical care and that healthcare professionals can make mistakes.[9-10]
- Accepting care from medical students, residents, and other trainees under appropriate supervision, if desired. Participation in medical education is to the mutual benefit of patients and the healthcare system.[9]
- Reporting illegal or unethical behavior by physicians or other healthcare professionals to the appropriate medical societies, licensing boards, or law enforcement authorities.
- Being financially responsible. Patients should discuss financial hardships with physicians.[9] Patients should be knowledgeable about personal health plan coverage and health plan options, including all covered benefits, limitations, and exclusions, rules regarding use of network providers, coverage and referral rules, appropriate processes to secure additional information, and the process to appeal coverage decisions.[9-10]
- Being respectful and showing respect for other patients and health workers.[10]
- Refraining from behavior that unreasonably places the health of others at risk. Patients should avoid being disruptive in the healthcare setting.[9-10] See **Figure 13.1**.

Healthcare Providers' Rights and Responsibilities

Healthcare providers have rights and responsibilities that are linked to health insurance plans.[12] For example, health insurance plans focus on evaluation of healthcare services, such as collecting the healthcare provider's data for cost/benefit analysis.[12] Healthcare providers have the right to advocate on behalf of a patient, file a complaint against the health insurance plan, and appeal a decision of the health insurance plan with the appropriate government body regarding the health insurance plan's actions. Also, healthcare providers have the right to advocate and inform patients regarding all treatments available for each patient's condition, including treatments that may not be covered by the health plan and filing a filing a complaint to an appropriate governmental body if the health provider believes the quality of care or access to care has been negatively impacted.[12]

Last, after reviewing the rights and responsibilities of patients and healthcare providers, it is time to blend the information to establish and maintain trust to support the patient-provider relationship.[13] The following points cover the details for reasonable healthcare provider/patient communication:

1. Communication is essential and impacts multiple aspects of health consequences:

   - Improved medical, functional, and emotional condition of the patient[13]
   - Better patient compliance with medical treatment[13]
   - Enhanced fulfillment of patient toward healthcare services[13]
   - Lesser risks of medical misconduct.[13]

2. Empathy is vital and enables the physician to understand the symptomatic experiences, quality of life, therapeutic effects, and needs of each patient.[13]

3. Trusting healthcare providers allows patients to effectively discuss health issues. Trust enables the patient to comply with the treatment plan to improve health.[13]

Four basic patients' rights

1) Dignity
   a. Ability to receive care and treatment without bias related to age, ethnicity/race, religion, language, socioeconomic status, and gender orientation.
   b. Care and instructions are given in the first language of the patient and at the appropriate literacy level is given with respect for cultural needs, spiritual beliefs, social and family support.
   c. Care is received in a safe environment and free of abuse, neglect, and harassment including financial, exploitation, unnecessary restraints, and intentional isolation.

2) Quality of care
   a. Provide the patient with understandable language and literacy level for diagnosis, treatment, prognosis along with care plans while in the hospital and outpatient discharge plans
   b. Provide pain management instructions and options for the treated condition.
   c. As unexpected events occur, the patient is informed of the change, treatment, and additional diagnosis and plan of care.
   d. Provide consults with additional physicians for a second opinion at the patient's request and cost.
   e. Respect the need for a Bioethics Committee consultation at the patient's or family's request.

3) Safety
   a. Respectful caregivers with proper licensure and free of known criminal charges
   b. Receive all conversations in the patients' language and at the appropriate literacy level; technology is commonly used
   c. Provide patients with information of interest regarding research clinical trials related to their diagnosis
   d. Receive notice of scheduled treatment and procedures that are not covered by the patient's health insurance policy
   e. Provide discharge planning to include safety measures and needed medical equipment, schedule physical therapy and other therapies as needed.

4) Respectful personal care
   a. Know the names of essential healthcare providers and caregivers
   b. Create legal Advanced Directives and assure that facility, family and staff follow the guidelines; if requested, complete documents for organ donation
   c. Obtain copies of medical records and charges; schedule a consult with Financial Services, if desired

Patient Responsibilities:

- Participate in healthcare by following instructions and asking questions to achieve greater understanding
- Provide accurate and detailed information about your health history
- Promptly report any changes to your healthcare provider, such as falls and vision changes
- Update any changes to your health insurance or financial situation
- Be respectful of other patient's medical information by stepping away from overhearing a conversation
- Follow the treatment plan as prescribed and ask questions for greater understanding as needed
- Update your Advanced Directives as events in your life change, such death of a spouse
- Keep your family members or health advocate updated as changes occur
- Comply with the rules that affect others, such as Turning Off Your Cell Phone or No Smoking sign on campus of hospital or within a healthcare facility

Figure 13.1 Patient Rights and Responsibilities

Data from Patient rights and responsibilities. Peace Health Web site. https://www.peacehealth.org/sites/default/files/patient_rights_and_responsbilities_hospitals_and_clinics_washington_updated_june_6_2020_revised.pdf. Accessed February 6, 2022.

4. Informed consent is based on the moral and legal arguments of the patient's autonomy to make independent decisions. The healthcare provider must be honest with the patient and families to provide a genuine risk and benefits for the suggested procedure or therapy.[13]

5. A breach in professional boundaries occurs when a healthcare provider's behavior disobeys the limits of the professionalism between the provider and patient. Also, patients should avoid frequent phone calls and unscheduled visits to show respect.[13]

Community Health Workers: Core Values, Code of Ethics, Rights, and Responsibilities

Before presenting the core values, rights, and responsibilities, it is useful to recall the various roles and tasks of CHWs. See **Figure 13.2** followed by **Table 13.2**.

After reviewing the various titles, tasks, and functions of CHWS, it is time to move into a discussion of the core values, code of ethics, responsibilities, and resources for the CHW profession.

Core Values

The profession of CHWs is defined by **core values**. The core values are divided into two categories: self-determination and community.

Self-determination:

- Empowerment among the CHW community to improve their individual skills as well as improve the CHW profession

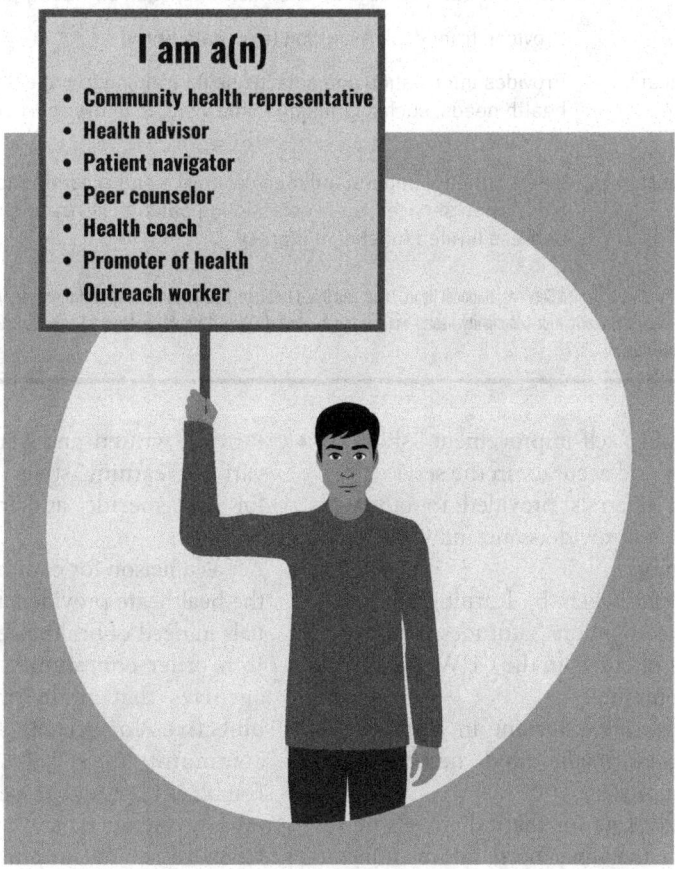

This is Miguel who is a CHW (Community Health Worker).
CHWs can be given different titles depending on where they work – insurance companies, clinics, hospitals, etc.

I am a(n)

- Community health representative
- Health advisor
- Patient navigator
- Peer counselor
- Health coach
- Promoter of health
- Outreach worker

Figure 13.2 A Day in the Life of a CHW

Table 13.2 Functions of CHWs

Function	Definition
Care coordination	Provides information and assistance to patients about receiving care from institutions and providers outside of primary care
Health coaching	Provides self-management support to patients through counseling, which involves collaborative goal setting, problem solving, and action planning
Providing social support	Provides a supportive, but nontherapeutic relationship, such as peer-based informational, emotional, or instrumental support
Health assessment	Performs clinical assessments within or outside of clinic appointments, such as blood pressure and weight
Resource linking	Helps patients access local services using standardized resources
Case management	Assesses patients' needs and provides personalized assistance
Medication management	Provides limited medication reconciliation without making recommendations
Remote primary care	Provides limited primary care services in remote areas (e.g., first aid, simple chronic disease care, follow-up care)
Follow-up	Monitors patients outside of office visits, such as weekly phone calls
Administration	Provides front desk reception (e.g., data entry)
Targeted health education	Provides information and didactic skills training to patients with specific health needs, such as making home visits to deliver curriculum with hands-on activities
Health literacy support	Helps patients understand medical advice and recommendations, including translation services, such as assisting patients in reading medical forms to address limited functional literacy

Data from U.S. Department of Health and Human Services, National Heart, Lung, and Blood Institute. Role of Community Health Workers. Available at https://www.nhlbi.nih.gov/health/educational/healthdisp/role-of-community-health-workers.htm#:~:text=CHWs%20offer%20interpretation%20and%20translation,such%20as%20first%20aid%20and. Accessed February 6, 2022.[15]

- Seek continuous self-improvement skills when in quality and accuracy in the services, resources, and referrals provided to other CHWs, healthcare providers and individuals in the community
- Enhance personal beliefs by learning about and accepting of opinions, attitudes, beliefs and differences of others in the CHW profession and the community
- Maintain quality improvement in technology skills, social media, and healthcare updatesCommunity:
- Support and advocate for the individuals in the community that may need information and assistance

- Provide written and verbal information in various learning styles and literacy levels for the specific audience of community members
- Act as a liaison for community members and the healthcare providers treating the individuals in need of healthcare services
- Join other community organizations and agencies that share the same goals and objectives for serving and improving the community
- Establish trust and respect among the community members and the healthcare providers to achieve improve health outcomes. See **Figure 13.3**.

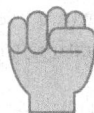

Self-empowerment

Promoting self-actualization and self-advocacy among community health workers.

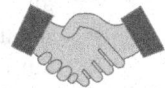

Social justice and equity

Ensuring fair treatment, access, opportunity advancement and outcomes for individuals and communities.

Self-determination

Promoting the efforts of the community health workers, and the communities in which they work to create a shared vision and direction for the future.

Dignity and respect

Building trusted relationships based on honoring the inherent value and contributions of every person irrespective of socio-economic class, religion, race, national origin, language spoken, immigration status, abilities or disabilities, age, sex, sexual orientation, and gender identity/expression.

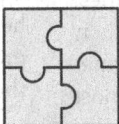

Unity

Encouraging collaboration among community health workers to promote a common professional identity regardless of job title or work-setting.

Integrity

Promoting and nurturing the authenticity and character of the community health worker profession and promoting the contributions made by Community Health Workers toward eliminating health disparities and advancing.

Figure 13.3 Summary of Core Values for CHWs

Reproduced from National Association of Community Health Workers. Our Values. Available at https://nachw.org/. Accessed February 8, 2022.[17]

Code of Ethics for CHWs

The responsibility of all CHWs is to strive for excellence by providing quality service and the most accurate information available to individuals, families, and communities.[17] Employers are encouraged to consider this code when creating CHW programs. The **code of ethics** is based upon commonly understood principals that apply to all professionals within the health and social service fields (e.g., promotion of social justice, positive health, and dignity).[17] The code, however, does not address all ethical issues facing CHWs, and the absence of a rule does not imply that there is no ethical obligation present. As professionals, CHWs are encouraged to reflect on the ethical obligations that they have to the communities that they serve and to share these reflections with others. The entire code of ethics for CHWs is provided in Appendix A at the end of this chapter.[17]

Based on the code of ethics, this section exhibits the professional rights and responsibilities for CHWs, including confidentiality, documentation, legal obligations, professional conduct, personal safety, and self-care.[17]

Professional Rights and Responsibilities

Article 4. Professional Rights and Responsibilities (Code of Ethics for CHWs)

The CHW profession is dedicated to excellence in the practice of promoting well-being in communities.[17] Guided by common values, CHWs have the responsibility to uphold the principles and integrity of the profession as they assist families to make decisions impacting their well-being. CHWs embrace individual, family, and community strengths and build upon them to increase community capacity.[17]

Confidentiality

1.2 Confidentiality (Code of Ethics for CHWs)

CHWs respect the confidentiality, privacy, and trust of individuals, families, and communities that they serve. They understand and abide by employer policies, as well as state and federal confidentiality laws that are relevant to their work.[18]

Documentation

By the nature of their role, CHWs manage sensitive information about clients and communities. CHWs rely on laws and protocols to guide their decisions about how to handle client information.[17] As discussed previously, one of the most important laws established to protect the privacy and confidentiality of health information is commonly referred to as HIPAA, also known as Health Insurance Portability Act.[4,17]

Legal Obligations

1.6 Legal Obligations (Code of Ethics for CHWs)

CHWs have a legal obligation to report actual or potential harm to individuals within the communities they serve to the appropriate authorities.[17] Additionally, CHWs have a responsibility to follow requirements set by states, the federal government, and/or their employing organizations. Responsibility to the larger society or specific legal obligations may supersede the loyalty owed to individual community members.[17]

Professional Conduct

Article 3: Interactions with Other Service Providers (Code of Ethics for CHWs)

CHWs maintain professional partnerships with other service providers to serve the community effectively.[17]

3.1 Cooperation: CHWs place the well-being of those they serve above personal disagreements and work cooperatively with any other person or organization dedicated to helping provide care to those in need.[17]

3.2 Conduct: CHWs promote integrity in the delivery of health and social services. They respect the rights, dignity, and worth of all people and have an ethical obligation to report any inappropriate behavior (e.g., sexual harassment, and racial discrimination) to the proper authority.[17]

3.3 Self-Presentation: CHWs are truthful and forthright in presenting their background and training to other service providers.[17]

Personal Safety and Self-Care

4.4 Wellness and Safety (Code of Ethics for CHWs)

CHWs are sensitive to their own personal well-being (physical, mental, and spiritual health) and strive to maintain a safe environment for themselves and the communities they serve.[17]

Resources for CHWs

As health care faces many challenges, including providing care to patients with complex illnesses, lowering healthcare costs, and advancing a population health framework, CHWs provide valuable services when working in a team-based approach to address all three issues.[18] This section offers some valuable resources for CHWs to improve as individuals and professionals to enhance their abilities to build trustworthy relationships and deepen communication between patients and providers. CHWs have an innate understanding of their communities through lived experience, which makes them uniquely qualified to address social and behavioral determinants of health.[19] For the most current CHW Certification Programs, see **Figure 13.4**.

When CHWs begin a new position, it is important to survey the community to determine what services and resources may be valuable to their clients. This section provides resources to consider when examining the community. Information related to services, days or hours of operation, address, website, phone numbers, cost, membership fees, age group focus (e.g., preschool children, afterschool services, or elderly) are all important community factors that implicate health and access to services. Keep in mind that each community has its own unique assets to discover with a focus on food, clothing,

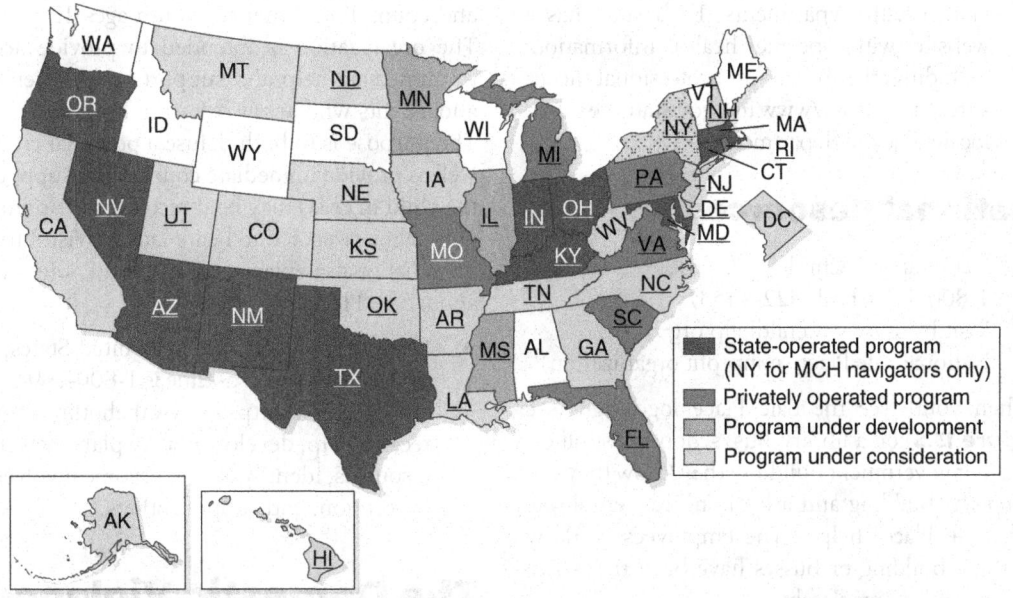

Figure 13.4 State Approaches to CHW Certification

Reproduced from Ever-Changing Picture: State Approaches to CHW Certification https://www.astho.org/topic/brief/state-approaches-to-community-health-worker-certification/

and shelter. Many community services require eligibility, proof of citizenship, a local address, and numerous other documents. A CHW must call to verify the eligibility requirements prior to providing a referral for services. Also, it is useful to the client if the CHW provides the name of a contact person.

City and County Services and Resources

- Health Department: services, vaccines, health care, prevention, and referrals
- Fire Departments: fires, emergencies, and services
- Police Departments: violence, motor vehicle accidents, assaults, and many other situations
- Libraries: story time for children, free classes for adults, check-out books as well as small appliances, free computer use and classes, open to public for warmth and air conditioning to reduce exposure to cold and heat
- Food banks and soup kitchens: eligibility, days, and hours of operation

- Faith-based communities and churches: multiple services and referrals.
- Community Recreation Center, YMCA, parks and recreation: childcare, family services, swimming, and free classes, such as aerobics and gymnastics for children

State Resources

- State elder abuse hotlines—elder protection center: If elder abuse, neglect, or exploitation is suspected, the CHW should contact the supervisor. The supervisor will call the state elder abuse hotline or reporting number. In an emergency, 911 or the local police are called.
- State insurance commissioner: A state insurance commissioner's department is a state government organization that enforces insurance laws. Every state has one. These departments exist to protect insurance policyholders from fraud or other unlawful actions. As regulators of the insurance industry, they make sure the insurance companies operating within the state are legitimate and law-abiding.[20]

- State health departments: Each state has a website with specific health information, including the board of professional licensure. Visit https://www.usa.gov/state-health to locate a health department.[21]

National Resources

- National Child Abuse Hotline: 1-800-4-A-Child (422-4453) Visit https://www.childhelp.org[22]
- National Safe Place (nonprofit organization)[23]

When youth see the Safe Place logo sign (see **Figure 13.5**) on a library, bus, school, post office, or other government building, they know they can enter the building and ask the nearest employee for "Safe Place" help.[23] The employees working in these building or busses have been trained to assist youth immediately.

National Safe Place is a nonprofit organization based out of Louisville, Kentucky. It originated in 1983 from an initiative known as "Project Safe Place," established by a short-term residential and counseling center for youth ages 12 to 17.[23] The organization is intended to provide access to immediate help and support for children and adolescents who are at risk or in crisis situations. The purpose is to both defuse a potential crisis as well as provide immediate counsel and support so the child in crisis may be directed to an appropriate shelter or accredited care facility. Visit https://www.nationalsafeplace.org/ to find out more about Safe Place.[23]

- Domestic violence: In the United States, the domestic violence hotline is 1-800-799-SAFE (7233). Visit https://www.thehotline.org/ to receive help, develop a safety plan, view local resources, identify abuse, become involved in prevention, and support others.[24]

The Domestic Violence Hand Signal

The domestic violence hand signal is a call for help.[25] The signal was formed during the

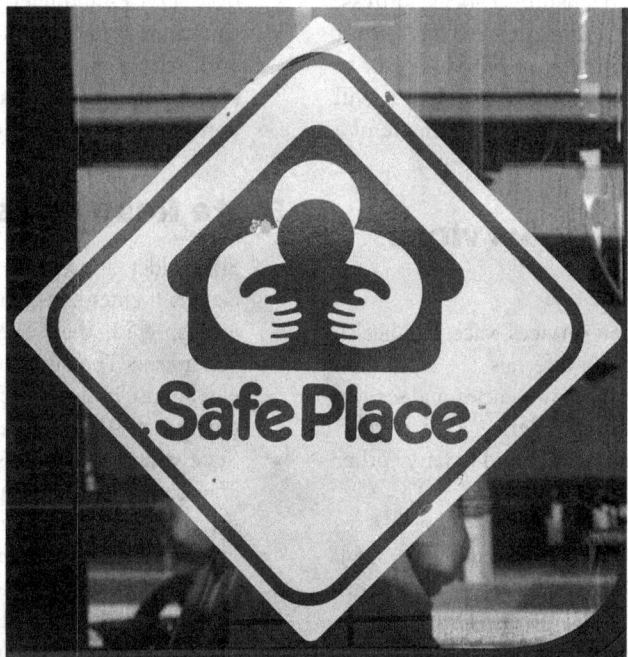

Figure 13.5 Safe Place Logo

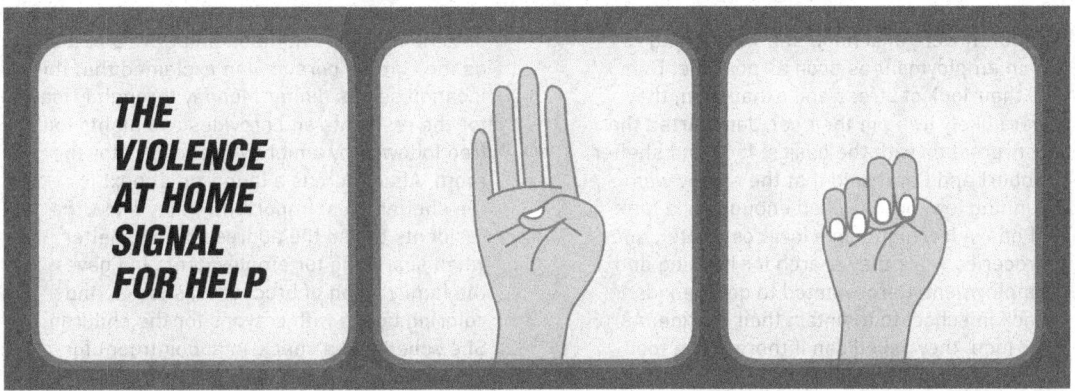

Figure 13.6 Domestic Violence Hand Signal
© Pokota Poco/iStock/Getty Images Plus/Getty Images.

pandemic as a means for men and women to tell others they were being abused while in lockdown. It can be used on virtual phone calls, FaceTime, in a car, restaurant, public area, movie theater, or behind your back while walking down a sidewalk.[25] During the COVID-19 lockdown, fears increased for children and spouses living in abusive households. They were now confined to their house or apartment with only their abuser and no way to communicate their situation to anyone.[25]

The hand signal was created to tell people that you are in trouble without speaking up and your abuser noticing.[25] The hand signal is an open palm, almost in a hello greeting, with the thumb curved in. A quick motion of folding the other four fingers over the thumb is the signal.[25] Everyone should be aware of this signal and seek help immediately. See **Figure 13.6**.

Chapter Summary

This chapter began with a discussion about health-care ethics, including the four main principles:

- Autonomy: respect and honor the patients right to make their own decision
- Beneficence: do good
- Nonmaleficence: do no harm
- Justice: be fair and equitable

The next section explained three commonly used acronyms by healthcare providers: HIPAA, EMR, and EHR. Each term was described for greater understanding and application for CHWs to use. Patient and Health Care Providers Rights and Responsibilities were examined in the detail. Last, the discussion turns to the role of CHWs including values, code of ethics, rights, responsibilities, and resources (See **Case Study 13.1**).

Case Study 13.1 Family in Need of Assistance

On Monday morning, a family of four (parents and two children: Josie, 9, and Joshua, 7) walked into the Health Department Clinic in search of community services. As they walked up to the receptionist window, Jan, the CHW, was pouring a cup of coffee. She noticed the family and went around the glass barrier to greet them. Since Jan had some paperwork to complete this morning but no appointments until 11:00 a.m., she invited the family in to follow her into the children's play area. Jan gathered some snacks and juice boxes for the children as they started playing. Jan offered the parents some coffee and snacks as she got acquainted with them. Robert introduced himself and explained that the family had been on the road a few days since he was laid off from a construction job in a neighboring state. He had been told that there might be construction jobs available in this county. His wife, Carol, had been working two part-time jobs as a waitress and hotel maid while the children were in school. She was hoping to gain employment as soon as possible. Due to their look of stress and exhaustion, they were likely living in their car. Jan started the conversation with the basics: food and shelter. Robert and Carol said that the money was running low, but they had enough for a tank of gas, a few nights in a low-cost motel, and groceries while they search for housing and employment. Carol wanted to get the kids back in school to maintain their routine. As for food, they asked Jan if there was a food bank or soup kitchen available. The children were hungry and needed a healthy, hot meal. Jan mentioned a few options and answered to their questions. Jan called a local faith-based community shelter. The day manager, Dave, said that they had one room with two double beds. Jan told Robert and Carol good news along with providing the address, directions, phone number, and Dave's name as the contact person. Jan explained that this location serves dinner Monday through Friday for the residents and provides two nights for free followed by a nightly cost of $15 for the room. Also, there is a laundromat next to the shelter. Most importantly, they allow the residents to use the address of the shelter when searching for employment. Jan gave the family a bag of brochures, snacks, and coloring books with crayons for the children. She scheduled a check-in appointment for the family in 3 days. Robert, Carol, and their children looked less stressed as they left the clinic.

Questions

1. As the CHW, where would you begin to assist this family at their next appointment?
2. As the CHW, what would be your top two priorities for this family?

References

1. How the four principles of health care ethics improve patient care. The Lawyers and Jurists Web site. https://www.lawyersnjurists.com/article/how-the-four-principles-of-health-care-ethics-improve-patient-care/. Accessed February 5, 2021.
2. Frequently asked questions: health care ethics. Vermont Ethics Network Web site. https://vtethicsnetwork.org/medical-ethics/frequently-asked-questions. Accessed February 5, 2022.
3. HIPPA vs. FERPA infographic 2018. Centers for Disease Control and Prevention Web site. https://www.cdc.gov/phlp/docs/hipaa-ferpa-infographic-508.pdf. Accessed February 5, 2022.
4. Summary of the HIPPA privacy rule. U.S. Department of Health and Human Services Web site. https://www.hhs.gov/hipaa/for-professionals/privacy/laws-regulations/index.html. Accessed February 5, 2022.
5. What is an electronic health record (EHR)? HealthIT.gov. https://www.healthit.gov/faq/what-electronic-health-record-ehr. Accessed February 5, 2022.
6. Benefits of EHRs. HealthIT.gov. https://www.healthit.gov/topic/health-it-and-health-information-exchange-basics/benefits-ehrs. Accessed February 5, 2022.
7. What are my health care rights and responsibilities? U.S. Department of Health and Human Services Web site. https://www.hhs.gov/answers/health-insurance-reform/what-are-my-health-care-rights/index.html. Accessed February 5, 2022.
8. Shah P, Thornton I, Turrin D, Hipskind JE. *Informed Consent.* Treasure Island, FL: Stat Pearls Publishing; 2021. Available from: https://www.ncbi.nlm.nih.gov/books/NBK430827/. Accessed February 5, 2022.
9. Patient responsibilities. American Medical Association Web site. https://www.ama-assn.org/delivering-care/ethics/patient-responsibilities. Accessed February 5, 2022.
10. Module 4: ethics and the law. Colorado Patient Navigator Training Program Web site. https://www.patientnavigatortraining.org/healthcare_system/module4/2_patient_responsibilities.htm. Accessed February 5, 2022.
11. Patient rights and responsibilities. Peace Health Web site. https://www.peacehealth.org/sites/default/files/patient_rights_and_responsbilities_hospitals_and_clinics_washington_updated_june_6_2020_revised.pdf. Accessed February 6, 2022.
12. Provider rights and responsibilities. New York State Web site. https://www.dfs.ny.gov/consumers/health_insurance/rights_responsibilities. Accessed February 6, 2022.
13. Smith Y. Doctor-patient relationship. News-Medical.net https://www.news-medical.net/health/DoctorPatient-Relationship.aspx. Accessed February 6, 2022.
14. A day in the life of a community health worker. Connecticut Health Foundation Web site. https://www.cthealth.org/wp-content/uploads/2019/02/r4-CHF-0039-Health-Infographic.pdf. Accessed February 6, 2022.

15. Role of community health workers. U.S. Department of Health and Human Services, National Heart, Lung, and Blood Institute Web site. https://www.nhlbi.nih .gov/health/educational/healthdisp/role-of-community -health-workers.htm#:~:text=CHWs%20offer%20 interpretation%20and%20translation,such%20as%20 first%20aid%20and. Accessed February 6, 2022.

16. Our values. National Association of Community Health Workers Web site. https://nachw.org/. Accessed February 8, 2022.

17. Florida Certification Board. *Certification Guidelines: Credential Standards and Requirements Table, Certified Community Health Worker (CCHW)*. https:// flcertificationboard.org/wp-content/uploads/CCHW -Standards-and-Requirements-Tables-January-2020.pdf. Accessed February 9, 2022.

18. Community health workers. Association of State and Territorial Health Officials Web site. https://www.astho .org/Community-Health-Workers/. Accessed February 10, 2022.

19. Association of State and Territorial Health Officials. *Community Health Workers: Evidence of Their Effectiveness*. https://www.astho.org/globalassets/pdf/community-health -workers-summary-evidence.pdf. Accessed February 10, 2022.

20. State insurance department. Insuranceopedia Web site. https://www.insuranceopedia.com/definition/4325/state -insurance-department. Accessed February 18, 2022.

21. State health departments. USA.gov. https://www.usa.gov /state-health. Accessed February 18, 2022.

22. Child help—prevent child abuse. Childhelp.org. https:// www.childhelp.org/. Accessed February 18, 2022.

23. We're a safe place and we want to help. Safe Place Web site. https://www.nationalsafeplace.org/. Accessed February 18, 2022.

24. Here for you. National Domestic Violence Hotline Web site. https://www.thehotline.org/. Accessed February 18, 2022.

25. Main N, Thomas T. Speak out—What is the domestic violence hand signal? The Sun Web site. https://www.the -sun.com/news/3871818/what-is-the-domestic-violence -hand-signal/. Accessed February 18, 2022.

26. Code of ethics for community health workers. Ingov Web site. https://www.in.gov/health/files/CHW_CodeofEthics _approvedfinalJune2008.pdf. Accessed February 18, 2022.

Appendix A: Code of Ethics for CHWs

A CHW is a frontline public health worker who is a trusted member of and/or has an unusually close understanding of the community she or he serves.[26] This trusting relationship enables the CHW to serve as a liaison/link/intermediary between health/social services and the community to facilitate access to services and improve the quality and cultural competence of service delivery. A CHW also builds individual and community capacity by increasing health knowledge and self-sufficiency through a range of activities such as outreach, community education, informal counseling, social support, and advocacy.[26]

Purpose of the Code

The CHW Code of Ethics is based on and supported by the core values adopted by the American Association of CHWs.[26] The Code of Ethics outlined in this document provides a framework for CHWs, supervisors, and employers of CHWs to discuss ethical issues facing the profession. Employers are encouraged to consider this Code when creating Community Health Worker programs.[26] The responsibility of all CHWs is to strive for excellence by providing quality service and the most accurate information available to individuals, families, and communities.[26] The Code of Ethics is based upon commonly understood principals that apply to all professionals within the health and social service fields (e.g., promotion of social justice, positive health, and dignity).[26] The Code, however, does not address all ethical issues facing CHWs and the absence of a rule does not imply that there is no ethical obligation present. As professionals, CHWs are encouraged to reflect on the ethical obligations that they have to the communities that they serve, and to share these reflections with others.[26]

Article 1. Responsibilities in the Delivery of Care

CHWs build trust and community capacity by improving the health and social welfare of the clients they serve.[26] When a conflict arises among individuals, groups, agencies, or institutions, CHWs should consider all issues and give priority to those that promote the wellness and quality of living for the individual/client. The following provisions promote the professional integrity of CHWs.[26]

1.1 Honesty

CHWs are professionals that strive to ensure the best health outcomes for the communities they serve. They communicate the potential benefits and consequences of available services, including the programs they are employed under.

1.2 Confidentiality

CHWs respect the confidentiality, privacy, and trust of individuals, families, and communities that they serve. They understand and abide by employer policies, as well as state and federal confidentiality laws that are relevant to their work.

1.3 Scope of Ability and Training

CHWs are truthful about qualifications, competencies, and limitations on the services they may provide, and should not misrepresent qualifications or competencies to individuals, families, communities, or employers.

1.4 Quality of Care

CHWs strive to provide high quality service to individuals, families, and communities. They do this through continued education, training, and an obligation to ensure the information they provide is up to date and accurate.

1.5 Referral to Appropriate Services

CHWs acknowledge when client issues are outside of their scope of practice and refer clients to the appropriate health, wellness, or social support services when necessary.

1.6 Legal Obligations

CHWs have an obligation to report actual or potential harm to individuals within the communities they serve to the appropriate authorities. Additionally, CHWs have a responsibility to follow requirements set by states, the federal government, and/or their employing organizations. Responsibility to the larger society or specific legal obligations may supersede the loyalty owed to individual community members.

Article 2. Promotion of Equitable Relationships

CHWs focus their efforts on the well-being of the whole community. They value and respect the expertise and knowledge that each community member possesses. In turn, CHWs strive to create equitable partnerships with communities to address all issues of health and well-being.

2.1 Cultural Humility

CHWs possess expertise in the communities in which they serve. They maintain a high degree of humility and respect for the cultural diversity within each community. As advocates for their communities, CHWs have an obligation to inform employers and others when policies and procedures will offend or harm communities or are ineffective within the communities where they work.

2.2 Maintaining the Trust of the Community

CHWs are often members of their communities and their effectiveness in providing services derives from the trust placed in them by members of these communities. CHWs do not act in ways that could jeopardize the trust placed in them by the communities they serve.

2.3 Respect for Human Rights

CHWs respect the human rights of those they serve, advance principles of self-determination, and promote equitable relationships with all communities.

2.4 Anti-Discrimination

CHWs do not discriminate against any person or group based on race, ethnicity, gender, sexual orientation, age, religion, social status, disability, or immigration status.

2.5 Client Relationships

CHWs maintain professional relationships with clients. They establish, respect, and actively maintain personal boundaries between them and their clients.

Article 3: Interactions with Other Service Providers

CHWs maintain professional partnerships with other service providers to serve the community effectively.

3.1 Cooperation

CHWs place the well-being of those they serve above personal disagreements and work cooperatively with any other person or organization dedicated to helping provide care to those in need.

3.2 Conduct

CHWs promote integrity in the delivery of health and social services. They respect the rights, dignity, and worth of all people and have an ethical obligation to report any inappropriate behavior (e.g., sexual harassment and racial discrimination) to the proper authority.

3.3 Self-Presentation

CHWs are truthful and forthright in presenting their background and training to other service providers.

Article 4. Professional Rights and Responsibilities

The Community Health Worker profession is dedicated to excellence in the practice of promoting well-being in communities. Guided by common values, CHWs have the responsibility to uphold the principles and integrity of the profession as they assist families to make decisions impacting their well-being. CHWs embrace individual, family, and community strengths and build upon them to increase community capacity.

4.1 Continuing Education

CHWs should remain up-to-date on any developments that substantially affect their ability to competently render services. CHWs strive to expand their professional knowledge base and competencies through education and participation in professional organizations.

4.2 Advocacy for Change in Law and Policy

CHWs are advocates for change and work on impacting policies that promote social justice and hold systems accountable for being responsive to communities. Policies that advance public health and well-being enable CHWs to provide better care for the communities they serve.

4.3 Enhancing Community Capacity

CHWs help individuals and communities move toward self-sufficiency to promote the creation of opportunities and resources that support their autonomy.

4.4 Wellness and Safety

CHWs are sensitive to their own personal well-being (physical, mental, and spiritual health) and strive to maintain a safe environment for themselves and the communities they serve.

4.5 Loyalty to the Profession

CHWs are loyal to the profession and aim to advance the efforts of other CHWs worldwide.

4.6 Advocacy for the Profession

CHWs are advocates for the profession. They are members, leaders, and active participants in local, state, and national professional organizations.

4.7 Recognition of Others

CHWs give recognition to others for their professional contributions and achievements.

Reference: Appendix A Adapted from:

Ingov., AMA. Code of Ethics for Community Health Workers. https://www.in.gov/health/files/CHW _CodeofEthics_approvedfinalJune2008.pdf. Accessed February 18, 2022.[26]

CHAPTER 14

The Community Health Worker Profession

LEARNING OBJECTIVES

1. Describe how community health workers influence health services in countries beyond of the United States.
2. Explains how community health workers improve health outcomes related to maternal and child health, micronutrient deficiencies, diarrhea, HIV, malaria, malnutrition, onchocerciasis (river blindness), and tuberculosis.
3. Examine the overview of community health workers programs, including some details related to the education qualification, certifications, curriculum, and a description of a community health worker job.
4. Review the techniques for writing a professional resume and developing professional interview skills.

KEY WORDS

human resources
Sustainable Development Goals (SDGs)

Introduction

This chapter starts with a global perspective of community health workers (CHWs), including how low-resourced countries are utilizing CHWs to the role of CHWs in the reduction of specific diseases. The next section describes the CHW influence in health systems in various countries, including India, Brazil, South Africa, Bangladesh, and Nepal and their contributions in improvement of health conditions. Then the discussion moves to the CHW workforce in the United States,

including programs, a curriculum example, and a job description. The chapter ends with techniques for developing your individualized CHW career by creating an excellent resume and learning professional interview skills.

Global CHWs

In every nation, **human resources** are an essential component needed to solve a health crisis. Human resources are one of the underlying factors in delivering effective health systems, or delivering ineffective ones. A human resource crisis is more critical in developing countries. For example, during the COVID pandemic, high-resourced countries have struggled with a shortage of healthcare workers in hospitals, but low-resourced countries lack well-equipped hospitals as well as adequate clinical workers.[1] The World Health Organization (WHO) reports evidence showing how CHWs contribute to efforts of improving health in communities that lack healthcare professionals. From a global perspective, the role of CHWs directly compliments the United Nation's **Sustainable Development Goals (SDGs)**, also known as the Global Goals.[2] The SDGs encompass 17 global goals composed of many targets that seek to eliminate poverty, hunger, and disease. These goals align with the role of CHWs who work directly within communities to provide holistic care and make valuable contributions to preventative care, improving access, capacity building, and serving diverse community members.[2] This section specifically describes how CHWs impact low-resourced countries. For impact indicators, the focus was on those related to maternal and child health, HIV/AIDS, TB, and malaria, as well as mental health conditions and noncommunicable diseases.[1]

CHW Influence in Global Health Systems

CHWs are recognized around the globe by prestigious organizations, such as the World Health Organization, the Global Health Workforce Alliance, and the United Nations. CHWs are recognized as an essential factor in the health care system in addressing community concerns including access to health care, equity, community referrals, and equality. Since CHWs are based in the community, they are trained in various ways depending on the resources of the community. Some CHW training is offered in a group, formal with competencies and offers a certificate of completion for the graduates. Other training is offered in a rural clinic or agency. This training is likely to be more on-the-job training and the CHW trainee is from the community. Some CHWs receive a salary, while others receive incentives, or work entirely on a voluntary basis depending on the community needs and resources. The following discussion covers examples of how CHWs programs assist in providing ways to improve measurable health outcomes in various countries.

India. In eastern Maharashtra, India, where the population is poor, CHW programs have helped to significantly decrease child and newborn mortality. This program started 20 years ago and served as an important model for work worldwide to reduce the infant mortality rates by using community-based strategies.

Brazil. Brazil employs over 220,000 CHWs. Each CHW visits approximately 150 families every month. By adopting the CHW program from India, Brazil has one of the fastest declining rates of infant and child mortality rates worldwide. CHW programs have expanded over the past thirty years. The CHWs work in teams along with other health care providers to service families in specific geographical locations. Other successful CHW programs in Brazil include decreasing rates of malnourished children, increasing immunization rates, increasing the number of pregnant women who received a minimum of four prenatal visits, meeting the demand for family planning, treatment for qualified women in order to avoid transmission of HIV from the mother to the child, cases of TB are detected with accuracy, improving drinking water coverage and better sanitation treatment, and the majority of AIDS patients receive their required medication.

South Africa. CHW programs have been established based on the CHW model that has been recognized as effective elsewhere in the world including India and Brazil.

Bangladesh. In Bangladesh, there are approximately 80,000 CHWs. Their services and accomplishments include delivering complete and inclusive community-based maternal and child health and family planning services, collecting TB sputum specimens from individuals with TB symptoms, making sure TB patients receive their daily treatments every day, and performing other needed services in their geographical location.

Other CHWs are trained to provide family planning services, vaccinations, as well as regular health care. Bangladesh reached its goal for lowering child mortality years ahead of schedule. CHW are seen as a major component of progress of maternal and child health and control of TB.

Nepal. In Nepal, the CHWs are recognized as one of the most significant contributors in Nepal for decreasing the child mortality rates in the world. Also, the CHW are responsible for the greatest coverage of vitamin A distribution. In Nepal, CHW receive two weeks of training and they serve as resources for family planning, identifying and treating childhood sicknesses, including pneumonia, and they offer in-home-based newborn and toddler care and breastfeeding support.

CHWs Contributions to Improvement in Health Conditions

Studies have demonstrated that the programs using CHWs make important contributions to improving health and nutrition behaviors, increasing utilization of key preventive and curative health services, and diagnosing and treating serious illnesses at the community level with beneficial effects on population health. Health programs rely on CHWs to provide a broad array of health services, including mother and child health and disease-control for HIV, TB, and malaria. See **Figure 14.1**.

Infant and Child Health. CHWs teach parents about healthy nutrition with the food that is available, since one out of every four children in developing countries suffer from malnutrition. In addition, infant and child mortality are linked to poor nutrition.

Breastfeeding. CHWs assist with the recommendation of only breastfeeding during the first six months of life. This recommendation improves health outcomes and prevents diarrhea for infants. CHWs provide valuable information for the mothers in the community on ways in which to identify moderately or severely malnourished children and help improve the nutritional status of the infants and children.

Micronutrient deficiencies. Micronutrient deficiencies are vitamins and minerals that are essential for healthy development and disease prevention. Most micronutrients are obtained

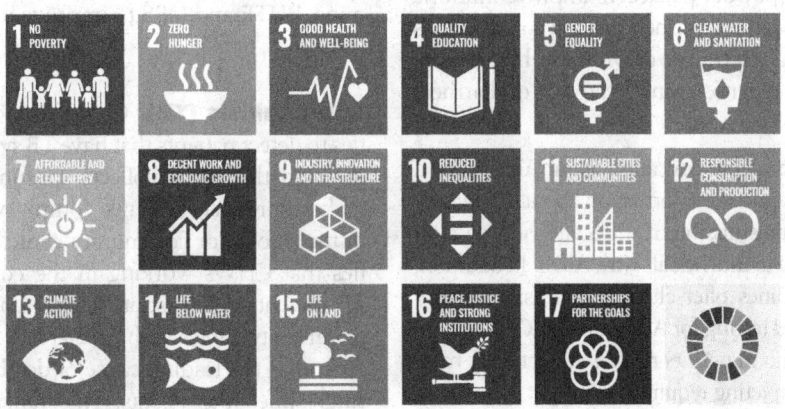

Figure 14.1 The United Nations Sustainable Development Goals

through eating the proper foods. There are six essential micronutrients:

- Iron is vital for children because it improves cognitive development and the ability to learn.
- Vitamin A is needed for healthy eye vision and the immune system.
- Vitamin D builds strong bones by helping the body absorb calcium. The body makes Vitamin D with exposure to sunlight. Too much sun light exposure leads to skin cancer.
- Iodine is found in fortified salt and is essential during pregnancy for the infant's cognitive development.
- Folate (Vitamin B9) is vital for cell development. During pregnancy, it is important to prevent neural tube defects in the spine of the infant.
- Zinc promotes healthy immune functions and is needed for healthy pregnancies.

CHWs are given the role of distributing packets of supplements in their communities to prevent and eliminate micronutrients among the entire community.

Diarrhea. In poor countries, diarrhea is the second leading cause of death for children under the age of five years. CHWs teach mothers in the communities about the importance of oral rehydration solution (ORS) and how to safely boil the water and mix the ORS powder into the boiled water. Zinc is added to ORS powder packets to improve immune function. It is well-established that the communities where CHWs teach the use of ORS have higher rates of prevention, diagnosis, and treatment of diarrhea.

HIV. CHWs promote education about AIDS-related risks as well as provide information about the behavioral risks of transmission of AIDS and how to offer supportive care to individuals with AIDS. In addition, some communities offer clinical services, voluntary counseling, and testing for AIDS and the CHWs have a role in promoting AIDS-related educational messages after completing required training.

Malaria. In Africa, CHWs provide education to the community about interventions to decrease

transmission of malaria and treat malaria cases. CHWs distribute and promote the use of insecticide-treated bed nets, teach families how to rapidly diagnose and treat malaria, and provide preventive therapy and antibiotics to pregnant women, infants, and children. CHWs provide a range of malaria control intervention programs for all age groups to help control and prevent outbreaks.

Malnutrition. CHWs are involved in the distribution of the provisions of ready-to-use therapeutic foods (RUTF) in the community with desperate and serious needs as well as providing food to hospitalized children in need. Often the CHWs serve as an essential role in organizing, distributing, and administering the RUTF programs.

Maternal Mortality (Death). CHWs are involved with improving maternal mortality by interventions such as home visits to educate expectant and post-partum mothers about good nutrition, danger signs of complications during pregnancy and childbirth, cleanliness during delivery, care of the newborn, and monitor newborns for signs of neonatal infection and referral.[3]

Onchocerciasis (River Blindness). CHWs distribute antibiotics to remote and isolated locations in Africa. This type of distribution is called the community directed interventions (CDI). It is also used for distribution of essential vitamins, RUTF, and ORS to improve infant and child health.

Tuberculosis (TB). CHWs work in communities to detect patients that have TB symptoms. Once detected the CHW collects sputum samples and makes sure that patients comply with treatment in their home or community clinic. Research verifies that CHWs working in the community with TB patients demonstrate higher compliance than community clinics without CHWS. Since TB ranks second as the leading cause of death globally from single infectious agents, HIV ranks first. CHWs play an essential role in TB programs globally.

CHWs have various roles and responsibilities across countries. However, CHWs do not have standardized training and certifications. There are recommendations to support standardized recommendations in governments, community agencies, international health non-government organizations (NGO), training facilities, such as hospital programs, community colleges, and independent schools. Whether urban or rural geographical locations, CHWs play an essential role in reaching every family and neighborhood and providing services, resources, and referrals to access health services. CHW programs are gaining recognition in health care systems to explore ways to shift expenditures to cost-effective interventions. They are trained in a short period of time. CHWs services are efficient and valuable due to their experience of living in the community in which they work including speaking the same language, respecting the culture, recognizing the traditions, and having the ability to serve as a liaison between the individual and the healthcare provider.

CHW Workforce in the United States

CHW training and certification programs offer some possible solutions as a supplement delivering services in community clinics and hospital systems. CHWs serve as a liaison between the healthcare providers, the patient and their families by addressing all aspects of the social determinants of health. These types of services reduce the number of readmissions and emergency department overuse. In addition, CHW services assist with meeting the needs of the elderly population as well as making appropriate resource referrals in their local community. Evidence shows that CHW programs save money, improve patient understanding and compliance, and improve patient health outcomes in their communities. See **Figure 14.2**.

In Figure 14.2, the CHW is part of a multidisciplinary care team that includes a variety of members.[6] The care team partners work with the patient to develop an implementation plan to address the issues and needs identified by the patient and care team. CHWs do not function independently, but rather under the direction of the team, while they address the goals and wishes of the patient. The CHWs are grounded and knowledgeable about the environment (home, social structure, relationships, financial capabilities) in which the patient functions.[6] The patient environment impacts how CHWs can be most effective in helping patients to achieve their goals. Because CHWs are part of the team that develops the interventions, they can ground the care team in what is realistic and will or will not work by providing the essential "reality check."[1] CHWs meet individual and community members at a convenient, comfortable place and address the whole person along with the family. This meeting

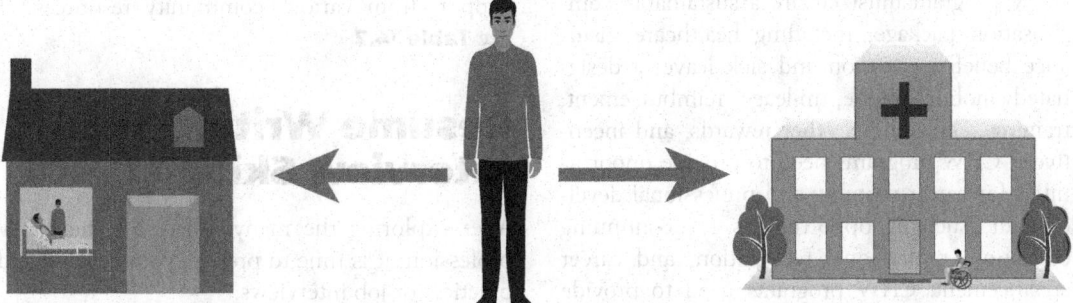

The CHW workforce is rapidly expanding in the United States

Figure 14.2 CHW Workforce in the United States

involves making referrals to address unmet social and/or emotional needs as well as social determinants of health, such as housing, early childhood development, and neighborhood conditions.[1,6]

CHWs have an appreciation and respect for the ethnic, linguistic, cultural, or experiential connections of the population they serve. CHWs are trusted and knowledgeable members of their communities and play a critical bridge role serving as cultural mediators and liaisons.[6] As members of healthcare teams, CHWs increase the team's cultural competence by helping the team better understand cultural norms and the beliefs of their community members, including basic cultural understanding, religious beliefs, and use of traditional herbs and medicines. CHWs work with vulnerable patients of all ages, typically from underserved, low-income communities in urban, suburban, and rural areas. They offer services prevention to helping people appropriately access care, such as outreach and education to increase immunization rates and screenings to chronic disease management.[1]

Overview of CHW Programs

This section includes information on the topics of CHW program design, education, certifications, curriculum, and a job description. First, CHW program designs are based on community needs.[1] Prior to starting a CHW program, a community health assessment is recommended to determine the needs and demographics. Generally, a new CHW program hires staff from the community who reflect the linguistic and cultural diversity of the population served. The funding for a new CHW program must ensure a sustainable compensation package, including healthcare insurance benefits, vacation and sick leave, a designated mobile phone, mileage reimbursement, training scholarships, other rewards, and incentives.[1] CHW programs need to provide opportunities for career mobility and professional development, such as opportunities for continuing education, professional recognition, and career advancement. CHW programs need to provide

core supplies and equipment for the CHWs to function in the community.[1]

Second, CHWs are required to have a minimum education of a high school diploma or General Education Diploma (GED). The 2007 Community Health Worker National Workforce Study reported that 32 percent of organizations required CHWs to hold a bachelor's degree.[7] University, community colleges, and community agency-based programs use core skills to develop the educational plan for their CHW workforce programs.[7-8] See **Table 14.1**.

Third, the CHW certifications are relevant to each state based on specific statutes and regulations. In some states, certification is required for reimbursement. After CHWs are brought on board, they are trained to strengthen the skills they had at the time of hiring and educated regarding skills and competencies they need for the specific program.[7] In 2014, federal Medicaid rules changed in support of CHWs.[6] See **Figure 14.3**.

Most CHWs are trained on the job through a mentoring process.[7-8] A lack of standardized training can lead to variations in the implementation of the role. A standard curriculum would aid in the recognition and integration of the CHW role across health care in all states.[8-10]

Fourth, job descriptions for CHWs offer a wide variety of the characteristics, depending on the place of employment and assigned duties. CHWs recruited from local communities have an enhanced impact on utilization, the creation of health awareness, and health outcomes. They can communicate the desired message, to liaise between clients and providers, and to garner support from various community resources.[7-10] See **Table 14.2**.

Resume Writing and Interview Skills

After exploring the many aspects of the CHW profession, it is time to prepare your resume and practice for job interviews.

Table 14.1 Sample of the Minnesota CHW Curriculum

The Minnesota CHW curriculum is based on the core competencies that incorporates health promotion competencies as an introduction to a broad range of individual, family, and population health needs. The internship is the centerpiece of the curriculum's practice competencies.[8]

Phase 1: Role of the CHW—Core Competencies

1. Role, Advocacy, and Outreach

This course focuses on the role of the CHWs personal safety, self-care, and personal wellness and the promotion of health and disease prevention for clients.

2. Organization and Resources: Community and Personal Strategies

The course focuses on the CHW's knowledge of the community and the ability to prioritize and organize work. Emphasis is on the use and critical analysis of resources and on problem solving.

3. Teaching and Capacity Building

This course focuses on the CHW role in teaching and increasing capacity of the community and of the client to access the healthcare system.

4. Legal and Ethical Responsibilities

This course focuses on the legal and ethical dimensions of the CHW role; included are boundaries of the CHW position, agency policies, confidentiality, liability, mandatory reporting, and cultural issues that can influence legal and ethical responsibilities.

5. Coordination, Documentation, and Reporting

This course focuses on the importance and ability of the CHW to gather, document, and report on client visits and other activities.

6. Communication and Cultural Competence

This course provides the content and skills in communication to assist the CHW in effectively interacting with a variety of clients, their families, and a range of healthcare providers.

Phase 2: Role of the CHW—Health Promotion Competencies

1. Healthy Lifestyles

This course focuses on the knowledge and skills a CHW needs to assist clients in realizing healthy eating patterns, controlling their weight, integrating exercise into their lives, taking their medications, talking with their health providers, controlling substances such as tobacco, managing stress, achieving life balance, and attaining personal and family wellness.

2. Heart Disease and Stroke

This course focuses on CHWs working with clients and community members in preventing heart disease and stroke as well as working with those who already have heart disease or have experienced a heart attack or stroke.

3. Maternal, Child, and Teen Health

This course emphasizes the needs and requirements to support the health of mothers, children, and teens. Issues such as sexuality, family planning, sexually transmitted diseases, substance abuse, and domestic violence as well as the resources needed by mothers and their children are also discussed.

(continues)

Table 14.1 Sample of the Minnesota CHW Curriculum   *(continued)*

4. Diabetes
This course focuses on the role of the CHW in working with clients with diabetes. The role of the CHW in diabetes prevention, control, resource identification, and education is also included.
5. Cancer
This course focuses on the role of the CHW when working with cancer patients and their families. Also covered is the role of CHWS to help identify resources, facilitate client access to those resources, as well as give aid and support to cancer clients and their families.
6. Oral Health
This course focused on a broad range of topics needed to understand and promote oral health, including dental anatomy, infection control, oral hygiene instruction and care, plus a guide for parents, use of fluoride and dental caries prevention, as well as nutrition required for good oral health.
7. Mental Health
This course provides CHWs with an introduction to mental health and illness. This course also provides opportunities for the CHW to promote the mental health of self, clients, families, and communities.

Phase 3: Practice Competencies—Internship: 72–80 hours of supervised practical experience that allows opportunities for the student to prepare for independent work in the CHW role.

Data from Minnesota Community Health Worker Alliance. Minnesota CHW Curriculum. Available at http://s472440476.onlinehome.us/wp-content/uploads/2013/05/EducationCurriculum.pdf. Accessed February 23, 2022.[8]
Minnesota Community Health Worker Alliance. Education. Available at https://mnchwalliance.org/education/#:~:text=MN%20CHW%20Curriculum%20Minnesota%20is%20the%20first%20state,high%20school%20diploma%20or%20GED%2C%20at%20a%20minimum. Accessed February 23, 2022.[9]
Minnesota Department of Health. Community Health Worker (CHW). Available at https://www.health.state.mn.us/facilities/ruralhealth/emerging/chw/index.htm. Accessed February 23, 2022.[10]

"Changes in Federal Medicaid Rules Effective January 2014 Allow Payment for Preventive Services by Non-licensed Individuals including CHWs." (Federal Register, July 15, 2013 [78 FR 135 p. 42306])

Preventive services "recommended by a physician or other licensed practitioner …

1. Prevent disease, disability, and other health conditions;
2. Prolong life; and,
3. Promote physical and mental health efficiency."

Figure 14.3 Changes to Federal Medicaid Rules
Federal Register, July 15, 2013 [78 FR 135 p. 42306]

Resume Writing

Over the past few years, the format of a new resume has changed because many companies utilize applicant tracking software to scan through the hundreds of applications, searching for the key words relevant to the job. If your resume does not include the correct terms, the software will reject your resume, and it will never be reviewed by a human.[12] The key terms are a must-add to any resume and are ideal for the "List of Reverent Skills" or "Areas of Expertise" section on your resume when competing in a globally competitive market. Key terms are found in the job description

Table 14.2 **Example of a CHW Job Description**

The desired qualifications for this CHW position include the following:

CHW Personal Qualities	a. Willingness to learn b. Compassion, caring about others c. Communication skills d. Cultural competence e. Professional experiences f. Commitment to serving the community g. Respect by peers in the community h. Shared values and experiences of the people being served i. Good personal health practices, attitudes, and self-esteem j. Ability to grow, change, and learn k. Recognition as a trusted community member
CHW Expectations	a. Constructive in interpersonal relationships b. Friendly, outgoing, sociable, culturally competent, patient, open-minded, and nonjudgmental c. Knowledge about health issues and the healthcare system d. Understand the importance of sharing that knowledge with family and friends e. Communication skills (speaking, listening, writing, teaching, bilingual ability) f. Ability identify and use resources g. Empowerment and leadership skills h. Ability to resolve conflicts i. Respectful and honest
CHW Support and Supervision	a. Provide support and supervision for CHWs within the structure and function of the health team b. Offer ongoing mentoring, support, and acknowledgment of their efforts so CHWs excel in their roles c. Support peer-to-peer to increase retention and motivation
CHW Rewards and Recognition	a. Recognize satisfaction in serving others b. Acknowledge the responsibility given to CHWs c. Value personal motivations for acquired new knowledge to improve the health of their own families d. Retain CHWs based on financial and nonfinancial incentives and benefits e. Reward ongoing mentoring, support, and certification

Data from Hometown Health Center. Community Health Worker Job Description. Available at https://hometownhealthcenter.org/wp-content/uploads/sites/61/2021/05/Community-Health-Worker-1222820.pdf. Accessed February 26, 2022.[11]

of the position of which you are applying. Also, notice that your education has moved to the end of your resume. Employers are more interested in your career goals, recent jobs, and relevant skills.[12]

Length. In today's job market, recruiters prefer two pages if you have enough information. If you are an entry-level candidate with limited information, leave it at one page. However, if you have years of experience, reduce your resume two pages. Generally, recruiters spend less than 10 seconds reviewing your resume.[13] It is essential to present a concise document that highlights your work history, skills, and education.

Contact Information. When choosing your contact information, make sure you consistently represent your name the same way on all materials, such as business cards, LinkedIn profile, and any other online portfolio.[14] Today companies use social media, particularly LinkedIn, to post job opportunities, search for candidates, and check potential hires. Putting your LinkedIn profile URL front and center on your resume with the rest of your contact information is one way to ensure that hiring managers have an easy time distinguishing you from all the other applicants.[14]

It is recommended that you to create an email address dedicated to your job-search activities. You do not want to miss an email message from a potential employer. Look closely at your email account address.[14-15] If you continue to use an outdated email account (e.g., Comcast, AOL, Hotmail, or other antiquated free email), the recruiter will assume that you are older than the desired age, regardless of your current skills and abilities.[14] Create a Gmail with your name: Joan. Fox@gmail.com. As for your phone number, only put your cell phone number. Again, landlines are outdated, and there is no reason to have more than one phone number on your resume.[15]

Format and Style. Current standards prefer a comprehensive format of essential information, including the removal of the objective statement and references, which leaves room to add your Career Summary and Areas of Expertise.[15] Think of your Career Summary as two to four lines that outlining your qualifications for the job. The Areas of Expertise are six to nine bullet points to highlight your relevant skills using the keywords from the job description. After these two sections, present your latest experiences up to 15 years with emphasis on why you are the best candidate. This format leaves room for your Education and Credentials section at the end. Last, the basic format is best, unless you are applying to a creative job. Avoid using any odd or fancy fonts and infographics.[15] Do not make your resume hard to read by using a column on the left with additional information. Any deviation from a simple format will confuse the reader. Stick to the basics because your skills and experience are what matter the most.[14-15]

If you are over 50 years old, you were probably taught to use two spaces after a period during your high school typing class.[14] However, this typing rule was created to make it easier to see the beginning of new sentences. Thanks to the advent of computers and proportionally spaced fonts, this practice is completely obsolete. The modern style is to put one space after all end punctuation.[14]

Technical Skills and Proficiencies. As a CHW, list the technical platforms and tools that you are proficient. For example, Microsoft Office would be a common requested skill for a CHW. However, if you are proficient with Word, know a little about PowerPoint, but not familiar with Excel and Access, you would not state Microsoft Office proficiency on your resume or during an interview.[15] Be specific, and the list can include social media platforms, electronic health record (EHR) systems, or project management systems. If you need to refresh your computer skills or medical terminology skills, you may check out adult education courses at your local community college or library.

Language Skills. For a CHW, language skills are a great selling point on your resume.[14-15] If you are proficient in several languages, be sure to list each language you speak and your proficiency level. For example:

- Spanish: written and speaking proficiency
- French Creole: speaking proficiency
- Korean: basic speaking

Professional Experience. Start with your most recent job and work your way backward within the past 15 years.[15] Your resume should describe all your professional positions. For example, if you served in the military or held a board position, list this experience as any other role in your work history. If you recently graduated from college, add your internships and any work experience that took place during college. Use the following template to list the information for each role:

- Company name and URL
- Job title: If your title is specific to your organization, add a description next to the job title.

- Start and end dates including the month and year for each entry.
- Job description: Describe your roles and responsibilities as they relate to your target role. This is especially important if you are in the process of changing careers.[15] For example, if you are applying for a CHW position, provide details such as how you worked with the public, computer skills used, supervision of other employees, the territories that you covered, and so on.
- Achievements: List your accomplishments and major contributions that benefited the organization during your employment. The number of achievements you provide will depend on how long you remained in that role and how relevant it is to your current job goals.[15] Quantify your accomplishments whenever possible; for instance, how did you help save the company money, generate revenue, improve customer satisfaction, increase productivity, and so forth?[15]

If you have employment gaps, be honest and explain yourself. There is no need to hide your past and employment gaps on your resume. If you have gaps, be prepared to explain the situation with what you gained from your time away and speak to that situation.[16] For example, you may have left your past position to become a full-time caregiver for your parents. Since you are applying for a CHW position, your employment gap gave you firsthand knowledge and experience for the CHW position.

Volunteer Work. Skills-based volunteering (SBV) is a great way to fill an employment gap or supplement your work history when you are trying to change careers. List any volunteer work, the name of the organization and its website URL, your involvement and contributions that are relevant to your current job goals in chronological order.[15] If you are new to the workforce, include any campus activities or clubs in which you were active.

Professional Affiliations. List any memberships in relevant professional organizations or affiliations that are not listed elsewhere on your resume.[15] For each entry, list the name and URL, when you became a member, what positions you held, your responsibilities and any notable achievements.[15]

Education and Professional Development. Create a record of your education.[15] Start with your most recent degree. List the institution, its location, the name of your degree, your major and minor, your graduation year, and any honors associated with the degree, such as summa or magna cum laude. Do the same for any relevant certifications you obtained or additional training opportunities or workshops you have attended that you did not state earlier on your resume.[15]

After you complete your basic resume, it useful to search online and gather a few job postings that represent the type of position you are targeting.[15] It does not matter about the location; the purpose of this exercise is to determine if your resume matches the job description and the qualifications. Print the description and then highlight or bold any requirements or desirable skills that you have on your resume. This exercise will identify which of your qualifications should be showcased throughout your resume.[15]

Last, read your resume aloud line by line. It will help you find grammar and spelling errors. Next ask a professional resume writer or instructor to help you incorporate some of the information found in the sample job descriptions into your resume to demonstrate your skills in the workplace.[15] See **Table 14.3** and **Figure 14.4**.

Interview Skills

Now that your resume is created, it is time to start thinking about your interviewing skills. It is important to prepare your interview skills prior to obtaining a job interview appointment. You want to be ready. This section covers some steps that will increase your chances of success at interviews including dress code, researching the company, list of questions, preparation for interview, day of interview, and after the interview.

Dress Code. Even if the company employees dress casual at work, you need to wear business

Table 14.3 How Do CHWs Compare to Other Frontline Roles?

	Work Setting	Formal Training	Duties	Median Hourly Wage
CHW	Community clinics, health departments, hospitals and integrated health systems, schools, social service agencies and other nonprofits, housing providers	Varies from on-the-job to community college certificate programs. High school diploma or GED required by many employers. No national standardized curriculum. Certification required for Medicaid reimbursement in select states.	Supervision varies depending on worksite. Culturally appropriate preventive services, patient education, outreach, and info referrals. Basic health screenings, such as vital signs*. Administrative duties, i.e., social services paperwork, insurance forms. *CHW is not a clinician and does not typically provide "hands on" care.	$18.45 per hour
Certified Nurse Assistant	Hospitals, nursing homes, and residential care facilities	Community colleges, vocational schools, technical schools, or universities. One-year program typically leading to a certificate or diploma. Certification required for Medicare/Medicaid reimbursable services.	Supervised by licensed nursing staff. Assistance with activities of daily living (ADLs). Maintain patient health records. Monitors changes in patient conditions.	$13.23 per hour
Home Health Aide	Homes and residential care facilities	No formal education requirements.	Supervised by case manager. Assists with activities of daily living (toileting, feeding, bathing, dressing, transfers). Light housekeeping. Simple rehabilitative and lifestyle counseling.	$11.16 per hour
Medical Assistant	Ambulatory settings such as provider offices, urgent and outpatient clinics	High school diploma or GED Community colleges, vocational schools, technical schools, or universities. One-year program typically leading to a certificate or diploma.	Supervised by medical doctor. Client history, vital signs, phlebotomy, injections. Administrative duties, schedule appointment, hospital admissions, prescription refills.	$15.61 per hour

Data from National Institute of Health, National Heart, Lung, and Blood Institute. Role of Community Health Workers. Available at https://www.nhlbi.nih.gov /education/heart-truth/CHW/Role#:~:text=Since%20CHWs%20typically%20reside%20in%20the%20community%20they,helping%20to%20reduce%20health%20 disparities%20in%20underserved%20communities. Accessed March 2, 2022.[17]

attire for the interview. Currently, business attire is gender neutral: a dark or neutral color suit, flat closed-toe shoes, dark socks, a freshly ironed shirt or blouse, a simple necklace or plain tie, a belt that matches the shoe color.[18] Your hair should be trimmed, and nails are short and clean. If desired, make-up is natural without flashy eyelashes, bright colors on eyes, lips, or fingernails. Remove all piercing jewelry (e.g., nose, lip, eyebrow, and multiple ear jewelry). One pair of simple earrings are appropriate. Simple rings are acceptable. Tattoos on arms and neck should be covered with clothing, when possible. Have your hair styled or pulled back so you will not be tempted to twirl your hair with your fingers when you get nervous. Specific clothing based on religious practices are appropriate. For example, a hijab (head scarf) is proper for women and a yarmulke, Koppel, or kippah (skull cap) or prayer shawl for men. Overuse of cologne, aftershave, or perfume is not appropriate for an interview or in the workplace. Also, you need to keep your breath fresh by using a mint or mouthwash. Remember that you wish to be remembered by the interviewer as the person most qualified for the position rather than the person that wore the bright red plaid jacket. Last, it is appropriate to carry a flat portfolio, envelope, or folder that contains several copies of your resume and business cards, your list of questions to ask during the interview, a copy of the company's website, and a pen.[18]

Research the Company. Before the interview, it is advisable to research the company by reviewing their website.[19] It will provide information about the healthcare agency, such as number of clinics nationwide, scope of healthcare services, annual revenue, mission statement and values, and number of years in business. Companies are proud of their websites.[19] A common initial interview question is, "Have you have had a chance to look at our website?" Your answer should reflect that you explored several areas of the website, not merely the front page. For example, your response could be, "I loved the slow-moving graphics on the front page.

It reflects a peaceful energy for the clinic. As I clicked on several different pages, I learned that there are several clinics in statewide and more nationwide. I was not aware that this healthcare agency started in Kentucky in 2004. I look forward to learning more from you." As you prepare for the interview, be mindful of the company's mission, vision, and culture. This information can help you adequately prepare for your interview. Additionally, you can creatively find ways to answer interview questions by customizing your responses to align with the mission, vision, values, and culture.[19]

While you are on the healthcare agency's website, get the address, directions, and main local phone number. If you do not have GPS, use a digital map search for directions and best routes. If times permits, it is good to take a test-run to the address.[19] This practice drive allows you to learn where to park and the location of the front entrance. It may sound basic, but if the building is surrounded by several tall buildings or on a large corporate campus, it is never easy to locate the building numbers and visitor parking. In fact, the main entrance of the company may be located off the elevator in a community multi-story parking garage.[19]

List of Questions. As you review their website, begin to write down a few questions that you may wish to ask during the interview. Your questions should not focus on topics, such as salary, benefits, personal time off, and other human resources information. Those kinds of questions are addressed after you are offered the position rather than during an interview.[19] The interview questions may include:

- I saw on the website that you have clinics in three locations in the state. Will I be expected to travel to the other locations?
- Have many CHWs are currently employed statewide with this agency?
- Since the clinic hours are 7:00 a.m. to 7:00 p.m. Monday to Saturday, would you please give me an example of a typical schedule that I might work?

Maria Jo Smith
Mobile phone: (703) 973-0000
MJSmith@gmail.com
www.linkedin.com/in/mjsmithgmailcom

Career Summary: While taking care of my grandmother, I enjoyed assisting her with scheduling medical appointments, arranging for the home health equipment and services, and explaining how to manage her prescriptions. Since I am fluent in Spanish, I translated for my grandmother, taught her health team about the culture of Costa Rica, and served as her liaison.

Areas of Expertise:

- Fluent Spanish: written and verbal
- Associate Degree in Health Science
- Certified Nursing Assistant
- EPIC Electronic Health Record System certified
- Advanced Cardiac Life Support Certification
- Medical Terminology
- Leadership and Teamwork Skills
- Experience assisting elderly individuals

Technical Skills and Proficiencies

2012   Certified Nursing Assistant
2012   Certified in EPIC Electronic Health Record System
2011   Advanced Cardiac Life Support
2011   Spanish Medical Terminology
2010   Medical Terminology
2009   Advanced Microsoft Office Suite Certificate
2009   Cardiopulmonary Resuscitation (CPR) certificate

Professional Experience:

Longview Waffle House (www.longviewwaffles.com)
1/2011 to 11/2011   Food Server   Owner: Phyllis Grainer (794) 837-0001.
Job description: Worked two 8-hour shifts on Saturday and Sunday. Food server, taking orders, customer service, cashier, cleaning, making coffee, training new servers, problem-solving when employee failed to come to work, translating for Spanish-speaking customers.
Achievement: Designed, translated, and printed the Spanish menu.

Goody Yogurt Shoppe (www.goodyyogurt.com)
6/2010 to 12/2010 Yogurt Server   Owner: Bill Johnson (794) 834-0000
Job description: Customer service, making yogurt, cashier, supervising new employees, balancing cash drawer at end of shift, cleaning at closing time.
Achievement: Designed a way to clean the yogurt machines faster after the shop closed.

Longview High School (longviewhs.com)
9/2009 to 5/2010   Co-Captain, Girls Volleyball Team   Coach: Ms. Wagner (794) 832-0020
Achievement: Team achieved 2nd place in the Regional Finals Tournament

Longview High School (longviewhs.com)
3/2008 to 4/2009   Team Capitan for Volunteers (2nd year of participation)
Job description: Spring Break Beach Clean-up Month: Clean-up kicked-off the week of spring break and continued each Saturday for the next six weeks.
Achievement: Two years as Team Capitan

Figure 14.4 Sample Resume for a CHW

YMCA Middle School Youth Group (ymcalongview.com)
8/2006 to 5/2010   Volunteer for Middle School Youth/Elderly Group at the YMCA
<u>Job description</u>: Worked with disadvantaged youth 4-hours per week; organized activities related to sports and crafts; assisted with homework.
<u>Achievement</u>: Initiated a youth and senior citizen activity once per quarter

Education and Professional Development

2010 to 2012   Associate Degree in Health Science
                       Lake County Community College, Fairfield, FL
2005 to 2010   Longview High School, Longview, FL

References
Tamara Samuels, RN, MPH
Instructor, Lake County Community College
(794) 832-0101
TSamuels@LCCC.org

Leslie Randolph, MD
Pediatrician
(794) 834-0202
LRandolphMD@gmail.com

Beth Walker, Associate Pastor
Spring of Life Community Church
(794) 832-0303
BWalker@SOLCC.org

Figure 14.4 (Continued)

Preparation of Interview. Preparation and practice are key to a successful interview.[19] Preparation for an interview is an excellent way to conduct a self-evaluation. Take time to think about what is important to you. Be prepared to answer the following questions:

- Tell me about yourself.
- How would your friends describe you?[19]
- How do your present and past experiences relate to the position?
- What are your current and future career goals?
- How do you deal with stress?
- Do you prefer a set schedule or a flexible schedule?
- Are you willing to drive to other locations within the state? Day trips or overnight trips?
- What did you like and dislike about a previous job?
  - Explain your reason for leaving your current job.

- Do you wish to work with a team of people or more by yourself?
- What do you value in a supervisor?[19]
- What appeals to you about this job and organization?
- What are your strengths and weaknesses related to this position, such computer skills?
  - When answering a question about your weakness, always mention what you are doing to diminish your weakness, such as enrolling in an online medical terminology course.
- What are the most important things to you in a job?
- What would you like me to know most that is not on your resume?
- Tell me about a time when a team you were working on was unable to proceed due to some interpersonal conflict. How did you respond, and what role did you play on the team?

- Give an example of a situation where you demonstrated leadership.
- What skills and experience do you have to offer this employer?
- What skills that you would like to develop or improve if you are selected for this job?[19]
- We are conducting interviews with three applicants. Why should we hire you?
- What questions do you have about the organization?
  - Questions for the interviewer are queries that usually focus on the culture or mission of the organization, and job responsibilities.

Keep in mind that interviews are a two-way communication process.[19] While employers are taking the opportunity to assess you for the job, you are accessing if the company is a good "fit" for your needs. In some cases, you both may determine that the position is not suitable for you currently. For example, if you wish to relocate to another state, the position may not fit your location, salary, and lifestyle priorities.

When practicing for an interview, consider asking a friend to act as an interviewer by asking you to answer the previously stated questions.[19] Practice several times until you feel comfortable answering each question. If you practice excessively, you will sound like you memorized your responses. During the practice interview, you may wish to wear the outfit that you plan to wear. You wish to feel comfortable in your outfit. Visual first impressions are important; if in doubt, always dress on the conservative side.[19]

Your responses should be concise and to the point. When applicants ramble when providing a response, it wastes time and suggests that you do not know the answer. You should never make negative comments about a previous employer or company; rather, find a way to give the experience a positive outcome, such as saying that you learned from the experience.[19] In addition, your responses must be truthful and be prepared to explain every fact on your resume. If you embellished your accomplishment, the interviewer may ask specific questions about that experience. Sometimes near the end of the interview, you may begin to feel comfortable with the interviewer. Stay in your professional role and avoid sharing any personal information. However, it is useful to find something that you have in common with the interviewer. For example, if you see a picture on the wall or in the background of the screen of a famous location where you have traveled, such as Paris or the Rocky Mountains. Be sincere about the connection and return to the interview. Avoid commenting on family photos.

Day of the Interview. The day has arrived. You are dressed and ready to leave early. Plan to arrive at least 20 minutes early to account to unexpected traffic or a last-minute stop for the restroom stop. Remember that first impressions take about 30 seconds.[19] A well-groomed, professional appearance is critical. After COVID, it is no longer necessary to greet individuals with a firm handshake. Let the interviewer take the lead on offering a handshake or not. A warm smile denotes confidence during the interview, and do not be afraid to use some hand animation while answering questions to show enthusiasm. If possible, request a business card from the interviewer and each member of the committee. After you are shown to your seat, remove the items from your folder or envelope.[19] You do not need to spread the items across the table space, but rather stack the papers neatly with your pen on top.

Virtual Interviews. Virtual interviews are popular due to improved technology, COVID, geographic location, travel costs, and divergent schedules. Also, a phone interview may be your initial contact with a recruiter prior to scheduling a virtual interview with the employer. The purpose of the phone interview is to gain an invitation for a virtual or personal interview. Prepare for the phone interview by having your resume, notepad, and pen on your desk. Speak clearly and answer questions with enthusiasm. Use this opportunity to talk about your skills and experience. When the phone interview is over, let the recruiter know that you are interested in scheduling an interview with the employer.[19]

For the virtual interview, here are a few ways to prepare:

- When the virtual interview is scheduled, ask the scheduler if you could test the virtual technology prior to the actual interview.[19]
- Wear the same outfit to the virtual interview as you would for an in-person interview. Have your hair styled or pulled back so you will not be tempted to twirl your hair with your fingers when you get nervous.
- Have your resume, list of questions, notepad, and pen on your desk prior to the scheduled interview.
- Verify that the background on your screen is a blank wall. You do not wish to have your unmade bed, a sink of dirty dishes, or a pile of clothes in the background.[19]
- Make sure that your location is silent during the virtual interview, meaning no music, people talking, traffic noise, or barking dogs.
- The questions asked in a virtual interview are like the questions for an in-person interview.
- If possible, write down the names of the committee members as they are introduced.
- If the interviewer signals the end of the interview and asks you for questions, it is reasonable to briefly mention some key points that you were unable to state and then ask one or two questions from your prepared list.[19]

Body Language. Body language is essential in both an in-person and virtual interview. Sit with good posture but no need to be rigid.[19] Look the interviewer and if there are several individuals in the room address your answers to the person that asked the question. Listen before answering the questions. Interviewers are impressed with someone who thinks about an answer before speaking. You may write down a few notes on the paper in your stack. For example, the question may be to list three of your strengths. Write down three words on your paper. If you did not understand the questions, ask for clarification. Speak clearly with assurance to show confidence, even if you are wearing a mask. In most interviews, the employer begins the interview, but you should be prepared with some opening statements related to the position.[19]

After the Interview. At the end of the interview, thank the interviewer and other committee members in the room or on the screen. Within a day, email thank-you letters to all the interviewers with whom you spoke. You will be able to locate their email addresses on the company website if you were unable to obtain their contact information in person or virtually.[19]

Last, go into the interview with a desire to obtain that job position. Even if your interest diminishes during the interview, do not give up, and use the interview as a practice session for your dream job. Not all interviews will lead to offers of employment, but every interview provides valuable skills.[19]

Accepting a CHW Position. During the interview process, you probably had a few questions that were not answered. Once you have been offered the CHW position, it is time to ask your questions prior to accepting the job offer.[20] Here are a few possible questions to ask your employer if they were not discussed during the duration of the initial interview:

- What are your expectations for me in this position?
- What will my schedule look like? Is it flexible?
- When is my official start date?
- What will be my wages? How often will I be paid?
- Will I earn overtime pay if I work more than 40 hours per week?
- What does the benefits package, e.g., health insurance, tuition, and retirement savings?
- What are policies regarding vacation, sick leave, and paid-time-off?
- Who will be my supervisor?
- Will I be reimbursed for mileage when I drive to and from community agencies?
- When do you need a decision on the job offer?
- What are the next steps?

Before you accept the CHW position, you must be sure you understand all the answers to your questions.[20]

Congratulations, you are employed as a CHW!

Chapter Summary

This chapter began with a global perspective of CHWs, including how low-resourced countries are utilizing CHWs and the role of CHWs in reducing specific diseases in India, Brazil, South Africa, Bangladesh, and Nepal, as well as CHW contributions to improving health conditions. Then the discussion moved to the CHW workforce in the United States, including programs, a curriculum example, and a job description. The chapter ended with techniques for developing your individualized CHW career by creating an excellent resume and professional interview skills.

CASE STUDY

Connecting the Role of CHWs to Other Frontline Occupations

Sonia was born in El Paso, Texas. For most of her childhood, her parents were farmworkers in Texas, Colorado, New Mexico, and California. Sonia and her two older brothers went to many different elementary schools. By the time the three children were in middle school, their parents had settled in Albuquerque, New Mexico, and they had higher paid employment opportunities. Jose, Sonia's dad, worked in the service department of a car large dealership. Maria, Sonia's mom, worked in a legal office as a translator for the refugee immigrants. The family was able to afford a modest home near Old Towne in Albuquerque, and the teens were able to attend the same high school from 8th to 12th grades. As the youngest, Sonia was able to attend one location for high school. After her brothers Alejandro, and Carlos graduated from high school, they attended college. By the time that Sonia was a senior in high school, Alejandro had graduated from the local community college with a double trade certification as a plumber and electrician. He was hired by a large construction company in Santa Fe. A few years later, Carlos earned an undergraduate degree in accounting from the University of New Mexico.

Since Sonia obtained her cosmetology license during her last year in high school, she was able to begin working soon after graduation. She had always loved her long dark hair and learned at a young age how to create new hair styles for herself, her mom, and her friends. Being a hair stylist was her dream job at age 18. Besides enjoying the opportunity to talk to her clients and learning about their interesting lives, she enjoyed making the weekly salary of $660 per week. She makes her own flexible schedule depending on her appointments and does not work 8 hours each day. Out of her earnings, she had to pay for her supplies (e.g., shampoo, conditioners as well as color and styling products) plus she did not have any benefits, such a sick leave, vacation time, or health insurance costs. The hair salon charges each stylist $150 per month to rent the booth space, and Sonia's supply costs were $120 per month. The hair salon was closed for the week between Christmas and New Year's and closed for one week from July 1 to July 8. Sonia had to pay for own health insurance, which was $118 per month, and does not accrue any benefits, such as sick leave, vacation pay, or retirement options.

After a few years, Sonia sustained a knee injury when she slipped while walking on ice outside her parent's home. She had surgery and several weeks of physical prior to returning to work. She found that standing all day caused her knee and back to hurt. She decided to take Alejandro's advice and schedule an appointment with a career counselor at the local community college.

Sonia enjoyed meeting Beth Richards, the career counselor. Beth started the appointment by asking Sonia what she liked about working in the hair salon. Sonia responded that she liked working with her clients, being able to speak English or Spanish as needed, helping the clients navigate through their life problems, making suggestions related to their hair style, giving advice, and getting to know each client over time from high school prom to wedding day. Beth laughed and told Sonia that she should become a CHW because Sonia had provided a brief description of what CHW workers do, except they do not have to stand most of the day.

Questions

1. What do you see as the similarities between hair stylist and CHW?
2. By reviewing **Table 14.2: Example of a CHW Job Description**, what differences do you recognize between Sonia's hair stylist position and a CHW position?
3. Use the information in **Table 14.3: How Do CHWs Compare to Other Frontline Roles?** to calculate Sonia's annual salary before taxes if she became a CHW.

References

1. World Health Organization, Global Health Workforce Alliance. *Global Experience of Community Health Workers for Delivery of Health-Related Millennium Development Goals: A Systematic Review, Country Case Studies, and Recommendations for Integration into National Health Systems.* https://www.who.int/news/item/02-06-2022-global-strategy-on-human-resources-for-health--workforce-2030 Accessed October 3, 2022.

2. Sustainable Development Goals (SDGs). World Health Organization Web site. https://www.who.int/health-topics/sustainable-development-goals#tab=tab_1. Accessed February 23, 2022.

3. Perry H, Zulliger R. *How Effective Are Community Health Workers?* Johns Hopkins Bloomberg School of Public Health; 2012. https://www.childhealthtaskforce.org/sites/default/files/2019-07/How%20Effective%20are%20CHWs_Evidence%20Summary%20Condensed%28JHSPH%2C%202012%29.pdf. Accessed February 23, 2022.

4. Hodgins S. Learning from community health worker programs, big and small. *Global Health: Science & Practice.* 2020;8(2):147–149.

5. Zwick S. Applying carbon standards to sustainable development goals. https://www.ecosystemmarketplace.com/articles/applying-carbon-standards-sustainable-development-goals/. Accessed February 23, 2022.

6. Brooks BA, Davis S, Frank-Lightfoot L, Kulbok PA, Poree S, Sgarlata L. *Building a Community Health Worker Program: The Key to Better Care, Better Outcomes & Lower Costs.* https://www.aha.org/system/files/2018-10/chw-program-manual-2018-toolkit-final.pdf. Accessed February 23, 2022.

7. Viswanathan M, Kraschnewski J, Nishikawa B, Morgan LC, Thieda P, Honeycutt A, Lohr KN, Jonas D. Outcomes of community health worker interventions. *Evidence Reports/Technology Assessments, Agency for Healthcare Research and Quality.* 2009;181. https://www.ncbi.nlm.nih.gov/books/NBK44604/. Accessed February 26, 2022.

8. Minnesota CHW curriculum. Minnesota Community Health Worker Alliance Web site. http://s472440476.onlinehome.us/wp-content/uploads/2013/05/EducationCurriculum.pdf. Accessed February 23, 2022.

9. Education. Minnesota Community Health Worker Alliance Website. https://mnchwalliance.org/education/#:~:text=MN%20CHW%20Curriculum%20Minnesota%20is%20the%20first%20state,high%20school%20diploma%20or%20GED%2C%20at%20a%20minimum. Accessed February 23, 2022.

10. Community health worker (CHW). Minnesota Department of Health Web site. https://www.health.state.mn.us/facilities/ruralhealth/emerging/chw/index.htm. Accessed February 23, 2022.

11. Community health worker job description. Hometown Health Center Web site. https://hometownhealthcenter.org/wp-content/uploads/sites/61/2021/05/Community-Health-Worker-1222820.pdf. Accessed February 26, 2022.

12. Elmers D. How to write a modern resume in 2021. https://www.topresume.com/career-advice/job-tips-for-a-modern-resume?pt=D2V9Ip0HgD4oi&msclkid=5fdfcec9448715badd8eaf25156a82de&utm_source=bing&utm_medium=cpc&utm_campaign=US%20-%20TopResume%20-%20Search%20-%20Top%20EM&utm_term=resume%20writing&utm_content=resume%20writing%20-%20skag%20-%20exact&adgroup=resume_writing_-_skag_-_exact&matchtype=e&geo=&Network=Search&device=c&msclkid=5fdfcec9448715badd8eaf25156a82de&utm_source=bing&utm_medium=cpc&utm_campaign=US%20-%20TopResume%20-%20Search%20-%20Top%20EM&utm_term=resume%20writing&utm_content=resume%20writing%20-%20skag%20-%20exact. Accessed February 28, 2022.

13. Ladders updates popular recruiter eye-tracking study with new key insights on how job seekers can improve their resumes. Ladders, Inc. Web site. https://www.prnewswire.com/news-releases/ladders-updates-popular-recruiter-eye-tracking-study-with-new-key-insights-on-how-job-seekers-can-improve-their-resumes-300744217.html. Accessed February 28, 2022.

14. Augustine A. 7 signs your resume is making you look old. https://www.topresume.com/career-advice/7-signs-your-resume-is-making-you-look-old. Accessed February 28, 2022.

15. Augustine A. 11 steps to writing the perfect resume. https://www.topresume.com/career-advice/11-tips-to-writing-perfect-resume. Accessed February 28, 2022.

16. Stanish I. Bad resume advice you should completely ignore. https://www.topresume.com/career-advice/bad-resume-advice-to-ignore. Accessed February 28, 2022.

17. Role of community health workers. National Institute of Health, National Heart, Lung, and Blood Institute Web site. https://www.nhlbi.nih.gov/education/heart-truth/CHW/Role#:~:text=Since%20CHWs%20typically%20reside%20in%20the%20community%20they,helping%20to%20reduce%20health%20disparities%20in%20underserved%20communities. Accessed March 2, 2022.

18. Interview dress code. Interview Cracker Web site. https://interviewcracker.com/interview-preparation/interview-dress-code/#:~:text=Interview%20Dress%20Code%201%20Dress%20Code%20of%20Interview.,formal.%20...%204%20Conclusion.%20...%205%20Suggested%20Articles%3A. Accessed March 2, 2022.

19. Interview skills. fip Web site. https://www.fip.org/files/ypg/Project%20Documents/career%20development/CareerDevelopment-Interviews.pdf. Accessed March 11, 2022.

20. Ariella S. How to accept a job offer with examples. https://www.zippia.com/advice/how-to-accept-a-job-offer/. Accessed March 19, 2022.

Appendix

In November 2018, the Association of State and Territorial Health Officials (ASTHO. summarized community health worker (CHW. core competencies from 18 states with CHW training standards. See this website for the full document: https://astho.org/Programs/Clinical-to-Community-Connections/Documents/CHW-Training-and-Core-Competencies-Chart/. **Table A.1** presents the Quality Matters format using the CHW Competencies and learning objectives from the chapters of this book.

Table A.1 Quality Matters format using the CHW Competencies and learning objectives

ASTHO CHW Competencies	Competencies Met in Chapter	Chapter Learning Objectives	Knowledge Acquisition
Communication Skills including but not limited to:		**Chapter 1** 1. Define public health and individual health. 2. Describe the history of community health workers. 3. Explain the roles, skills, and responsibilities of community health workers.	Determined by the instructor including quizzes, exams, papers, group presentations, role playing, demonstration with return demonstration, PowerPoint slide presentations, resume writing, and practice interviews.
a. Culturally aware; respectful written, verbal, and nonverbal expression; health literacy.	2a, 2c, 3d, 3e	**Chapter 2** 1. Define literacy. 2. Provide a definition and example for each of the five types of literacy: verbal, written/reading, digital, numerical, and health. 3. Create health documents that support plain language and lower literacy levels. 4. Explain effective listening skills. 5. Demonstrate teaching techniques for the learning styles including visual, auditory, reading/writing, and kinesthetic.	
b. Conflict resolution; rights and responsibilities of CHW and client; Health Insurance Portability and Accountability (HIPAA) and ethical guidelines.	13a, 13b, 13c	**Chapter 3** 1. Define the terms: health equity, health inequities, race, and ethnicity. 2. Describe the terms: equality, diversity, and inclusion. 3. Explain the five categories in the social determinants of health. 4. Illustrate examples of cultural competencies. 5. Demonstrate the link between cultural competencies and health literacy.	
Interpersonal and Relationship–Building Skills including but not limited to:		**Chapter 4** 1. Define social justice. 2. Describe self-advocacy and community advocacy. 3. Categorize effective community resources. 4. Determine access and barriers to community resources.	

a. Explain how plans for supporting individuals and families relate to wider social factors that influence health.	12a, 12b, 12c, 12d, 12e, 12f, 12g	**Chapter 5** 1. Explain the health hazards of climate effects, water, air, and noise pollution affect health. 2. Describe the mental health impact and various influence of stress related to climate. 3. Discuss the negative effects of water pollution on human health. 4. Examine three types of air pollution and the consequences on health. 5. Describe how noise pollution causes the deterioration of health. 6. Define risk factors and protective factors in relationship to health.
b. Use a variety of strategies, such as role-modeling, to support clients in meeting objectives, depending on challenges, and changing conditions.	2d	**Chapter 6** 1. Explain the major body systems with examples to specific diseases. 2. List common prefixes and suffixes from medical terminology with examples. 3. Define leading causes of death in the United States. 4. Explain behaviors for chronic disease prevention.
Service Coordination and Navigation Skills including but not limited to:		**Chapter 7** 1. Identify and define the four categories of infectious diseases. 2. Explain why antibiotics resistance is so challenging and important. 3. Explain the risk factors and transmission of acquiring infectious diseases. 4. Describe the four steps of food safety. 5. Demonstrate how to properly use personal protective equipment. 6. Explain herd immunity and how it is achieved.
a. Update information about health insurance, social services, public health programs, and additional resources.	11a, 11b, 11c, 11d, 11e	**Chapter 8** 1. Explain how addressing community safety is impacted by communication skills, basic need assessments, activities of daily living, falls, and home safety. 2. Describe how the signs and symptoms of elder abuse are linked to the safety and care of the elderly. 3. Describe how to prepare for natural disasters and arrange emergency plans for the elderly. 4. Describe ways that community health workers manage stress, utilize body mechanics to avoid injuries, use personal protective equipment, and resolve conflicts.

(continues)

Table A.1 Quality Matters format using the CHW Competencies and learning objectives

(continued)

ASTHO CHW Competencies	Competencies Met in Chapter	Chapter Learning Objectives	Knowledge Acquisition
b. Maintain appropriate boundaries that balance professional and personal relationships, recognizing dual roles according to agency policy.	14c	**Chapter 9** 1. Define "elderly" and describe the cultural views of the elderly across countries. 2. Explain three reasons why elderly adults need to receive an annual physical examination. 3. Describe four physical body systems, including how each body system changes with aging. 4. Define the symptoms and care management of Alzheimer's disease. 5. List two positive and two adverse behaviors that are affected by aging. 6. List the common economic difficulties that affect the financial aspects of aging.	
Capacity Building Skills including but not limited to:		**Chapter 10** 1. Compare and contrast the landmark cases of Karen Quinlan, Nancy Cruzan, and Terry Schiavo. 2. Describe the differences and similarities between palliative care and hospice care. 3. Examine the aspects of end-of-life planning including cultural and religious beliefs, pain management, language barriers, and communication. 4. Describe three burial options that are available in most U.S. states. 5. Define the difference between grief and bereavement.	
a. Build, maintain networks, and collaborate with community partners in capacity building activities.	4a, 4b, 4c, 4d, 5a, 5b, 5c, 5d	**Chapter 11** 1. Discuss the history of health insurance in the United States. 2. Explain an overview of the various types of health insurance in the United States. 3. Describe the reasons for the uneven coverage of health insurance in the United States. 4. Define the most common terms used in health insurance. 5. Identify and define the most common types of U.S. health insurance.	

b. Apply principles and skills needed for identifying and developing community leadership.	14c	**Chapter 12** 1. Describe the difference between an urgent care clinic and the emergency department in a hospital. 2. Identify four types of physician practices. 3. Define federally funded nonprofit health centers (FQHC). What services do FQHCs offer? 4. Describe six types of integrative therapies including the benefits of each therapy. 5. Identify practical ways for seniors to age in place. 6. Explain the difference between assisted living facilities and nursing home/skilled nursing facilities. 7. Describe the five signs when family members may wish to begin the process of exploring memory care centers.
Advocacy Skills including but not limited to:		**Chapter 13** 1. List and define the four main principles of healthcare ethics. 2. Define the Health Insurance Portability and Accountability Act (HIPAA) and explain the purpose of protecting patient health information. 3. Explain three professional rights and responsibilities for community health workers.
a. Encourage clients to identify and prioritize their personal, family, and community needs; advocate for clients and communities to attain needed care and resources in a timely fashion.	2e, 4a, 4b, 4c, 4d	**Chapter 14** 1. Describe how community health workers influence health services on countries outside of the United States. 2. Explains how community health workers influence the improved health outcomes related to maternal and children health, micronutrient deficiencies, diarrhea, HIV, malaria, malnutrition, onchocerciasis (river blindness), and tuberculosis. 3. Examine the overview of community health worker programs, including some details related to the education qualification, certifications, curriculum, and a description of a community health worker job. 4. Review the techniques for writing a professional resume and developing professional interview skills.

(continues)

Table A.1 Quality Matters format using the CHW Competencies and learning objectives

(continued)

ASTHO CHW Competencies	Competencies Met in Chapter	Chapter Learning Objectives	Knowledge Acquisition
b. Promote health equity and efforts to reduce health disparities through engagement with clients, professional colleagues, and community partners.	3a, 3b, 4a, 4b, 4c, 4d		
Education and Facilitation Skills including but not limited to:			
a. Use data and evidence-based practices in efforts to support clients in reaching their goals; learning styles.	2b, 2d, 2e		
b. Promote efforts to prevent injury and disease, including those that require policy changes, and support effective use of the healthcare system.	5a, 5b, 5c,		
Individual and Community Assessment Skills including but not limited to:			
a. Gather and combine information from different sources to better understand clients, their families, and their communities; social determinants of health.	3c		
b. Assess barriers to accessing health care and other services; protective and risk factors.	5d		

Outreach Skills including but not limited to:	
a. Develop and implement outreach plans in collaboration with colleagues, based on individual, family, and community needs, resources, and strengths.	12a, 12b, 12c, 12d, 12e, 12f, 12g
b. Use a range of outreach methods to engage individuals and groups in diverse settings.	10a, 10b, 10c, 10d, 10e
Professional Skills and Conduct including but not limited to:	
a. Comply with reporting, record keeping, and documentation requirement in one's work; use appropriate technology and update skills according to employer requirements; resume writing.	14a, 14b, 14c, 14d
b. Handle ethical challenges as they address legal and social challenges facing the clients and communities served.	13a, 13b, 13c
Evaluation and Research Skills including but not limited to:	
a. Share community assessment results with colleagues and community partners to inform planning and health improvement efforts.	1c, 1d, 7a, 7b, 7c, 7d, 7e

(continues)

Table A.1 Quality Matters format using the CHW Competencies and learning objectives

(continued)

ASTHO CHW Competencies	Competencies Met in Chapter	Chapter Learning Objectives	Knowledge Acquisition
b. Continue assessment as an ongoing process, considering changes in client circumstances and the CHW-client relationship.	8a, 8b, 8c, 8d, 9a, 9b, 9c, 9d, 9e, 9f		
Knowledge Base including but not limited to:			
a. Know and promote health information about common chronic diseases; simplify medical terminology for clients and community.	5c, 6a, 6b, 6c, 6d, 6e		
b. Know the core functions of public health and applications to communities; definition and history of CHW.	1a, 1b, 14a, 14b, 14c, 14d		

Data from Association of State and Territorial Health Officials (2018). https://www.astho.org/globalassets/pdf/chw-training-and-core-competencies-chart_nov-2018.pdf

Glossary

activities of daily living (ADLs) five basic categories are personal hygiene, dressing, eating, maintaining continence, and transferring/mobility.

acupuncture a technique for balancing the flow of energy through pathways (meridians) in the body by inserting tiny, thin needles into specific points along these meridians. Many Western practitioners view the acupuncture points as places to stimulate nerves, muscles, and connective tissue to stimulate the body's natural painkillers.

advanced directive individuals plan for their future health care.

adverse childhood experiences (ACEs) traumatic experiences in childhood and throughout the teenage years that increase the child's risk of exposure to violence, chronic health problems, mental illness, and substance abuse in adulthood.

advocacy derived from the Latin language where "ad" = to, and "vocare" = means to call or speak for someone.

alcohol use disorder involves a pattern of problems controlling consumption of alcohol, preoccupation with alcohol, continued use of alcohol even when it causes problems, consuming more to get the same effect, or experiencing withdrawal symptoms without alcohol consumption.

all-payer system providing a universal health insurance; available in Germany, Japan, and France.

ambulatory surgery centers (ASC) facilities that perform surgeries and procedures that do not require hospital admission; provide cost-effective services and a convenient environment that is less stressful compared to hospitals.

annual mental status examination important for people over 70 years old. Most tests take about 30 minutes to administer and assess orientation, short-term memory, long-term memory, basic math or computational skills, word finding, attention and concentration, naming objects, following commands, writing, spatial orientation, abstract reasoning, and judgment.

antibiotic resistance happens when bacteria and fungi develop the ability to defeat the drugs that were initially designed to kill them.

antibiotic kills bacterial infection; discovered by Alexander Fleming in 1928.

art therapy includes drawing, painting, sculpture, clay modeling, and a variety of other creative outlets.

autonomy respect and honor the patients right to make their own decision.

bacteria can live in almost any type of environment, from extreme heat to intense cold, and some can even survive in radioactive waste; enter the body through droplets into the mouth, genitals, open wounds, nose, and eyes and can be transmitted via bodily fluids, skin-to-skin contact, contaminated items, or airborne particles or droplets. After entering the body, they begin to multiply, causing an infection.

beneficence do good.

bereavement the period after loss and includes the time where grief is experienced, and mourning occurs.

birth center a home-like facility within a healthcare system with a program of care designed in the wellness model of pregnancy and birth.

body mechanics ways to move oneself or perform daily activities with ease and without sustaining injuries.

calendar quarter the three calendar months ending on March 31, June 30, September 30, or December 31.

cardiovascular system includes the circulation of blood, which transports gases, nutrients, hormones, and wastes.

chiropractic care a healthcare profession that focuses on the spine, various joints of the body, and the connection to the nervous system. Certain diagnoses related to the spine and joints may benefit from manipulative treatment to prevent the onset of additional disorders that would affect nerves, muscles, and organs. The focus is on prevention, diagnosis, and conservative care of spine-related disorders and other painful joint issues.

code of ethics ethical obligations that CHWs have to the communities that they serve and to share these reflections with others.

coinsurance percentage of costs of a covered healthcare service that the insured pays after paying the deductible.

community advocacy involves speaking for individuals or identifying an issue or cause to initiate the change of a policy or program to improve conditions for a specific people group or for the entire community needs related to age, race, ethnicity, disabilities, and sexuality.

community health workers (CHWs) a frontline public health worker who is a trusted member of and/or has an unusually close understanding of the community served, which enables the worker to serve as a liaison/link/intermediary between health/social services and the community to facilitate access to services and improve the quality and cultural competence of service delivery; builds individual and community capacity by increasing health knowledge and self-sufficiency through a range of activities such as outreach, community education, informal counseling, social support, and advocacy.

conflict resolution to dissolve tensions and maintain a safe environment for all.

copayment form of medical cost sharing in a health insurance plan that requires the insured person to pay a fixed dollar amount when a medical service is received.

core values access, acceptance, advocacy and education, excellence, learning, partnership, self-determination, social justice, strength, trust, and unity.

cultural competency capacity to value, understand, and consider diversity across various domains, learn about cultural knowledge, adapt to diverse cultures, and incorporate all cultural aspects into community practice and policies.

deductible fixed dollar amount during the annual benefit period that the insured pays before the insurer starts to make payments for covered medical services.

dialysis centers feature an effective staff-to-patient ratio. Staff members include registered nurses, certified chronic hemodialysis technicians, a renal dietitian, and a renal social worker, all under the direction of a dedicated nephrologist, a physician with 2 to 3 years of specialized training in nephrology.

dialysis type of renal replacement therapy that is used to provide an artificial replacement for inadequate or lost kidney function.

digital learning gap causing distinct differences in how individuals in the United States access and use technology to improve learning opportunities and outcomes.

digital literacy defined as the knowledge and ability to use computers and related technology devices efficiently.

direct contact includes person-to-person or skin-to-skin contact with bodily or sexual fluids, such as blood or saliva.

discrimination finding positive or negative differences between two similar outlooks, actions, or treatment.

diversity empowering people by respecting, recognizing, and appreciating what makes them different, in terms of age, sexual orientation, ethnicity, religion, disability, education, and national origin.

elder abuse abuse may include many forms, including domestic violence, emotional abuse, financial abuse, theft, and neglect.

elderly someone over 65 years old who has functional impairments.

electronic health records (EHR) a centralized, shareable record of a patient's entire medical history.

electronic medical records (EMR) digital version of the paper charts in the clinician's office;

contains the medical and treatment history of the patients in one practice; does not travel across various medical offices.

emotional stress involves relationships, such as divorce, domestic violence, housing eviction, loss of property, loss of family members via child protection removal, foster care, incarceration, mental health conditions, suicide, homicide, and the lack of adequate treatment of disease or delay of diagnosis.

employee health programs a coordinated and comprehensive set of health promotion and protection strategies implemented at the worksite and include programs, policies, benefits, and environmental supports to encourage health and safety for all employees.

employer-based health insurance health insurance that is contracted by employers for their employees.

endocrine system ensures the regulation of body processes through hormone production; composed of glands located throughout the body.

end-of-life decisions A legal document that states a person's wishes at their end-of-life, such as Do Not Resuscitate orders and pain management desires.

end-of-life planning decisions after tragic circumstances.

environmental protective factors include social support and physical (e.g., clean air and water, safe outdoor space, access to resources and health care); more protective factors lead to improved health outcomes and decreased development of chronic disease.

environmental risk factors include the social environment and physical environment (e.g., poor air and water quality and noise pollution).

environmental stress caused by multiple factors related to climate change, wildfires, air quality, water pollution, extreme weather conditions, noise, traffic, and poor quality of housing.

equality equal opportunities and protection of individuals from discrimination due to various reasons including age, sexual orientation, disability, race, ethnicity, religion, marital status, and pregnancy.

ethnicity cultural identity of an individual, which includes language, religion, nationality, ancestry, dress, and customs; members of a particular ethnicity tend to identify with each other based on these shared cultural traits.

executor the person named to carry out the directions of a will.

fall-related injuries represent the leading cause of injury related deaths among individuals aged 65 years and older.

Federally Qualified Health Centers (FQHC) provide primary care services to these populations using a sliding scale model where the fee is based on the individual's ability to pay.

fee for service the doctor and other healthcare providers are paid for each service performed.

flexible spending accounts (FSA) These accounts are offered and administered by employers and provide a way for employees to set aside, out of their paychecks, pretax dollars to pay for the employee's share of insurance premiums or medical expenses not covered by the employer's health plan, such as eyeglasses, dental expenses, and medical products not covered by the health insurance policy.

functional literacy able to read simple signs.

functional medicine a systems biology–based approach that focuses on identifying and addressing the root cause of disease; an individualized, patient-centered, science-based approach to health care that looks beyond symptom resolution to identify why illness occurs and address those root causes to restore health.

fungus decompose and absorb organic matter using an enzyme; almost always reproduce by spreading single celled spores.

grief experienced in many ways and affects everyone differently; can vary between emotional and psychological well-being due to cultural beliefs, relationship to the deceased, or attachment to the loss. The level of suffering due to grief is subjective and unique to the experiences of the individual.

group practice two or more physicians who all provide medical care within the same facility.

health equity the achievement when each person has the opportunity to attain his or her full health potential and no one is disadvantaged from achieving this potential because of social position or other socially determined circumstances.

health inequities quality and length of life, rate and severity of disease, disability, and death, and access to health care and treatment.

Health Insurance Portability and Accountability Act (HIPAA) federal law that required the creation of national standards to protect patient health information from being disclosed without the patient's consent or knowledge via the Privacy Rule.

health maintenance organization (HMO) health insurance plans that typically cost the least but offer a limited number of providers and facilities. The benefits are faster appointments times in most cases and ease of referrals to specialty physicians within the network.

health a state of complete physical, mental, and social well-being and not merely the absence of disease or infirmity.

healthcare ethics ethical obligation to the patient of autonomy, beneficence, nonmaleficence, and justice.

healthcare power of attorney appoints a close family member or other trusted person as one's health care agent. This person may make healthcare decisions for the person when they can no longer speak for themselves or no longer have decisional capacity.

herd immunity occurs when a large percentage of the population is immune to a specific disease.

hospice focuses on the care, comfort, and the quality of life related to a total person with a serious illness.

hospitalists a physician is assigned to care for patients admitted to the hospital; may or may not work closely with the patient's primary care physician.

human resources the department of a business or organization that deals with the hiring, administration, and training of personnel

hysterectomy surgery to remove a woman's uterus, and perhaps the ovaries, because of pain, bleeding, fibroids, or other reasons.

immune system recognizes normal, healthy cells and unhealthy cells. Cells are unhealthy due to infection or damage, such as sunburn, cancer, or congenital immune deficiency. The immune system recognizes a problem and responds.

inclusion an individual's experience in the workplace, community, and society; viewed as the extent to which the individual feels as an active participant rather than merely invited, but not given an equal voice.

indirect contact characterized by transmission that occurs when there is no direct human-to-human contact.

individual health relates to health care and clinical disciplines (i.e., medicine, nursing, pharmacy, physical therapy, clinical psychology, dental, vision, hearing, and others) in which licensed professionals examine, diagnosis, and treat the health of one person at a time.

infusion center is an outpatient facility that is certified to administer infusion therapy.

instrumental activities of daily living (IADLs) include basic communication skills, transportation, meal preparation, shopping, housework, managing medications, and managing personal finances.

justice be fair and treat all persons alike.

lifetime maximum dollar limit the maximum dollar amount that a health insurance company agrees to pay on behalf of a member for covered services during the course of his or her lifetime.

literacy the capacity to communicate through verbal, written, numeric, reading, and digital/technological formats.

living will document provides the instructions about life-sustaining treatment and other end-of-life care that the individual desires to be followed when they can no longer speak for themselves.

local health departments (LHDs) governmental entities and obtain their authority and responsibility from the state and local laws.

locum tenens derived from the Latin phrase for "to hold the place of," refers to physicians who travel to or relocate to geographical areas in need of healthcare professionals, such as during the COVID-19 pandemic or following a natural disaster.

longevity expected length of a person's life.

lymphatic system a network of vessels and tissues composed of extracellular fluid and lymph nodes. The primary function of this complex system is to collect the excess fluid from tissues, vessels, and cells and return it to the blood stream to be recirculated.

managed care plans generally provide comprehensive health services to their members and offer financial incentives for patients to use the providers under the plan.

Maslow's hierarchy of needs the well-known psychological theory is depicted as a pyramid with five levels that build upon each other.

mastectomy surgery to remove all breast tissue from a breast as a way to treat or prevent breast cancer.

medical tourism international travel for the purpose of receiving medical care.

mindful meditation stress reduction practice that offers secular, intensive mindfulness training to assist people with stress, anxiety, depression, and pain.

morbidity sickness; reference to having a specific illness, disease, or condition.

morbidity rate is the frequency or proportion with which a disease appears in a population

mortality death; the relative frequency of deaths in a specific population.

mortality rate typically expressed in units of deaths per 1,000 individuals per year.

muscular system primary function is to permit movement of the body, maintain posture, support the skeletal system, and circulate blood throughout the body.

negative stress also known as distress, is a more complex, intricate topic because everyone responds to negative stress differently; response to a stressor is unique based on their past experiences, genetics, trauma, coping mechanisms, and behavioral patterns.

nervous system the processing center for sensory input and using the input to produce appropriate body responses.

nonmaleficence do no harm.

numerical literacy the ability to use and understand mathematics to solve basic problems in real-world situations.

obesity a medical condition in which excess body fat may have a negative effect on health. Symptoms include above average body weight, trouble sleeping or sleep apnea, enlarged veins in the legs, skin problems as moisture accumulates in skin folds, gallstones, and osteoarthritis in hip and knee joints.

organizational health literacy the degree to which organizations equitably enable individuals to find, understand, and use information and services to inform health-related decisions and actions for themselves and others.

palliative care specialized medical care that focuses on providing patients relief from pain and other symptoms related to a serious illness or condition, regardless of the diagnosis or stage of disease.

parasites living organisms that are capable of laying eggs in the host while undetected; attach to the host, lay eggs, and then symptoms occur once the eggs hatch and infection has taken place.

personal barriers any obstacle that impedes personal basic care needs.

personal health literacy the degree to which individuals can find, understand, and use information and services to inform health-related decisions and actions for themselves and others.

personal protective equipment (PPE) mask, face shield, disposable gown, gloves.

personal protective factors linked to an individual's knowledge, skills, experience, personal behavior, and lifestyle; a greater number of protective factors (e.g., healthy weight, nutritious food, never smoking, and routine exercise) decreases likelihood of developing a chronic illness or disease.

personal risk factors linked to an individual's knowledge, skills, experience, personal behavior, and lifestyle; the greater number of risk factors in an individual's life, the greater the chance of developing an illness, disease, or injury.

physical stress short term or long term. In short-term situations, the body has a fight-or-flight response that is a natural, life-saving system that allows the muscles to move quickly and effectively.

plain language grammatically correct language that includes complete sentence structure and accurate word usage.

positive stress also known as eustress, is natural, and biological reaction to a specific demand or event in which the individual faces or chooses to accept.

preadmission certification authorization for hospital admission given by a healthcare provider to a group member prior to their hospitalization.

pre-admission testing the process of pre-screening to help achieve the optimal surgical outcome by ensuring the patient is prepared in every way for the schedule surgery and the recovery process.

preferred provider organization (PPO) a network of healthcare providers that offer medical care at a certain rate. Unlike HMO, a PPO offers the freedom to receive care from any healthcare provider in or out of your network.

primary care provider (PCP) the healthcare provider that isa responsible for dealing with the majority of a patient's routine healthcare issues and for coordinating care with specialists that may be needed.

productive health communication Communication that occurs when the healthcare provider and the patient have a conversation in the language of the patient and at the health literacy level of the patient to yield the greatest possible understanding and ability to ask questions regarding diagnosis and treatment plan for best health outcomes.

prostatectomy surgery that removes all or part of a man's prostate because of cancer or an enlarged prostate.

protective factors positive assets; two kinds of protective factors are personal and environmental.

proxy person who is designated and legally permitted to make healthcare decisions for a specific individual.

public health considers all aspects of health in an entire community including social, education, economic, housing, environmental, and so on.

quality of life refers to the degree in which an individual is healthy, comfortable, and able to participate in or enjoy life events; refers to both the experiences and living conditions in an individual's life.

quantity of life refers to number of days in an individual's life. Using statistics, an individual's life span is estimated based on the available data including gender, age, ethnicity, geographical location, co-morbidities, environmental exposures, occupation, and numerous other variables.

race physical characteristics of an individual including skin color, eye color and shape, facial structure, and hair color, texture, and curl; the diverse qualities or attributes among populations, including evident genetic differences.

radiation therapy center a freestanding facility or linked to a clinic or hospital. It provides radiation therapy services to patients.

reading literacy the ability to understand and use the written language required by society.

registered dietitian nutritionists (RDN) food and nutrition experts who have met the following criteria to earn the RDN credential, which includes obtaining a minimum of a bachelor's degree at a U.S. regionally accredited university or college and completing course work accredited or approved by the Accreditation Council for Education in Nutrition and Dietetics (ACEND) of the Academy of Nutrition and Dietetics.

rehabilitation center or facility an inpatient or outpatient facility that offer a set of interventions designed to optimize functioning and reduce disability in individuals with health conditions in interactions with their environment.

reproductive system produces reproductive cells that generate offspring.

risk factors negative, personal, or environmental indicators.

second opinion the opinion of a physician other than the patient's current physician; the second opinion physician reviews the patient's medical records and gives an opinion about the patient's health problem and how it should be treated.

self-advocacy speaking for yourself and effectively communicating with others about your emotional, physical, and mental needs regardless of a known health condition.

sepsis the body's extreme response to an infection.

single-payer system the government acting as the single administrator to collect all healthcare fees and pays out all associated healthcare costs; available in Canada, Denmark, Taiwan, and Sweden.

skeletal system includes the bones, joints, ligaments, tendons, and cartilage; the internal framework of the body.

social cohesion the strength of relationships and the sense of community among the members.

social determinants of health the conditions in which individuals are born, grow, live, work, and age.

social justice equal rights, equal opportunities, and equal treatment for all.

Social Security Disability Insurance (SSDI) also known as Social Security Disability (SSD) A U.S. federal government program that provides benefits to disabled or blind persons who have previous worker's contributions to Social Security; musty meet Social Security's disability criteria; and benefits are based on earning records.

social stress caused by living in neighborhoods with poor quality housing and schools, exposure to institutional racism, low-income employment opportunities, neighborhood violence, lack of law enforcement protection, and discrimination based on ethnicity, religious beliefs, gender, disability, age, and sexual orientation.

societal barriers barriers related to conditions in which people are born, grow, live, learn, work and age or social determinants of health that can contribute to decreased functioning among people with disabilities.

stress management identifying what causes stress, how stress impacts health, and what strategies are useful to adequately reduce stress.

suicide attempt when someone harms themselves with any intent to end their life, but they do not die because of their actions.

suicide a form of intentional self-harm and death caused by severely injuring oneself with the intent to die.

Supplemental Security Income (SSI) pays benefits based on financial need; these modest payments make a difference in meeting basic needs when an individual is unable to work but may or may not be a lifetime benefit. If a person recovers from the injury and can obtain gainful employment, the benefit would not continue.

Sustainable Development Goals (SDGs) 17 global goals developed by the United Nations targeting the elimination of poverty, hunger, and disease.

systemic infections infections throughout the body.

Tai chi type of energy or breath skill (Qigong) practiced by millions of people worldwide. Although originally a martial art, it is mainly practiced today as an excellent form of exercise with many health benefits that utilize breathing, visualizations, and movements to work the entire body all at once.

travel clinics educate travelers about the known health risks associated with traveling abroad.

urgent care clinics the middle ground between the primary care provider (PCP) and the Emergency Department (ED); appropriate for a minor injury (sprain or cut) or an illness without other symptoms, such as a sore throat or cough, and no major underlying medical conditions. Typically staffed with physician assistants, nurse practitioners, and nurses; can order basic labs and imaging tests, such as X-rays, to provide diagnoses and develop treatment plans; have set hours and an established list of conditions treated; often less expensive and have shorter wait times than EDs.

urinary system the organs the urinary system includes the kidneys, renal pelvis, ureters, bladder and urethra; the purpose of the urinary system is to eliminate waste from the body, regulate blood volume and blood pressure, control levels of electrolytes and metabolites, and regulate blood pH.

usual, customary, and reasonable (UCR) charges a physician's usual fee for a service that does not exceed the customary fee in that geographic area and is reasonable based on the circumstances.

utilization review process of reviewing the appropriateness and quality of care provided to patients; may take place before, during, or after services are rendered.

vaccination a preparation that is used to stimulate the body's immune response against disease; vaccines are usually administered through needle injections, but some can be administered by mouth or sprayed into the nose.

VARK learning styles visual, auditory, reading/writing, and kinesthetic.

verbal literacy speaking and listening that occurs in every aspect of daily life.

virus a simple microorganism that infects cells and may cause disease.

Worker's compensation a type of business insurance that provides benefits to employees who suffer work-related injuries or illness.

wound care center (or clinic) a medical facility for treating wounds that do not heal easily.

Index

Note: "Page numbers followed by *b*, *f* or *t* indicate material in boxes, figures, or tables, respectively."